Advances in Cardiopulmonary Rehabilitation

Jean Jobin, PhD
Hôpital Laval
Québec, Canada

François Maltais, MD
Hôpital Laval
Québec, Canada

Pierre LeBlanc, MD
Hôpital Laval
Québec, Canada

Clermont Simard, PhD
Physical Education Department
Laval University
Québec, Canada

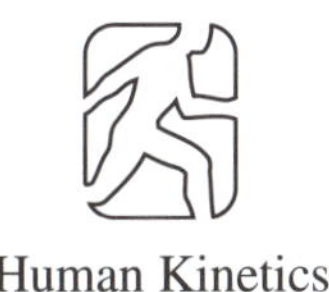

Human Kinetics

Library of Congress Cataloging-in-Publication Data

Advances in cardiopulmonary rehabilitation / Jean Jobin . . . [et al.], editors.
p. ; cm.
Includes bibliographical references and index.
ISBN 0-7360-0312-6
1. Cardiopulmonary system--Diseases--Patients--Rehabilitation. I. Jobin, Jean, 1949- II. Québec International Symposium on Cardiopulmonary Rehabilitation (1st : 1999 : Québec, Québec)
[DNLM: 1. Heart Diseases--rehabilitation--Congresses. 2. Exercise Therapy--Congresses. 3. Heart Diseases--drug therapy--Congresses. 4. Lung Diseases--drug therapy--Congresses. 5. Lung Diseases--rehabilitation--Congresses. WG 200 A2457 2000]
RC702 .A387 2000
616.1′206--dc21

99-059589

ISBN: 0-7360-0312-6

Acquisitions Editor: Loarn D. Robertson, PhD; **Developmental Editor:** Spencer J. Cotkin, PhD; **Assistant Editors:** Amanda S. Ewing, Mark Zulauf; **Copyeditor:** Kelly Winters; **Proofreader:** Erin Cler; **Indexer:**Marie Rizzo; **Permission Manager:** Heather Munson; **Graphic Designer:** Fred Starbird; **Graphic Artist:** Kathleen Boudreau-Fuoss; **Cover Designer:** Robert Reuther; **Printer:** Versa Press; **Binder:** Dekker & Sons

Printed in the United States of America 10 9 8 7 6 5 4 3 2 1

Human Kinetics
Web site: http://www.humankinetics.com/

United States: Human Kinetics, P.O. Box 5076, Champaign, IL 61825-5076
1-800-747-4457
e-mail: humank@hkusa.com

Canada: Human Kinetics, 475 Devonshire Road Unit 100, Windsor, ON N8Y 2L5
1-800-465-7301 (in Canada only)
e-mail: humank@hkcanada.com

Europe: Human Kinetics, P.O. Box IW14, Leeds LS16 6TR, United Kingdom
+44 (0)113-278 1708
e-mail: humank@hkeurope.com

Australia: Human Kinetics, 57A Price Avenue, Lower Mitcham, South Australia 5062
(08) 82771555
e-mail: liahka@senet.com.au

New Zealand: Human Kinetics, P.O. Box 105-231, Auckland Central
09-523-3462
e-mail: humank@hknewz.com

Contents

List of Contributors

J. Beyene; Department of Public Health Sciences, University of Toronto, Toronto, Ontario, Canada

Sonia Boivin; Université du Québec à Montréal, Montréal, Québec, Canada; and Institut de Cardiologie de Montréal, Montréal, Québec, Canada

Jean Bourbeau; Respiratory Epidemiology Unit and the Respiratory Division, McGill University Health Centre, and Research Scholar, Fonds de la Recherche en Santé du Québec, Montréal, Canada

Richard Casaburi; Division of Respiratory and Critical Care Physiology and Medicine, Harbor-UCLA Medical Center, Torrance, California, USA

William A. Dafoe; University of Ottawa Heart Institute, Ottawa, Canada

Richard Debigaré; Hôpital Laval, Institut Universitaire de Cardiologie et de Pneumologie de l'Université Laval, Québec, Canada

Jean-François Doyon; Hôpital Laval, Institut Universitaire de Cardiologie et de Pneumologie de l'Université Laval, Québec, Canada

Serge Dumont; École de Service Social, Faculté des Sciences Sociales, Université Laval, Québec, Canada

Gilles Dupuis; Université du Québec à Montréal, Montreal, Québec, Canada; and Institut de Cardiologie de Montréal, Montreal, Québec, Canada

Anne-Marie Étienne; Université de Liège, Liege, Belgium

Ovide Fontaine; Université de Liège, Liege, Belgium

Barry A. Franklin; Cardiac Rehabilitation and Exercise Laboratories, William Beaumont Hospital, Royal Oak, Michigan, USA; and Professor of Physiology, Wayne State University, School of Medicine, Detroit, Michigan, USA

Victor Froelicher; Cardiology Division, Palo Alto Veterans Affairs Health Care Systems, Palo Alto, California, USA

Déborah Fuchs-Climent; Département de Physiologie, Université Montpellier, Hôpital Arnaud de Villeneuve, Montpellier, France

Véronique Gautier-Dechaud; Département de Physiologie, Université Montpellier, Hôpital Arnaud de Villeneuve, Montpellier, France

Pantaleo Giannuzzi; Division of Cardiology, Medical Center of Rehabilitation, Veruno, Italy

Roger S. Goldstein; Department of Medicine, University of Toronto, Toronto, Ontario, Canada

Gordon Guyatt; Department of Medicine and Department of Clinical Epidemiology and Biostatistics, McMaster University, Hamilton, Ontario, Canada

Larry F. Hamm; Toronto Rehabilitation Centre, Cardiac Rehabilitation and Secondary Prevention Program, Toronto, Ontario, Canada

Jean Jobin; Hôpital Laval, Institut Universitaire de Cardiologie et de Pneumologie de l'Université Laval, Québec, Canada

Martin Juneau; Department of Medicine, Montreal Heart Institute, Montréal, Québec, Canada

Terence Kavanagh; Toronto Rehabilitation Centre, Cardiac Rehabilitation and Secondary Prevention Program, Toronto, Ontario, Canada; and Department of Medicine, and Faculty of Physical Education and Health, University of Toronto, Toronto, Ontario, Canada

Takayuki Kawamura; Department of Exercise and Sports Science, University of Wisconsin-LaCrosse, LaCrosse, Wisconsin, USA

Johana Kennedy; Toronto Rehabilitation Centre, Cardiac Rehabilitation and Secondary Prevention Program, Toronto, Ontario, Canada

Yves Lacasse; Hôpital Laval, Institut Universitaire de Cardiologie et de Pneumologie de l'Université Laval, Québec, Canada

Marie-Hélène LeBlanc; Hôpital Laval, Institut Universitaire de Cardiologie et de Pneumologie de L'Université Laval, Québec, Canada

Pierre LeBlanc; Hôpital Laval, Institut Universitaire de Cardiologie et de Pneumologie de l'Université Laval, Québec, Canada

François Maltais; Institut Universitaire de Cardiologie et de Pneumologie de l'Université Laval, Québec, Canada

Dany-Michel Marcadet; Clinique Bizet, Paris, France

Donald J. Mertens; Toronto Rehabilitation Centre, Cardiac Rehabilitation and Secondary Prevention Program, Toronto, Ontario, Canada

Markku Ojanen; Department of Psychology, University of Tampere, Finland

Neil Oldridge; Schools of Allied Health Sciences and Medicine, Regenstrief Institute for Health Care, Indiana University, Indianapolis, Indiana, USA

Magali Poulain; Département de Physiologie, Université Montpellier, Hôpital Arnaud de Villeneuve, Montpellier, France

Christian Préfaut; Département de Physiologie, Université Montpellier, Hôpital Arnaud de Villeneuve, Montpellier, France

Andrew L. Ries; Professor of Medicine University of California, San Diego, California, USA

Roy J. Shephard; Faculty of Physical Education and Health, University of Toronto, Toronto, Ontario, Canada; Cardiac Rehabilitation and Secondary Prevention Program, Toronto, Ontario, Canada; Department of Public Health Sciences, University of Toronto, Toronto, Ontario, Canada

Clermont Simard; Départment d'Éducation Physique, Université Laval, Québec, Canada

Martin J. Sullivan; Department of Medicine, Duke University Medical Center, Durham, North Carolina, USA

Marie-Christine Taillefer; Université du Québec à Montréal, Montréal, Québec, Canada; and Institut de Cardiologie de Montréal, Montréal, Québec, Canada

Pier Luigi Temporelli; Division of Cardiology, Medical Center of Rehabilitation, Veruno, Italy

Alexandra Von Turk; Université de Lausanne, Lausanne, Switzerland

Philip K. Wilson; Department of Exercise and Sports Science, University of Wisconsin-LaCrosse, LaCrosse, Wisconsin, USA

Eric Wong; Department of Medicine, University of Alberta, Edmonton, Alberta, Canada

Acknowledgments

The editors wish to thank Dr. Jean Deslauriers for his outstanding work as ad hoc editor of the original manuscripts. We also want to acknowledge the excellent work of Mr. Réjean Lamontagne as coordinator and technical assistant in the preparation of this book. We extend our thanks to Mrs. Cécile Bilodeau for creating the original artwork of the heart-lung design of the cover page of this book.

Introduction: Current and Future Issues in Cardiopulmonary Rehabilitation

Jean Jobin, François Maltais, Clermont Simard, and Pierre LeBlanc

Preamble

Cardiopulmonary rehabilitation is not new; its origin can be traced back to the 18th century (1). Since the beginning of the 20th century, however, it has evolved from simple exercise to multidimensional programs that now integrate biological and psychosocial features (2,3). During the same period, the incidence of cardiovascular (4) and pulmonary (5) diseases has also increased not only because people live longer, but also because they benefit from new biomedical developments. In this context, why is enrollment in cardiopulmonary rehabilitation programs more or less at a standstill, and why is it well below 50% of eligible patients (6-12)? Why can't every heart or pulmonary disease patient enjoy the benefits of rehabilitation? It is perhaps time to reflect on what cardiopulmonary rehabilitation is, what it means, and where it should be heading.

This volume features a series of articles reviewing some of the most controversial issues in the field of rehabilitation. By looking at our beginnings and our current position, we should be able to conceptualize what the future might be. This is one of the reasons why the historical analysis discussed in the first two chapters of this book is challenging and likely to provide the necessary background for an in-depth reflection on where we want to go.

The evolution of cardiac and pulmonary rehabilitation has been influenced not only by new economic standards but also by a multitude of other factors, some of them well known but others poorly identified. Cardiopulmonary rehabilitation has always been considered a "minor partner" of medicine and consequently, it has received inadequate funding and poor support from the medical profession. Further, rehabilitation is often misunderstood by the general public, which is more inclined to rely on health specialists, instead of on self-care. Most contemporary people seem to overestimate their own power over their health. As a result, the enrollment of cardiac patients in North American rehabilitation programs is still in the range of only 20% to 50% of eligible patients (6-10). In some regions, it is even estimated to be below 10% (11). In Canada, recruitment of pulmonary patients is only 1% of eligible patients (12).

To increase their effectiveness, cardiac rehabilitation programs have attempted to become more diversified or more tantalizing by adopting the secondary prevention paradigm or by including primary prevention patients. But will the secondary prevention paradigm be a choice of tomorrow? Chapter 2 discusses the potential sociological consequences of this paradigm as well as the limitations inherent to the funding of health prevention programs in industrialized and postindustrialized societies.

If funding and reimbursement remain at a lower level and if resources are still limited, voluntary restriction through selective recruitment as discussed in chapter 5 might be envisioned. But is it the solution or should resources and funding be increased? Why is physician referral so low? Why do so few referred patients actually enroll once they have been referred? Because there are still some doubts that pulmonary rehabilitation has a significant physical impact on patients, why fund programs that have only subjective and nonmeasurable effects?

Over the past few years, it has been clearly demonstrated that exercise benefits the physiology of patients suffering from chronic obstructive pulmonary disease (COPD) or congestive heart failure (CHF) (13,14), but enrollment has not significantly increased. Section IV of this volume helps us understand the benefits of cardiopulmonary rehabilitation despite the absence of direct effects on cardiovascular or pulmonary function. At another level, low referral or enrollment is probably not surprising, considering the perceived dangers of exercise by physicians, health professionals, and the lay public. Chapters 11,12, and 13 scrutinize the foundations of this problem. Perhaps the real problem in funding and reimbursement is simply that the economics of cardiopulmonary rehabilitation are poorly understood, and that rehabilitation does not appear to be cost effective. This issue is discussed at great length in chapter 18.

One of the difficulties in convincing the medical community and the lay public of the efficacy of cardiopulmonary rehabilitation may be at least partly related to the absence of a simple outcome that would measure its efficacy. Physiological or psychosocial benefits are numerous but the response to rehabilitation varies from patient to patient, as reviewed in chapters 19 and 20. Quality of life appears to be an excellent measure of the global response to rehabilitation. Will a better mix of medical technology and self-care as advocated by the newly developing integrated medicine make cardiopulmonary rehabilitation the cornerstone of a more holistic approach to the treatment of heart and lung disease? This question is addressed in chapter 22.

As envisioned by Wenger (15), cardiopulmonary rehabilitation is a still-evolving science, and one can oversee that in the future its role among other health services might be difficult to determine. The complexity of the situation is reflected by the wide spectrum of chapters included in this volume, by the diversity of topics, and by the way the authors have chosen to discuss the issues. Although the majority of chapters are review articles, some authors have elected to present their original study because they felt it was a better way to cover the topic. Each manuscript is challenging through its discussion of important controversies.

The editors have decided to invite specialists in cardiac and pulmonary rehabilitation to contribute to this volume because many of the topics are common to both fields. Thus, one question is likely to come to the reader's mind: Why are there so few programs involving both patient populations and why are facilities, professional resources, and funding so limited? Further, can we learn from each other by discussing common problems, sharing recipes for success, and benefiting from each other's mistakes?

About This Book

The contents of all chapters included in this book have been presented at the First Québec International Symposium on Cardiopulmonary Rehabilitation held in Québec City, Canada, May 12-14, 1999. More than 30 of the most renowned specialists in cardiac and pulmonary rehabilitation were invited to submit topics relating to the theme "Cardiopulmonary Rehabilitation: Challenges of the Third Millennium." Among the 40 different topics submitted to the editors, 22 were selected for presentation at the meeting. Thereafter, authors were asked to write a manuscript to be published in this volume. Each manuscript was reviewed by one of the authors uninvolved in its initial writing, by the four editors, and by an ad hoc independent editor. The editors are thankful to Dr. Jean Deslauriers for his high-quality work as the ad hoc editor and to Mr. Réjean Lamontagne for his excellent technical support in the preparation of this book.

Each paper was then allocated to one of eight sections reflecting the reality of cardiopulmonary rehabilitation at the beginning of the third millennium. Part I, titled "Historical Perspectives on the Evolution of Cardiopulmonary Rehabilitation," summarizes the history and actual status of rehabilitation and where it is heading. In the first chapter, Wilson and Kawamura review the past as it leads to the future, whereas the second chapter by Dumont presents the philosophical evolution of cardiac rehabilitation. The following sections present the general sequence in which patients are integrated within cardiopulmonary rehabilitation programs. Optimizing medical treatment is the first step (part II, "Pharmacological Treatment of Congestive Heart Failure and Chronic Obstructive Pulmonary Disease: An Update"), followed by current and upcoming issues related to the selection and recruitment of candidates (part III). The most recent advances in cardiac and pulmonary rehabilitation are regrouped in part IV, "Peripheral Components of Exercise Intolerance: Implications for Cardiopulmonary Rehabilitation." Part V discusses exercise as the cornerstone of any rehabilitation intervention, and partVI includes three chapters presenting some psychosocial aspects of rehabilitation, including economic impact. Part VII covers issues concerning quality of life, which is considered to be a key outcome in rehabilitation. Finally, part VIII presents "Cardiopulmonary Rehabilitation in the Third Millennium."

References

1. Heberden, W. 1992. Some accounts of a disorder of a chest. *Med Trans Coll Phys* 2:59.
2. Wenger, N.K., E.S. Froelicher, L.K. Smith, and the Cardiac Rehabilitation Panel. 1995. Cardiac rehabilitation. *Clinical Practice Guideline No. 17.* Rockville, MD: U.S. Department of Health and Human Services, Public Health Services, Agency for Health Care Policy and Research, and the National Heart, Lung, and Blood Institute. AHCPR Publication No. 96-0672.
3. American Association of Cardiovascular and Pulmonary Rehabilitation (AACVPR). 1998. *Guidelines for Pulmonary Rehabilitation Programs,* 2nd ed. Champaign, IL: Human Kinetics.
4. Pashkow, F.J. 1993. Issues in contemporary cardiac rehabilitation: a historical perspective. *JACC* 21:822-834.
5. Lacasse, Y., D. Brooks, and R.S. Goldstein. 1999. Trends in the epidemiology of COPD in Canada, 1980 to 1995. *Chest* 116(2):306-313.
6. Evenson, K.R., W.D. Rosamond, and R.V. Luepker. 1998. Predictors of outpatient cardiac rehabilitation utilization: the Minnesota Heart Survey Registry. *J Cardiopulm Rehab* 18:192-198.
7. Ades, P., M. Waldmann, D. Polk, and J. Coflesky. 1992. Referral patterns and exercise response in the rehabilitation of female coronary patients aged >62 years. *Am J Cardiol* 69:1422-1425.
8. Ades, P., M. Waldmann, W. McCann, and S. Weaver. 1992. Predictors of cardiac rehabilitation participation in older coronary patients. *Arch Intern Med* 152:1033-1035.
9. Armstrong, K.L., L.A. Wolfe, and M.C. Amey. 1994. Cardiovascular rehabilitation in Canada. A national survey. *J Cardiopulm Rehab* 14:262-272.
10. Thomas, R.J., N.H. Miller, C. Lamendola, K. Berra, B. Hedback, J.L. Durstine, and W. Haskell. 1996. National survey on gender differences in cardiac rehabilitation programs. Patient characteristics and enrollment patterns. *J Cardiopulm Rehab* 165(6):402-412.
11. Walling, A., G.J.L. Tremblay, J. Jobin, J. Charest, F. Delage, M. H. LeBlanc, Y. Tessier, and I. Villa. 1988. Evaluating the rehabilitation potential of a large infarct population: adverse prognosis for women. *J Cardiopulm Rehab* 8(3):99-106.

12. Brooks, D., Y. Lacasse, and R.S. Goldstein. 1999. Pulmonary rehabilitation programs in Canada: national survey. *Can Respir J* 6:55-63.

13. Coats, A.J.S., A.L.Clarck, M. Piepoli, M. Volterrani, and P.A. Poole-Wilson. 1994. Symptoms and quality of life in heart failure: the muscle hypothesis. *Br Heart J* 72(suppl.):S36-39.

14. Maltais, F., P. LeBlanc, C. Simard, J. Jobin, C. Berube, J. Bruneau, L. Carrier, R. Belleau. 1996. Skeletal muscle adaptation to endurance training in patients with chronic obstructive pulmonary disease. *Am J Respir Crit Care Med* 154:442-447.

15. Wenger, N.K. 1995. Future directions in cardiac rehabilitation. In Heart Disease and Rehabilitation, ed. M.L. Pollock and D.H. Schmidt. 3rd ed. Champaign, IL: Human Kinetics.

PART I

Historical Perspectives on the Evolution of Cardiopulmonary Rehabilitation

CHAPTER 1

Historical Review of Cardiopulmonary Rehabilitation and Implications for the Future

Philip K. Wilson and Takayuki Kawamura
Department of Exercise and Sports Science, University of Wisconsin-LaCrosse, LaCrosse, Wisconsin, USA

It has been said that the future is a result of the past; therefore, we can only have a good view of the future by carefully looking at the past. Cardiopulmonary rehabilitation, within the practice of North American cardiovascular medicine, began in the early 1970s and is still in its infancy. In contrast, the first description of the cardiovascular system dates back to Greek physicians in 384 B.C.E. (1).

History of Cardiopulmonary Rehabilitation

This section provides a review of the findings and discoveries of past centuries and of more recent years that have directly or indirectly contributed to the practice of cardiopulmonary rehabilitation as we know it today.

Before 1800

Although Galen stated in the year 131 that exercise "strengthens" the body (2), it was not until 1665 that Viseussens described the coronary circulation (3), and only in 1679 was occlusion of a coronary vessel documented by Bonnetus as a cause of death (1). In 1772, Heberden recommended that his "cardiac" patients exercise 30 minutes a day (4), and in 1789, Lavoisier conducted the first cardiovascular physiology experiment, in which oxygen uptake was measured at rest, after eating a meal, and during exercise (5).

1800-1900

Beddoes opened the Pneumatic Institute for the study of heart disease and asthma in 1800 (6), and shortly afterward, Heberden described angina pectoris (7). Regular exercise and walking were prescribed to cardiac patients in 1854 by both Stokes and Ortel (8). In the mid-1800s, Hilton prescribed bed rest for patients with cardiac conditions (9,10). Toward the end of the century (1870), Fick described the "Fick equation" for cardiac output, and in 1896, Williams developed fluoroscopy (11). Britain described the "athlete's heart" in 1895 (12).

1900-1950

Einthoven developed the first electrocardiograph in 1903 (1) and in 1912, Herrick reported the occlusion of a coronary artery as a cause of death (13). In 1916, a hospital was designated in England for the study of heart disease (14).

The 1930s and 1940s were significant in the development of current-day cardiopulmonary rehabilitation. In 1930, Barach, still considered the "father of respiratory therapy," began treating pulmonary patients with an oxygen tent (6) and in 1930, Sjostand developed the first cardiovascular exercise physiology laboratory in Sweden (9). At about the same time, Schneider reported a 24% increase in endurance following a 12-week exercise program for cardiac patients (2), and Gemmll recommended endurance exercise for his cardiac patients (9). In 1935, White became increasingly concerned about the negative effects of bed rest in the recovery process of cardiac patients (15), and the National Aeronautics and Space Administration (NASA) published a study documenting the negative effects of bed rest (16). In 1938, Bishop published the first article encouraging exercise for cardiac patients (17), and by the early 1940s, pulmonary rehabilitation became the accepted treatment for asthma, bronchitis, and emphysema (2).

The late 1940s were also a significant period for cardiac care and rehabilitation. Beck, Prichard, and Feil developed the defibrillator in 1947 (18), and in 1948, the National Heart Institute became a section of the National Institutes of Health. The American College of Cardiology was created one year later.

1950-1960

Interest in and documentation of the benefits of cardiopulmonary rehabilitation continued to increase with each successive decade. Whereas the 1930s and 1940s marked the beginning of research and the emergence of new cardiopulmonary treatment programs involving exercise, actual programs that resemble current cardiopulmonary rehabilitation programs were first designed in the 1950s. During that period, the work of Hellerstein and Goldston (19) in work classification units, cardiovascular exercise testing, assessment of patients' emotional and social needs, and vocational aptitudes and skills was very significant. In 1952, Levine and Lown examined the possibility of preventing coronary thrombosis by moving patients from bed to chair (20). In 1952, Newman et al. developed a walking program, which patients began four weeks after a myocardial infarction (21).

Millar reported on the value of exercise testing for pulmonary patients in 1952 (22), and in 1953, Morris et al. documented the relationship between physical activity and cardiovascular fitness (23). In 1957, Karvonen published his research on the effects of training on heart rate (24). Karvonen's research indicated that as training levels increased and as the individuals' conditioning level also increased, the heart rate level for a given amount of exercise decreased.

The 1960s

Growth and more widespread acceptance of cardiopulmonary rehabilitation continued in the 1960s. Komblueh and Micheal presented their exercise program for cardiac patients in 1961 (25), and Cain, Frasher, and Stiuelman began monitoring the intensity of daily activities of cardiac patients via ECG recordings (26). In 1968, Gottheimer further documented the benefits of exercise in the rehabilitation of cardiac patients (27). Saltin et al. reported their classic research on bed rest and its resulting decrease in cardiovascular performance levels in 1968 (28), and Cooper's book *Aerobics* became a best seller in 1968 (29). In 1969, Cantwell and Fletcher reported on cardiovascular complications and death in two joggers (30). The findings of Cantwell and Fletcher indicated the cause of death as a rhythm disturbance (arrhythmia) or a congenital heart defect.

The 1970s

In 1971, Kaufinan reported his work on walking programs for cardiac patients in which patients' cardiovascular level of conditioning improved via participation in a walking program (31), and in 1972, the American Heart Association published *Exercise Testing and Training of Apparently Healthy Individuals: A Handbook for Physicians* (32). In 1973, Wenger and colleagues reported on her inpatient cardiac rehabilitation program (33), and in 1974, Petty released material defining pulmonary rehabilitation (34). In 1975, the American College of Sports Medicine published the first edition of the *Guidelines for Graded Exercise Testing and Exercise Prescription* (35), and also in 1975, the American Heart Association published *Exercise Testing and Training of Individuals With Heart Disease or at High Risk for Its Development: A Handbook for Physicians* (36). The American College of Sports Medicine released its position statement on the recommended quantity and quality of exercise for developing and maintaining fitness in healthy adults in 1978 (37), and Haskell documented the low risk of complications during exercise training of cardiac patients (38).

The 1980s

In the 1980s, additional research funding became available, and cardiovascular research programs throughout North America continued to develop. The American Association of Cardiovascular and Pulmonary Rehabilitation was created in 1985. Probably the most significant report on the value of exercise for the general public was Paffenbarger et al.'s study of Harvard alumni, which documented that the risk of mortality decreased as the amount of exercise increased (39). In 1988, the Health and Public Policy Committee of the American College of Physicians published a position paper on cardiac rehabilitation (40), and Oldridge et al. published their investigation of the benefits of cardiopulmonary rehabilitation (41).

The 1990s

In the 1990s, cardiopulmonary rehabilitation became widely accepted as a valued service. The 1990s were also a period of continued growth and influence by the American Association of Cardiovascular and Pulmonary Rehabilitation. Universities began to offer specialized graduate programs in education and training in cardiopulmonary rehabilitation, and health professionals became more aware of the need for specialized staff in the cardiopulmonary rehabilitation process. Despite the growth in research and increased support by professional organizations, the arrival of managed care led to a decrease in available funds for cardiopulmonary rehabilitation. These difficulties with funding and third party reimbursement continue today.

What does the future offer for cardiopulmonary rehabilitation? Will the profession remain a viable service offered to cardiac and pulmonary patients in the years 2005, 2010, and beyond? Does the past provide us with any trends or information that would allow us to predict the path of our profession over the coming decades?

The Future of Cardiopulmonary Rehabilitation

The following predictions are related to general and specific concerns with cardiopulmonary rehabilitation. They are the result of multiple conversations with authorities in the field, as well as a review of the pertinent literature.

Areas Related to Cardiac Rehabilitation

Several factors, including a more healthy lifestyle, improved nutrition, and health screening, will lead to improved cardiovascular health for many people.

Healthy Lifestyle

Opportunities to exercise will become even more available. Corporate fitness programs will continue to be available and are likely to increase in number. Recent reports indicate that participants in corporate fitness programs have an increased awareness of wellness, less absenteeism and employee turnover, and greater productivity than employees who do not participate in the programs. It has also been reported that health care costs decrease for participating employees (42).

Growth of hospital-based wellness programs will continue, as will growth in health and fitness clubs. It is estimated that during the next few decades, hospital wellness facilities will experience a 70% growth, commercial facilities will grow 47%, corporate facilities will grow 39%, and not-for-profit facilities will grow 22% (43). Experts also predict that most health clubs will use some form of heart rate monitors. For cardiopulmonary patients, supervision via the Internet and/or transtelphonics (telephone monitoring) will be provided by ECG monitoring from local hospitals or private clinics. In short, health and fitness facilities will become major players in the health care system (44).

Nutrition

Changes of attitude toward nutrition are likely to have a major influence. The American Heart Association and other similar organizations will emphasize that obesity represents a major and primary risk factor for cardiovascular disease (45). Food products meeting individual nutritional needs will be more available for purchase via the Internet and in health clubs. They will also be available at hospitals and private clinics. The use of food supplements will increase, with particular interest in botanicals and phytochemicals.

Dieters will be more concerned with total number of calories than with fat calories. However, for the individual with high cholesterol levels, the impact of a low-fat diet will still be important. The science (and business) of lipid management will become more widely known, and the reduction of coronary events via lipid-lowering techniques will become accepted. Interest in cholesterol-lowering drugs will continue. The search for a safe "fat blocker" drug will also continue.

Screening

New health screening techniques will be introduced, and screening will be conducted in health clubs (46). The guidelines developed by the American College of Sports Medicine and the American Heart Association in 1998 (47) will have a tremendous impact not only on screening and identification of individuals at risk for cardiovascular problems, but also on staffing of health facilities. Hospital-based and private clinic–based screening techniques will continue to be developed. Myocardial perfusion imaging during the graded exercise test (treadmill or stationary bicycle) will become common practice. Computerized tomography or electron-beam computerized tomography (EBCT) used to identify, locate, and determine the degree of calcium deposits in the coronary arteries will become less expensive and more practical.

Procedures

New and improved procedures will have a major influence on prevention and treatment of cardiovascular conditions.

Drug Therapy

Drug treatment for the cardiopulmonary patient may include a "super aspirin," another form of platelet reception blockers to prevent clotting, or a new and improved medication to protect the myocardium from immediate and long-term infarction damage. Both "clot buster" techniques, such as percutaneous transluminal coronary angioplasty (PTCA), and β-blocker utilization are currently underutilized to either reverse the effect of a stroke or heart attack or for the treatment of heart failure, but in the future they will be more widely used.

Chelation therapy, with its possible effect on the calcium located within the arteriosclerotic plaque, is an interesting and potentially useful method. The main chemical agent of chelation therapy is ethylenediemine tetraacetic acid (EDTA), which is believed to bind with and remove calcium. Through an increased emphasis on education, the number of persons untreated for hypertension may significantly decrease, resulting in a decrease in related cardiovascular problems.

Surgery

From reoperation for coronary or valvular disease, to catheter blasting of channels in the inner wall of the heart to stimulate blood vessel growth and reduce angina, to implanted defibrillators, the surgical area of cardiovascular medicine will continue to expand in the next century. Not only will new surgical techniques be developed for both coronary artery and valve disease but new surgical techniques for electrical problems will be developed. Arrhythmias will be treated with radio frequency catheter utilization to destroy the unwanted electrical pathway. For selected patients, these types of procedures will eventually eliminate the need for arrhythmia drug therapy.

Gene Therapy

Gene therapy will have significant effects on cardiovascular medicine. The use of gene therapy to grow collateral coronary vessels will become common practice, although patients eligible for gene therapy are likely to be nonsurgical candidates. Many gene therapy patients will be those who have experienced repeated unsuccessful angioplasty procedures.

Increased Length of Life

Length of life will be a major factor in cardiovascular medicine during the next century. Our current understanding of the aging process and the effect of medical advancements will result in many more people becoming "cardiac patients" in their later life. Life expectancy is now 75-76 years for men and 82-83 years for women, but the life expectancy of a girl born in the United States will soon be approaching 100. Finally, between 1990 and 2020, the population aged 65-74 years is expected to grow 74% (48). Obviously, one effect of increased life expectancy will be an increase in cardiovascular procedures and treatments—which will ultimately result in further lengthening of life.

Cardiopulmonary Rehabilitation

Changes in administration and funding of cardiopulmonary rehabilitation programs, as well as new treatment philosophies, will have a great effect on both providers and patients.

Administration

As currently practiced, cardiac and pulmonary rehabilitation will no longer be available within the next 5 to 10 years. Major modifications in rehabilitation procedures and practice must take place before the reimbursement system will allow either cardiac or pulmonary rehabilitation, as currently practiced in many hospitals, to exist. What is necessary is a major reevaluation of goals and objectives, and new policies and procedures to reach those goals and objectives. In the next 5 to 10 years, the staff involved in these new programs will be highly skilled *clinical exercise physiologists,* with responsibilities beyond cardiopulmonary rehabilitation. Disease management will be a primary responsibility, and will include the management of diseased patients other than those with cardiac and pulmonary conditions. Certification of staff will be the rule, with procedures directly provided by these staff and billing from the provider (clinical exercise physiologist) to the payer. Finally, cardiopulmonary rehabilitation programs will need to be certified, or third party reimbursement will not be provided. Universities and colleges that educate and train clinical exercise physiologists will also need to be certified, or their graduates will not be eligible to take the board certification examination.

Treatment

The primary cardiopulmonary treatment procedures in the 21st century will be based on risk reduction therapy (49). Patients' risk tendencies will be identified and the appropriate treatment will be provided. In most cases, exercise will be the foundation of treatment methods and procedures that will be provided to patients in order to reduce their individual risk factors. Goals will be established by involved professional organizations, in companion with federal agencies, followed by directed activity to reach those goals (50). Techniques necessary to reach established goals will be refined far beyond techniques and procedures currently available (51). Other research on patient compliance will provide answers to questions regarding how to maintain individuals in programs (52). This research will be a combined effort of hospitals, clinics, and universities, and will benefit not only those in rehabilitation programs but patients of all types, since compliance is equally important to all therapy programs.

Summary

The plan of action for the American Heart Association for the period of 1998-2008 involves a further commitment to reduce disability and death from cardiovascular disease. Two major commitments have been established:

> "The basic need to reduce disability and death from heart disease and stroke by providing credible information for effective prevention and treatment with SPECIAL EMPHASIS ON THOSE AT RISK,"

and

> "By 2008, the AHA will reduce coronary heart disease, stroke and risk by 25%." (53)

These commitments are significant. However, will cardiopulmonary rehabilitation exist in the year 2008? With adjustments and modifications in step with advancements in cardiovascular medicine, the answer is: Yes! Those involved in cardiopulmonary rehabilitation must adapt to the needs of the patient as well as involved medical personnel. Multifactor rehabilitation, secondary rehabilitation, preventive cardiology clinics, and high-risk programs are all on the horizon for cardiopulmonary rehabilitation. The future of cardiopulmonary rehabilitation mandates that as a service, it must be provided by the exercise physiology department and staff. Exercise physiology as the basic body of knowledge and exercise physiologists as providers will be the foundation of the development of cardiopulmonary rehabilitation into and beyond the 21st century.

> *Eating alone will not keep man well; he must also take exercise. For food and exercise, while possessing opposite qualities, yet work together to produce health. For it is the nature of exercise to use up material, but of food and drink to make deficiencies. And it is necessary, as it appears, to discern the power of various exercises both natural exercises and artificial, to know which of them tends to increase flesh and which to lessen it; and not only this, but also to proportion exercise bulk of food, to the constitution of the patient, to ages of the individual, to the season of the year, to the changes of the winds, to the situation of the region in which the patient resides, and to the constitution of the year.*
>
> Hippocrates, 400 B.C.E. (54)

Acknowledgments

The authors thank the following people for assistance with this manuscript: Kathleen Berra, MSN, ANP; Kristine Clark, PhD, RD; Carl Foster, PhD; Barry A. Franklin, PhD; Linda K. Hall, PhD; Daniel J. Lynch, MS; and John P. Porcari, PhD.

References

1. Schmidt, J.E. 1959. *Medical Discoveries.* Springfield, IL: Thomas Publishers.
2. Berra, K. 1991. Cardiac and pulmonary rehabilitation: historical perspectives and future needs. *J Cardiopulm Rehabil* 11:8-15.
3. Harvey, W. 1958. *De Circulatione Sanguinis.* Oxford, England: Blackwell Scientific Publications.
4. Heberden, W. 1772. Some accounts of a disorder of the chest. *Med Trans Coll Phys* 2:59.
5. Dill, D.B. 1967. The Harvard fatigue laboratory: its development, contributions and demise. In *Physiology of Muscular Exercise,* ed. C.B. Chapman. New York: American Heart Association.

6. Barach, A.L. 1998. *Physiologic Therapy in Respiratory Diseases.* Philadelphia: J.B. Lippincott.
7. Heberden, W. 1802. *Commentaries on the History and Care of Disease.* London: T. Payne.
8. Stokes, W. 1854. *Disease of the Heart and Aorta.* Philadelphia: Lindsay.
9. Licht, S. 1961. *Therapeutic Exercise.* 2d ed. New Haven, CT: E. Licht.
10. Garrison, F.H. 1963. *An Introduction to the History of Medicine.* 4th ed. Philadelphia: W.B. Saunders.
11. Fye, W.B. 1984. Coronary angioplasty: it took a long time! *Circulation* 7:781-787.
12. Park, R.J. 1995. History of research on physical activity and health: selected topics, 1867 to the 1950s. *Quest* 47:274-287.
13. Herrick, J.B. 1912. Clinical features of sudden occlusion of the coronary arteries. *JAMA* 59:2015-2020.
14. Berryman, J.W. 1995. *Out of Many, One: A History of the American College of Sports Medicine.* Champaign, IL: Human Kinetics.
15. White, R.D, H.A. Rusk, and B. Williams, et al. 1957. *Cardiovascular Rehabilitation.* New York: McGraw-Hill.
16. Vogt, F.B., W.A. Spencer, and D. Cardus, et al. 1965. *NASA Contractor Reports: The Effects of Bedrest on Various Parameters of Physiological Functions.* Washington, DC: NASA.
17. Bishop, L.F. 1938. Exercise in the treatment of chronic cardiovascular disease. *Arch Phys Ther* 19:415-418, 435.
18. Beck, C.S., V. M. Prichard, and H.S. Feil. 1947. Ventricular fibrillation of long duration abolished by electric shock. *JAMA* 135:985-986.
19. Hellerstein, H.K., and E. Goldston. 1954. Rehabilitation of patients with heart disease. *Postgrad Med* 1 5:265-278.
20. Levine, S.A., and B. Lown. 1952. Armchair treatment of acute coronary thrombosis. *JAMA* 148:1365-1369.
21. Newman, L.B., M.S. Andrews, M.O. Koelish, and L.A. Baker. 1952. Physical medicine and rehabilitation in acute myocardial infarction. *Arch Intern Med* 89:552-561.
22. Millar, W.F. 1958. Physical therapeutic measures in the treatment of chronic bronchopulmonary disorders. *Am J Med* 24:929.
23. Morris, J.N., J.A. Heady, P.A. Raffle, C.G. Roberts, and J.W. Parks. 1953. Coronary heart disease and physical activity of work. Lancet 2:1053-1057.
24. Karvonen, M.J. 1957. The effects of training on heart rate: a longitudinal study. *Ann Med Exp Biol Fenn* 35:307.

25. Komblueh, I.H., and E. Micheal. 1961. Outline of exercise program for patients with myocardial infarction. *Pa Med* 60:1575-1578.

26. Cain, H.D., W.G. Frasher, and R. Stiuelman. 1961. Graded activity program for safe return to self-care following myocardial infarction. *JAMA* 177:111-115.

27. Gottheimer, V. 1968. Long-range strenuous sports training for cardiac reconditioning and rehabilitation. *Am J Cardiol* 22:426-435.

28. Saltin, B.G., J.H. Blomquist, and R. Mitchell, et al. 1968. Response to exercise after bed rest and training. *Circulation* 38 (suppl.) 7:71-78.

29. Cooper, K.H. 1968. *Aerobics.* New York: Bantam Books.

30. Cantwell, J.D., and G.F. Fletcher. 1969. Cardiac complications while jogging. *JAMA* 210:130-131.

31. Kaufinan, J.M. 1971. Early walking not harmful in uncomplicated myocardial infarction. *Int Med News* 3:5.

32. American Heart Association. 1972. *Exercise Testing and Training of Apparently Healthy Individuals: A Handbook for Physicians.* New York: American Heart Association.

33. Wenger, N.K., H. K. Hellerstein, H. Blackburn, and S.V. Castranova. 1973. Uncomplicated myocardial infarction. Current physician practice in patient management. *JAMA* 224:511-514.

34. Petty, T.L. 1974. *Pulmonary Rehabilitation. Basics of RD.* New York: American Thoracic Society.

35. American College of Sports Medicine. 1975. *Guidelines for Graded Exercise Testing and Exercise Prescription.* Philadelphia: Lea and Febiger.

36. American Heart Association. 1975. *Exercise Testing and Training of Individuals With Heart Disease or at High Risk for Its Development: A Handbook for Physicians.* Dallas, TX: American Heart Association.

37. American College of Sports Medicine. 1978. Position statement: the recommended quantity and quality of exercise for developing and maintaining fitness in healthy adults. *Med Sci Sports Exerc* 10:7-10.

38. Haskell, W. 1978. Cardiovascular complications during exercise training of cardiac patients. *Circulation* 57:920-924.

39. Paffenbarger, R.S., Jr., R.T. Hyde, A.L. Wing, and C.C. Hsieh. 1986. Physical activity, all-cause mortality, and longevity of college alumni. *N Eng J Med* 314:605-613.

40. Health and Public Policy Committee, American College of Physicians. 1988. Position paper. Cardiac rehabilitation services. *Ann Intern Med* 109:671-673.

41. Oldridge, N.B., G.H. Guyatt, M.E. Fischer, and A.A. Rimm. 1988. Cardiac rehabilitation after myocardial infarction: combined experience of randomized clinical trials. *JAMA* 260:945-950.

42. Shephard, R.J. 1999. Do work-site exercise and health programs work? *Phys Sports Med* 2:50-70.

43. McGough, S. 1999. Fitness 2000. *Fitness Management* 1:6-7.

44. Durak, E.P., and A.J. Palmieri. 1998. Opportunities in managed care. *Fitness Management* 10:48-50.

45. American Heart Association. 1999. Obesity is a major risk factor for heart disease. *Heart Stroke News* (winter): 2.

46. McInnis, K.J., and G.J. Balady. 1999. Higher cardiovascular risk clients in health clubs. *ACSM Health Fitness J* 1 / 2:19-24.

47. American Heart Association/American College of Sports Medicine. 1998. Recommendations for cardiovascular screening, staffing, and emergency policies at health and fitness facilities. *Med Sci Sports Exerc* 1009-1018.

48. U.S. Census Bureau. 1999. *USA Today.* March 17:7D.

49. Paul-Lavrador, M., P. Vongvanich, and C.N. Merz. 1999. Risk stratification for exercise training in cardiac patients: do the proposed guidelines work? *J Cardiopulm Rehab* 19:118-125.

50. Hall, L.K. 1998. Will my cardiac rehabilitation program survive in the new managed care era? The road map will be drawn by measured objectives. *J Cardiopulm Rehabil* 18:9-16.

51. Franklin, B.A., L.K. Hall, and G.C. Timmis. 1997. Contemporary cardiac rehabilitation services. *Am J Cardiol* 79:1075-1077.

52. Hershberger, P.J., K.B. Robertson, and R.J. Markert. 1999. Personality and appointment-keeping adherence in cardiac rehabilitation. *J Cardiopulm Rehabil* 19:106-111.

53. American Heart Association. 1999. Plan of action for 1998-2008. *Heart Stroke News* (winter):6.

54. Pitts, E.H. 1999. Redefining health redefines. *Fitness Management* (February): 6.

CHAPTER 2

Cardiovascular Rehabilitation: A Concept in Search of Its Identity

Serge Dumont
Université Laval, Institut Universitaire de Cardiologie et de Pneumologie, Hôpital Laval, Québec, Canada

Cardiovascular rehabilitation is part of the recent history of biomedicine. Over the last two decades, it has been in the process of defining its identity within the continuum of cardiology care. This chapter focuses on the issues related to this search for identity. First, we present the major paradigms[1] that have successively influenced clinical cardiology practices in North America, and more specifically, in Québec.

Paradigms in Clinical Cardiology

Four paradigms can be identified on the basis of a retrospective analysis of practices for treating coronary heart disease: bed rest, armchair, early mobilization, and secondary prevention. Each of these paradigms has had a significant impact on changes in the social representation[2] of cardiac patients and heart disease. At the same time, they have influenced, and continue to influence, the development of cardiology practice and rehabilitation programs in the field.

Bed Rest

The bed-rest paradigm largely determined clinical cardiology practices until the mid-20th century. It ensued from a very generalized principle in medicine that a diseased organ had to be put to rest to promote healing. Therefore, confinement to bed and prolonged rest were central to treating victims of cardiac events. "When the heart is diseased, the only feasible application of the principle of rest is the attempted diminution of cardiac load. Rest in a bed has been traditionally regarded as tantamount to optimal rest for the heart" (1). Thus, myocardial infarction patients were confined to bed for a period of 3-6 weeks.

During that period, knowledge of the physiopathology of infarction was based mainly on a description of coronary thrombosis from the work of Obrastzows and Straschesko published in 1910 (2) and studies carried out by Herrick in 1912 (1). From the outset, the scholarly (or scientific) discourse coincided with commonly held representations of the cardiac patient. In both discourses, cardiac patients were defined as chronic invalids confined to rest for the remainder of their lives. This social representation was deeply embedded in the collective imagination, and, even today, the stigma attached to myocardial infarction patients compromises their social and professional reintegration.

Armchair

Clinical observation of heart disease patients confined to bed rest led some physicians to question the therapeutic effect of prolonged bed rest for that category of patients. Levine and Lown (3) observed a deterioration in the physical and psychological condition of patients confined to bed rest. The main negative effects of prolonged bed rest were inanition, constipation, thrombophlebitis, osteoporosis, negative nitrogen balance, hypostatic pneumonia, atelectasis, prostate difficulties, and psychological distress among patients and members of their families (4). As a result, Levine and Lown (3) suggested transferring patients as quickly as possible from the bed to an armchair, arguing that a sitting position with the feet on the ground is less demanding on the heart and facilitates recovery. This assertion was based on a better understanding of cardiac hemodynamics. However, this development in the treatment of myocardial infarction had little influence on the social representation of the cardiac patient, who continued to be viewed as weakened and unfit for physical effort. That representation was largely responsible for a sociocultural process that had the effect of systematically disabling patients.

Early Mobilization

Early mobilization is the third paradigm that gradually transformed hospital-based cardiology practices during the 1970s (5). This paradigm resulted from the development of new knowledge in the field of human physiology. The heart was perceived less and less as an isolated organ; physicians recognized that it was first and foremost a muscle whose functioning was intimately connected to all the body's other muscles and to pulmonary functions. The heart was seen to be sensitive not only to the effects of deconditioning of its own structure, but also to the more generalized deconditioning of the body's musculature as a whole. A hypothesis was put forward that confinement to a bed or an armchair led to deconditioning of the heart and of all the muscular system, which appeared likely to compromise the patient's rehabilitation. Under this paradigm, patient rehabilitation found its first true purpose: getting patients to a better fitness level.

The restrictive nature of this first definition of cardiovascular rehabilitation may appear surprising, because in 1964, the World Health Organization gave the following definition: "The sum of activity required to ensure cardiac patients the best possible physical, mental and social conditions so that they, by their own efforts, regain as normal as possible a place in the community and lead an active life" (6). The resistance to engage patients with myocardial infarction in activities demanding a certain physical effort could be explained by the social representation of heart patients as vulnerable and fragile. However, an important change in this representation was observed during this period. Increasingly, in the collective imagination, myocardial infarctions were associated with hard-working, devoted people who push themselves at work. This transformation in the social representation of heart patients was part of a broader social movement in which work became valued as a source of personal and social accomplishment. It also coincided with an important research trend that attempted to identify a psychological makeup that could be associated with the development of coronary heart disease. On the basis of such research, two behavior profiles were identified: type A and type B (7). Type A individuals were described as ambitious, overinvolved in their work, and preoccupied by a chronic sense of time urgency. Type B individuals, on the other hand, were characterized as more flexible, rarely in conflict with others, and relatively unconcerned with time constraints.

At the beginning of the 1980s, exercise tests during the first days after an infarct were introduced into routine clinical evaluations. These tests led to the development of protocols of risk stratification (8,9). These protocols made it safer for physicians to recommend that patients progressively resume their daily activities. It also reinforced the idea that the majority of patients could resume a relatively normal life and return to work. To ensure that they recovered, they were encouraged to exercise by walking during their hospitalization. However, the new ideas that were progressively penetrating the world of health care came into conflict with stigmas associated with heart disease and the persistent representation that patients were fragile. Consequently, only a limited number of cardiovascular rehabilitation programs were established in treatment centers during this period, in spite of the fact that new knowledge on human physiology and psychology clearly supported such programs.

Unfortunately, the first studies of the effects of rehabilitation gave inconsistent results. They were criticized for their many methodological weaknesses (10). For instance, many subjects were excluded from early studies due to fears of submitting supposedly fragile patients to physical training programs whose safety had not yet been sufficiently demonstrated. Furthermore, the concept of cardiovascular rehabilitation went through an interesting development and increasingly incarnated the multidimensional perspective referred to by the World Health Organization 30 years earlier. The rehabilitation of heart patients was defined as a process by which patients recover their optimal physical, psychological, and social capacities.

> Short-term objectives included physical reconditioning sufficient for resuming customary activities, educating patients and family about the disease

> process, and providing psychological support during the early recovery phase of the illness. Long-term objectives included identifying and treating risk factors that influenced the progression of disease, teaching and reinforcing the health behavior that improved prognosis, optimizing physical conditioning, and facilitating a return to occupational and avocational activities. (11)

Although the clinical indications for cardiovascular rehabilitation were initially recommended for myocardial infarction patients, they were progressively extended to other categories of heart disease patients. As a result, rehabilitation is currently recommended for patients who have undergone coronary artery bypass grafting or heart transplantation as well as angioplasty. It is now recognized that even some patients with significant left ventricular dysfunction and low work capacity, who used to be viewed as poor candidates for rehabilitation, can benefit from rehabilitation (12,13,14).

Secondary Prevention

The fourth paradigm ensues from important developments observed in the field of epidemiological research on ischemic heart disease, which began in 1948 in the United States with Framingham's prospective study (15). It was soon followed by a number of similar studies in Europe and elsewhere in the United States, most notably the Seven Countries Study (16), the French Belgium Collaborative Group Study (17), and the Multiple Risk Factor Intervention Trial (18). Toward the end of the 1970s, these longitudinal studies led to the sanctioning of the concept of coronary risk factor, that is, a factor that is statistically linked to the later manifestation of a coronary event. The first three factors that were suspected to be intimately connected to heart disease were age, hypertension, and tobacco consumption, and more recently, diabetes, hypercholesterolemia, and lack of exercise. Obesity and a type A personality are still in question as independent risk factors.

This fourth paradigm, which progressively took root in the mid-1980s, has had a determining effect on recent developments in clinical cardiology. It reinforced the legitimacy of cardiovascular rehabilitation, whose effectiveness in reducing certain risk factors such as smoking, high cholesterol, lack of exercise, and obesity is increasingly recognized in the scientific literature (19).

This new epidemiological knowledge came at a time when many industrialized countries began questioning the effectiveness of their health care systems, which were putting more and more strain on public funds. Modern epidemiological research gave public health authorities the tools to identify more clearly the risk factors for certain diseases, to characterize high-risk populations, and to verify the effectiveness of strategies for reducing the incidence of certain diseases. The contribution of epidemiological research to the development of modern medicine became more and more determining.

Within the paradigm of secondary prevention, a discourse has developed over the last 10 years to the effect that government decision makers and clinicians must emphasize strategies that aim to reduce the risk factors that are statistically related to morbidity and mortality. From its beginnings, cardiovascular rehabilitation was based on this approach, and the new discourse has only reinforced its legitimacy.

Cardiovascular Rehabilitation as Secondary Prevention: Opportunity or Pitfall?

The paradigm of secondary prevention can, in some ways, jeopardize the development and establishment of rehabilitation programs in clinical settings. In the second half of this article, we present the arguments that justify this apprehension.

Health Care Organization

The secondary prevention paradigm introduced the concept of prevention. Although it can find a comfortable place in the world of public health, it clashes with the concept of curing in the field of biomedicine. The issues related to the debate (indeed the duality) between prevention and cure are well known, and the discourse on secondary prevention is no exception. The need for preventive action is indisputable and recognized by all. However, we are far from reaching a consensus on the portion of the health care budget that should be earmarked for it. That question is crucial in a health care system such as that in Québec or Canada, where resources are allocated according to a ration system. Alongside this debate is the issue of responsibility. Who is responsible for curing? Who is responsible for prevention? Although the answer to the first question appears clear, the answer to the second one is much less obvious. Moreover, beyond the budgetary division between curing and prevention is the issue of who is responsible. Prevention generally, and secondary prevention more specifically, involve many people from a wide variety of organizations not only in the field of health care, but also in education, the environment, municipal affairs, and other pursuits. This diversity, however, does not encourage the different authorities to become involved or to take responsibility for certain aspects of prevention. Moreover, hospital workers do not feel particularly concerned by the preventive mission, whether primary or secondary. To the contrary: The financial constraints that they have faced in recent years pressure them to concentrate their meager resources on the curative mission that must take priority in their work.

In summary, since the paradigm of secondary prevention inevitably engages the curative/preventive debate, the development of cardiovascular rehabilitation is subject to the same underfunding as the preventive mission with which it tends to be associated. Hospitals where cardiac patients are treated do not perceive themselves as having a specific mandate to offer rehabilitation services to their patients.

In fact, many people believe that this duty should fall to perihospital or community organizations. The question raises a crucial issue concerning the development of cardiovascular rehabilitation programs.

Treatment of Cardiac Patients

The growing influence of the secondary prevention paradigm on the treatment of cardiac patients can be observed in the changes in the discourse of Canadian medical authorities. The Canadian Cardiovascular Society's (CCS) 1997 Consensus Conference document on the evaluation and treatment of ischemic heart diseases (20) lies within a different perspective than its consensus report published in 1995 (21), which revised the guidelines formulated by the CCS in 1991 with respect to the treatment of myocardial infarction patients. Whereas the 1991 and 1995 documents supported their main recommendations for treating patients on the basis of clinical considerations, the 1997 guidelines were justified almost completely by epidemiological data on the effects of treatment on morbidity and mortality.

Furthermore, the 1995 report uses the World Health Organization's definition of cardiovascular rehabilitation, emphasizing that it eases the symptoms of heart disease, increases cardiac output, and improves quality of life among patients. The 1997 consensus document does not mention cardiovascular rehabilitation, but states: "It has recently been shown that regular exercise reduces morbidity and mortality among patients who suffer from chronic ischemic heart disease" 20).

These observations raise concerns about the progressive replacement of the concept of rehabilitation by an approach that focuses mainly on treatment strategies that are recognized to reduce morbidity and mortality from a population perspective. This kind of shift could be detrimental to the development of cardiovascular rehabilitation programs that focus first and foremost on the individual. Investigators who attempt to demonstrate their effectiveness in reducing morbidity and mortality will always come up against important methodological difficulties. Convincing demonstration in this area requires very large homogeneous samples recruited from multiple centers, and this kind of protocol in the field of cardiac rehabilitation is practically unfeasible.

Social Representation of the Cardiac Patient

Under the secondary prevention paradigm, new elements enter into the process of constructing the social representation of the cardiac patient. Within this paradigm, cardiac patients are defined as individuals with health problems that put them at risk (hypertension, diabetes, obesity, hypercholesterolemia); they are recognized as having high-risk habits (smoking, lack of exercise, overeating, noncompliance with prescriptions, work addiction); and they are considered to belong to a high-risk population. They are also described as persons who cost a lot in terms of health care, social, and financial resources. In other words, they are a burden to their fellow citizens, and their habits must be changed to comply to new social norms regarding healthy living.

Inevitably, this perspective raises the specter of social control. From high-performance workers in the preceding paradigm, cardiac patients are demoted to social delinquents. Despite its initial pretentions, the discourse related to secondary prevention risks being party to a process of normalization or acculturation in which the social representation of patients is based on the notion of deviance with respect to new norms. Not only does this discourse make heart disease patients feel guilty and take away their sense of initiative, it hides the fact that ischemic heart diseases are above all "diseases of civilization," which are mainly the result of modern lifestyles. According to the rationale behind the secondary prevention discourse, responsibility for the disease falls mainly on those who have it, and health care authorities are mandated to develop treatment strategies aiming to change high-risk habits among individuals in the identified populations.

This discourse, which revolves around the notion of risk, is reminiscent of the phenomenon of the medicalization of pregnancy and childbirth. Mothers-to-be progressively became labeled as high-risk patients simply because they were pregnant. The unexpected effect of this initially well-intentioned approach was that women's bodies were appropriated by the medical system; the standard number of radiodiagnostic examinations multiplied; and in some senses, women became removed from the experience of childbirth, which had become highly medicalized (22).

In a slightly different perspective, the current secondary prevention paradigm also carries the seed of a disinvolvement of patients and a disappropriation of their experience. It is worth pointing out that the establishment of norms based on scales such as the body mass index (BMI), the atherogenic index, and others, indirectly introduces criteria of deviance. Thus, initiatives aiming to modify "inappropriate" behavior in a group of individuals can all too easily lapse into a cultural construction of blame and, in that sense, they raise unavoidable ethical issues. It will be interesting to follow the work of the Réseau d'éthique clinique chez l'humain (Network of Clinical Human Ethics) as far as this approach is concerned. The network is funded by the Fonds de recherche en santé du Québec (a Quebec health research fund) and recently adopted a mandate to reflect on the importance and the foundations of ethical issues in public health (23).

Finally, we must acknowledge that there is a potential ideological conflict between the secondary prevention paradigm and the philosophy generally put forward in cardiovascular rehabilitation programs. That philosophy insists on the unique character of the individual and the value of independence, indeed even self-determination. Its main goal is improving the person's quality of life. In the field of rehabilitation, patients are defined as persons with needs, whereas in the secondary prevention paradigm, patients are viewed as high-risk individuals, targets for change. This distinction is fundamental.

Cardiovascular Rehabilitation: A Laborious Search for Identity

Cardiovascular rehabilitation has searched for its identity under the influence of the last two paradigms, which have progressively succeeded each other in the field of ischemic heart disease treatment. Its first real legitimacy came under the early mobilization paradigm. The current paradigm of secondary prevention has reinforced this legitimacy while renewing discourses that, in some ways, may compromise its actual effectiveness in clinical settings. However, attention must be paid to the concept of rehabilitation itself in the field of ischemic heart disease treatment. Within the early mobilization paradigm, rehabilitation was defined mainly as a way to help infarction patients recover. Treatment was aimed at physical recovery, with a growing emphasis on psychological and social recovery. Although this first definition was restrictive, it did have the advantage of coinciding with the more general definition of the concept of rehabilitation, which refers to treatments that enable individuals to resume the activities and habits that they had to interrupt during a certain period of time due a health problem.

However, more recent developments in the field demonstrate the significant therapeutic effect of multidimensional rehabilitation programs on coronary atherogenesis. Henceforth, the impact of such programs goes beyond their primary goal (patient recovery) and contributes to treating the disease itself. This new reality raises etymological and practical issues. Can we still speak of rehabilitation? Should we be calling it "treatment?" Are the interventions related to secondary prevention, or are they therapeutic interventions that address both the causes and the consequences of the disease? Does the concept of cardiovascular rehabilitation accurately translate the reality it is meant to define? Does it adequately reveal the meaning and scope of that reality?

These questions are all the more relevant because in the field of post-trauma physical deficiencies and disabilities (spinal injuries, cranial trauma, amputation, stroke, etc.) the concept of rehabilitation is increasingly confined to its original definition, that is, "a series of medical-social means enabling a handicapped person to have a social and professional life that is as close as possible to normal."[3] This definition (which by the way excludes action regarding the causes of the disability) refers to the notion of "handicap," which is rather foreign to the world of heart disease. Finally, it is interesting that the concept of rehabilitation is also widely used in the field of delinquency and substance addiction.

Conclusion

Today, there is a broad consensus on the definition of cardiovascular rehabilitation, both among specialists in the field and in scientific circles (19,21). However, cardiovascular rehabilitation remains on a rather dangerous path as it seeks to define its identity. The more or less forced association between cardiovascular rehabilitation and the world of prevention, and the difficulty that the concept of rehabilitation has in demonstrating its curative value, are detrimental not only to its search for identity but also to its acceptance in clinical settings. It is particularly distressing to realize that, at the dawn of the third millennium, only a very small percentage of cardiac patients have access to true rehabilitation programs.

This analysis of what is at stake in the identity definition process would be incomplete if it did not open onto new perspectives.

First, our analysis suggests that we need to be more aware of the fact that practices in the field of cardiovascular rehabilitation are dependent on discourses that are elaborated on the basis of knowledge from both scientific research and the collective imagination. It is worth remembering that words have the dual power to define reality in all its uniqueness and to reduce or even distort its meaning.

Similarly, we should remain particularly alert to the unexpected or undesirable consequences of the paradigm of secondary prevention and the discourse underlying it. It would most definitely be wise not to consummate the marriage between rehabilitation and secondary prevention too quickly. Respectful cohabitation would no doubt be wiser.

Finally, we need to assess the relevance of including all cardiovascular rehabilitation interventions in what could eventually become a new category of care called "post-acute care in coronary heart disease." Such interventions would become recognized as an integral part of the continuum of clinical cardiology care. As Dr. William A. Dafoe stated, "Cardiac rehabilitation should be perceived as a part of the continuum of care for the cardiovascular patient" (24). "Post-acute care in coronary heart disease" is a term that could reflect both the multidimensional needs of patients and the interdisciplinary characteristics of the global approach that patients require. Moreover, it is in logical continuity with the notion of "acute care in coronary heart disease." This proposal is in keeping with recent developments in the field of medical terminology, in which interventions are categorized according to therapeutic sequences: intensive care, postoperative care, palliative care, and so forth.

Last, within this perspective, rehabilitation activities become an integral part of the continuum of curative care, where the future of rehabilitation is, in our view, more secure.

Notes

1. Paradigms are conceptual frameworks of reference that orient research and action in a given field of activity.
2. "Social representation" refers to a form of common knowledge, known as common sense. It is elaborated socially from information, knowledge, and forms of thought that are passed on in a given cultural context through

tradition, education, and social communication. (Jodelet, D. 1993. *Les représentations sociales.* Paris: Presses universitaires de France. Translation by the author.)

3. Le Petit Larousse illustré 1999 (Larousse, 1998, translation by the author).

References

1. Herrick, J.B. 1912. Clinical features of sudden obstruction of the coronary arteries. *JAMA* 59:2015.
2. Obrastzows, W., and P. Straschesko. 1910. Zur kenntnis der thrombose der Koronararterien des heizen. *Z Kin Med* 71-116.
3. Levine, S.A., and B. Lown. 1952. Armchair treatment of acute coronary thrombosis. *JAMA* 148:1365-1369.
4. Dock, W. 1944. Evil sequelae of complete bed rest. *JAMA* 125:1083.
5. Bloch, A., J.P. Maeder, and J.C. Haissly, et al. 1974. Early mobilization after myocardial infarction: a controlled study. *Am J Cardiol* 34:152-157.
6. World Health Organization Expert Committee. 1964. *Rehabilitation of Patients With Cardiovascular Diseases.* Technical Report Series No. 270. Geneva: World Health Organization.
7. Roseman, R.H., and M. Friedman. 1994. Neurogenic factor in pathogenesis of coronary heart disease. *Med Clin N Am* 58:269-279.
8. Debusk, R.F. 1989. Specialized testing after recent acute myocardial infarction: a review. *Ann Intern Med* 110:470-481.
9. The Multicentre Postinfarction Research Group. 1983. Risk stratification and survival after myocardial infarction. *N Engl J Med* 309:331-336.
10. Shanfield, S.B. 1990. Return to work after an acute myocardial infarction: a review. *Heart Lung* 19:109-117.
11. Dennis, C. 1991. Rehabilitation of the patient with coronary artery disease. In *Heart Disease,* ed. E.B. Braunwald. 4th ed. Philadelphia: W.B. Saunders, 1991.
12. Pashkow, F.J. 1993. Issues in contemporary cardiac rehabilitation: a historical perspective. *JACC* 21:822-834.
13. Gattiker, H., and C. Dennis. 1992. Cardiac rehabilitation: current status and future directions. *West J Med* 156:183-188.
14. Dafoe, W.A. 1992. Cardiac rehabilitation: an essential part of treatment. *Med N Am* (November):4600-4606.
15. Kannel, W.B. 1990. Contribution of the Framingham heart study to preventive cardiology. Bishop lecture. *J Am Coll Cardiol* 15:206-211.

16. Keys, A. 1970. Coronary heart disease in seven countries. *Circ Res* (suppl.) 41:11.

17. French Belgium Collaborative Group Study. 1982. Ischemic heart disease and psychological patterns: prevalence and incidence studies in Belgium and France. *Adv Cardiol* 29:25-30.

18. Stamler, J., D. Wentworth, and J.D. Neaton. 1986. Is the relationship between serum cholesterol and risk of premature death from coronary heart disease continuous and graded? Results in 356,222 primary screenees of the Multiple Risk Factor Intervention Trial (MRFIT). *JAMA* 256:2823.

19. Agency for Health Care Policy and Research and National Heart, Lung, and Blood Institute. 1995. Cardiac Rehabilitation. In *Clinical practice guideline 203*. Rockville, MD: U.S. Department of Health and Human Services, Public Health Service, Agency for Health Care Policy and Research, National Heart, Lung, and Blood Institute.

20. Conférence consensuel 1997 de la Société canadienne de cardiologie. 1998. Sur l'évaluation et le traitement des cardiopathies ischémiques chroniques. *Can J Cardiol* 14C:4C-24C.

21. Fallen, L.F., P. Armstrong, J. Cairns, and W. Dafoe, et al. 1995. Traitement des patients ayant subi un infarctus du myocarde: rapport consensuel—révision des lignes de conduites de la SCC formulées en 1991. *Can J Cardiol* 11:659-669.

22. Saillant, F., and M. O'Neill. 1987. Accoucher autrement: repères historiques, sociaux et culturels de la grossesse et de l'accouchement au Québec, Montreal: Éditions Saint-Martin.

23. Dubuc, M. 1997. *Pleins feux sur l'éthique clinique*. Québec: Recherche Santé, Fonds de recherche en santé du Québec.

24. Dafoe, W.A. 1992. Cardiac rehabilitation: an essential part of treatment. *Medicine North America*, November: 4600-4606.

PART II

Pharmacological Treatment of Congestive Heart Failure and Chronic Obstructive Pulmonary Disease: An Update

CHAPTER 3

Current Pharmacological Therapy for Congestive Heart Failure

Marie-Hélène LeBlanc

Section Insuffisance Cardiaque et Transplantation, Institut Universitaire de Cardiologie et de Pneumologie de l'Université Laval, Québec, Canada

Congestive heart failure (CHF) is a major health problem in Canada and throughout the world. In 1999, between 5 million and 7 million North Americans were afflicted by this disease, as were another estimated 20 million people in the rest of the world.

In Canada, more than 1% of the population is suffering from CHF, and it is the most common cause of hospitalization of people over 65 years of age. The incidence and prevalence of CHF will likely continue to rise as the population ages.

Recent data suggest that the CHF mortality rate may be as high as 40% to 50% after only 2 years of treatment. Moreover, acute decompensation of CHF results in high hospital readmission rates and increased health care costs. Overall, the cost of hospitalization for heart failure is twice that for all forms of cancer (1,2).

Angiotensin-Converting Enzyme (ACE) Inhibitors

The treatment of congestive heart failure has been facilitated with the introduction of angiotensin-converting enzyme (ACE) inhibitors in the 1980s. Because of them, congestive heart failure has become the subject of intense clinical research. They are now well established as first-line drug therapy in the treatment of CHF.

ACE inhibitors are indicated in all stages of symptomatic heart failure resulting from systolic cardiac dysfunction, because of their proven mortality benefits and effects on disease progression (3).

The SOLVD study showed that ACE inhibitors administered to asymptomatic patients with ejection fraction below 35% can reduce the development of heart failure and related hospitalizations compared to placebo treatment (4). ACE inhibitors can restore the cardiac and hormonal response to volume overload and thus reduce natriuresis in mild heart failure (5). They cannot act as a substitute for diuretics when a patient has a tendency toward fluid retention. These agents work by decreasing the production of angiotensin II through the renin-angiotensin-aldosterone system, which results in improved hemodynamic function. They also provide a therapeutic benefit as vasodilators because they reduce cardiac loading conditions. This has been well demonstrated in the SAVE study (6).

Many questions remain unanswered, particularly concerning the optimal individual doses and the extent to which angiotensin II formation is prevented during chronic treatment. With the currently available data, it would seem prudent to aim for the target dosages used in large clinical trials, although only a small minority of patients treated with ACE inhibitors are receiving these doses. No long-term randomized study to evaluate the effects of ACE inhibitor dosage on survival has been published.

The adverse effects of ACE inhibitors can be related to angiotensin suppression (hypotension, potassium retention, and worsening renal function) and to kinin potentiation (cough and angioedema).

Angiotensin II Receptor Blockers

The angiotensin II receptor antagonists block the action of angiotensin II at the At_1 level more completely than do ACE inhibitors. Many questions, however, remain unanswered. What is the optimal individual dose and to what extent is angiotensin II formation prevented during chronic treatment? Angiotensin II can be formed through alternative pathways, such as via angiotensin I chymases, which are not affected by ACE inhibitors. Furthermore, angiotensin II antagonists have no effect on bradykinin pathways. Bradykinin induces the release of nitric oxide in the endothelium, thereby helping to improve endothelial function and vasodilatation. Bradykinin is also responsible for some of the adverse effects associated with ACE inhibition, such as cough and angioedema. It is possible that many of the benefits of ACE inhibitors may be associated with the accumulation of kinins.

Several ongoing studies are evaluating the role of angiotensin II receptor antagonists in monotherapy or in combination with ACE inhibitors in the treatment of CHF. No evidence currently indicates that angiotensin II receptor antagonists are equivalent or superior to ACE inhibitors in the treatment of heart failure (7,8). The Elite II study comparing the effects of losartan and captopril on mortality and morbidity in heart failure patients is under way. They are as likely as ACE inhibitors to produce hypotension, worsening renal function, and hyperkalemia and should be prescribed only in patients who are intolerant to ACE inhibitors because of intractable cough or angioedema.

Diuretics

The goal of diuretic therapy in congestive heart failure is the improvement of congestive symptoms. Diuretics reduce the preload and may prevent hospitalization resulting from volume overload (9,10). Loop diuretics are generally used in CHF patients because they are efficacious even when the patient has impaired renal function. Diuretics may alter the efficacy and toxicity of many drugs used for the treatment of CHF. Under- or overdosing is a frequent risk, and every effort should be made to find the proper dose for each patient.

Digitalis

The combined results of the PROVED (11) and RADIANCE (12) studies indicate that digoxin increase the ejection fraction of the left ventricle more in the idiopathic dilated cardiomyopathy (IDC) than in ischemic cardiomyopathies. The withdrawal of digoxin in IDC patients worsens their clinical condition.

In the DIG (13) study, although there was no effect on overall survival, there was a significant reduction in the number of deaths or hospitalizations for progression of heart failure higher for IDC patients.

Digitalis alleviates symptoms and improves clinical status in CHF patients, and those with severe heart failure (NYHA class III-IV) seem to benefit the most from a long-term treatment.

β-Blockers

β-blockers as therapeutic agents in heart failure have been investigated for the past 20 years. They are now at the forefront of research on treatments for CHF. Their inhibition of the sympathetic nervous system is a unique method of limiting the progression of heart failure.

The therapeutic effect of β-blockers is obtained by gradually and slowly increasing the dose in patients with mild to moderate CHF, who have already been treated with an ACE inhibitor and diuretics. Initially, the patient's condition may become worse, but after treatment for 2-6 months, there is considerable improvement of the patient's functional class as well as of the left ventricular ejection fraction.

Clinical studies have shown that beta blockers, in particular carvedilol, metoprolol, and bucindolol, can improve exercise tolerance, hemodynamic abnormalities, and left ventricular function in patients with ischemic or nonischemic heart failure (14). The degree of benefit appears to be related to the degree of disability before treatment.

Four multicenter trials were conducted with carvedilol in the United States. The combined data demonstrate that carvedilol therapy is associated with a 65% decrease in risk of death and with a 27% reduction in the risk of hospitalization.

Carvedilol (15) and bisoprolol (16) reduce the mortality associated with ischemic or nonischemic dilated cardiomyopathy. Metoprolol (17) has improved the prognosis of patients with nonischemic dilated cardiomyopathy.

Whether multiple-receptor blockade has advantages over single-receptor blockade is now being evaluated in the Comet trial (Carvedilol or Metoprolol European Trial). The results of this study should be available by the year 2001. In the meantime, the difference in mortality rates related to the use of selective or nonselective β-blockers is unknown.

Will there be an advantage to using β-blockers as the first intervention instead of ACE inhibitors? The CARMEN study will evaluate carvedilol versus enalapril, versus carvedilol plus enalapril in patients with mild heart failure. The results of the BEST (bucindolol) and COPERNICUS (carvedilol) studies will let us know the effect of β-blocker therapy in patients with advanced (class IIIB-IV) heart failure.

New Neurohormonal Modulators

New neurohormonal modulators, such as endothelin receptor antagonists and renin antagonists, are now being investigated for use in patients with CHF.

Endothelin Receptor Antagonists

Endothelins are endogenous peptides with patent vasoconstrictor and vasopressor properties. At least three subtypes of endothelins are known to exist. In patients with moderate CHF (NYHA class III), elevated plasma concentrations of endothelin-1 have been observed. Investigators have found a direct correlation between elevated endothelin-1 level, functional class, and left ventricular end diastolic volume, as well as an inverse correlation with the ejection fraction and cardiac index (18,19). Bosentan is an orally active endothelin receptor antagonist. A few studies are currently under way to investigate its effects in patients with moderate to severe CHF.

Renin Antagonists

Renin antagonists are more specific modulators of the renin-angiotensin-aldosterone system than are ACE inhibitors. However, their oral bioavailability is limited (20).

As more therapeutic options are developed, there are reasons to think that individualized drug selection for CHF patients might become possible. An early and precise diagnosis of the etiology of heart failure could be of particular importance in the initiation of a selective drug therapy. Moreover, an individualized drug regimen based on different criteria (clinical status and laboratory exams) could lead to improved efficacy and better long-term drug tolerance. CHF is a progressive condition, and patients remain at risk for worsening disease despite the optimal use of current first-line medication.

Summary

Significant progress has been achieved in the treatment of cardiovascular diseases since the early 1980s. Despite medical management, the incidence and prevalence of congestive heart failure are still increasing, and the mortality associated with this disease is extremely high. In recent years, neurohormonal activation has emerged as one of the main mechanisms in heart failure treatment. Both ACE inhibitors and β-blockers have been shown to improve the prognosis as well as the clinical course of heart failure.

Although angiotensin II receptor blockers appear promising, their use cannot be endorsed for heart failure patients until several multicenter, randomized, controlled clinical trials have been completed.

Several new neurohormonal modulators are being investigated with the hope that in the near future, drug selection for patients with congestive heart failure may be individualized.

References

1. O'Connell, J.B., and M.R. Bristow. 1994. Economic impact of heart failure in the United States: time for a different approach. *J Heart Lung Transplant* 13:S107-112.
2. Ghali, J.K., R. Cooper, and E. Ford. 1990. Trends in hospitalization rates for heart failure in the United States, 1973-1986: evidence for increasing population prevalence. *Arch Intern Med* 150:769-773.
3. The SOLVD Investigators. 1991. Effects of enalapril on survival in patients with reduced left ventricular ejection fractions and congestive heart failure. *N Engl J Med* 325:293-302.
4. The SOLVD Investigators. 1992. Effect of enalapril on mortality and the development of heart failure in asymptomatic patients with reduced left ventricular ejection fractions. *N Engl J Med* 327:685-691.
5. Volpe, M., C. Tritto, and N. DeLuca, et al. 1992. Angiotensin converting enzyme inhibition restores cardiac and hormonal response to volume overload in patients with dilated cardiomyopathy and mild heart failure. *Circulation* 86:1800-1809.
6. Pfeffer, M., E. Braunwald, and L.A. Moye, et al. 1992. Effect of captopril on mortality and morbidity in patients with left ventricular dysfunction after myocardial infarction. *N Engl J Med* 327:669-677.
7. Pitt, B., R. Segal, and F.A. Martinez, et al. on behalf of the ELITE Study Investigators. 1997. Randomized trial of losartan versus captopril in patients

over 65 with heart failure (Evaluation of Losartan in the Elderly Study, ELITE). *Lancet* 349:747-752.

8. Pitt, B., and M.A. Konstam. 1998. Overview of angiotensin II-receptor antagonists. *Am J Cardiol* 82(10A):47A-49S.
9. Cody, R.J. 1993. Clinical trials of diuretic therapy in heart failure: research directions and clinical considerations. *J Am Coll Cardiol* 22 (suppl. A):65A-71A.
10. Dyckner, T., and P. Wester. 1986. Salt and water balance in congestive heart failure. *Acta Med Scand* 707 (suppl.):27-31.
11. Uretsky, B.F., J.B. Young, and F.E. Shahidi, et al. 1993. Randomized study assessing the effect of digoxin withdrawal in patients with mild to moderate chronic congestive heart failure: results of the PROVED trial. *J Am Coll Cardiol* 22:955-962.
12. Packer, M., M. Gheorghiade, and J.B.Young, et al. 1993. For the RADIANCE study. Withdrawal of digoxin from patients with chronic heart failure treated with angiotensin converting enzyme inhibitors. *N Eng J Med* 329:1-7.
13. The Digitalis Investigation Group. 1997. The effect of digoxin on mortality and morbidity in patients with heart failure. *N Eng J Med* 336:525-533.
14. Frishman, W.H. 1998. Carvedilol. *N Eng J Med* 339:1759-1765.
15. Packer, M., M.R. Bristow, and J.N. Cohn, et al. 1996. The effect of carvedilol on morbidity and mortality in patients with chronic heart failure. *N Eng J Med* 334:1349-1355.
16. The CIBIS Investigators and Committees. 1994. A randomized trial of β-blockade in heart failure: the Cardiac Insufficiency Bisoprolol Study. *Circulation* 90:1765-1773.
17. Engelmeier, R.S., J.B. O'Connell, R. Walsh, N. Rad, P.J. Scanlon, and R.M. Gunnar. 1985. Improvement in symptoms and exercise tolerance by metoprolol in patients with dilated cardiomyopathy: a double-blind, randomized, placebo-controlled trial. *Circulation* 72:536-546.
18. Wei, C.M., A. Herman, and R.J. Rodeheffer, et al. 1994. Endothelium in human congestive heart failure. *Circulation* 89:1580-1586.
19. Ferro, C.J., and D.J. Webb. 1996. The clinical potential of endothelin receptor antagonists in cardiovascular medicine. *Drugs* 51:12-27.
20. Lin, C., and W.H. Frisman. 1996. Renin inhibition: a novel therapy for cardiovascular disease. *Am Heart J* 131:1024-1034.

CHAPTER 4

Pharmacological Treatment of Patients With Chronic Obstructive Pulmonary Disease: Update and Future Directions

Jean Bourbeau

Respiratory Epidemiology Unit and the Respiratory Division, McGill University Health Centre; and Research Scholar, Fonds de la Recherche en Santé du Québec, Montréal, Canada

Chronic obstructive pulmonary disease (COPD) is not a single entity but results from varying combinations of airway disease and emphysema, which share the feature of slowly progressive airflow limitation, in large part irreversible (1,2,3). Pharmacological treatment in COPD aims at

1. preventing further lung damage;
2. optimizing lung function, symptoms, and health status; and
3. preventing and treating COPD exacerbations.

By optimizing the pharmacological management of COPD, it may be possible to prevent exacerbation and to reduce symptoms sufficiently to permit patients to gradually increase their levels of activity as a form of self-directed respiratory rehabilitation.

Pharmacological Therapy to Prevent Further Lung Damage

Preventing further lung damage should be a priority in managing COPD patients.

Smoking Cessation and the Progression of Lung Disease

Fletcher and Peto (4) showed that 15%-20% of smokers demonstrate an increased susceptibility to tobacco smoke, and that smoking cessation could modify the rate of decline of forced expiratory volume in 1 second (FEV_1). More recently, the Lung Health Study I (5) showed that smoking cessation was a major benefit for all participants regardless of age, lung function, and gender. Early detection of COPD, followed by smoking cessation results in the best clinical outcome.

Pharmacological Approach to Smoking Cessation Medical practice is the ideal context in which to assist smokers. A key element in smoking cessation is identifying the readiness of the smoker to stop smoking. The Stages of Change Model developed by Prochaska (6,7) recognizes that at any one time, smokers are either not ready (40%), unsure (40%), or ready (20%) to stop smoking. A brief intervention should be appropriately targeted to each group's needs and concerns, rather than providing the same approach for all smoking patients. Recent advances in neurobiological science have shown evidence of specific functional and neurochemical commonalities between nicotine and well-known addictive drugs (8,9,10). Although people smoke cigarettes for a number of reasons, addiction is a major factor in maintaining the habit. Two pharmacological approaches as aids to smoking cessation have been shown to enhance the quit rates over physician advice alone. Nicotine replacement therapy (5,10,11) is designed to permit the smoker to give up smoking without going through the full syndrome of nicotine withdrawal. Because most formulations deliver nicotine much more slowly than a cigarette does, the nicotine replacement formulations are not as psychoactive and therefore not as reinforcing. The three most popular methods of replacement include nicotine gum, transdermal nicotine systems, and nicotine spray. They approximately double quit rates achieved with behavioral intervention alone (5,11). The choice in nicotine replacement depends on an individual's needs and coping abilities. Other pharmacological approaches include bupropion, an antidepressant of the aminoketone class, chemically unrelated to tricyclic antidepressants or nicotine replacement agents. To date, the mechanisms by which bupropion enhances smoking cessation and decreases some of the withdrawal symptoms are unknown. The efficacy of bupropion as an aid to smoking cessation was demonstrated in two placebo-controlled, double-blind trials in nondepressed chronic cigarette smokers (12,13). Bupropion was more effective than the nicotine transdermal system or placebo in helping patients maintain abstinence at 12 months. Bupropion combined with a nicotine transdermal system resulted in the highest rate of continuous abstinence throughout the study.

Does Long-Term Pharmacological Therapy Alter the Progression of Disease?

Several studies have been conducted to determine whether long-term pharmacological therapy can alter the progression of disease.

Progressive Lung Disease and Bronchodilator Therapy In the Lung Health Study I (5), in the ipratropium bromide intervention group, the initial improvement in lung function was followed by a progressive rate of decline that was identical to that in the placebo group. Thus, ipratropium bromide administered chronically neither improved nor accelerated the rate of decline of lung function. The effect of other bronchodilators, other dosages, or combinations of bronchodilators are unlikely to give different results, although these effects remain to be determined.

Airway Inflammation, Progressive Lung Disease, and Corticosteroid Therapy It is thought that the pathological and inflammatory processes associated with COPD lead to progressive airflow obstruction. In the last few years, steroids have been a subject of discussion regarding their potential effect in modifying the rate of decline of FEV_1. Results of major studies investigating the role of inhaled steroids in the long-term treatment of COPD have recently been reported at various international scientific meetings, but they all have not been published. The Copenhagen City Study (14), which included patients with very mild disease (postbronchodilator FEV_1 of about 2.4 L, 86% predicted), was not able to show any difference in the crude declines in postbronchodilator FEV_1. The two other long-term studies, EUROSCOP (15), which included patients with mild disease (prebronchodilator FEV_1 of 2.5 L, 77% predicted), and ISOLDE (16), which included patients with moderate to severe disease (postbronchodilator FEV_1 of 1.4 L, 50% predicted), have demonstrated acute, short-term improvements of mean FEV_1 in the first 3-6 months but the subsequent rate of decline was similar to that in patients treated with inhaled steroids or placebo. The studies are in keeping with a model of acute improvement with inhaled steroids, but with no change in the decline or underlying lung disease. The clinical significance of this acute improvement remains to be shown.

Proteinase Inhibitors, Progressive Lung Disease, and Pharmacological Therapy The hereditary disorder α1-antitrypsin deficiency, seen with Z, S, and other variants, is characterized by development of severe emphysema at an early age with smoking being the most significant additional risk factor. Commercial α1-antitrypsin replacement has, for some years, been licensed for general use in α1-antitrypsin deficient patients. Even though α1-antitrypsin replacement may indeed have proven biochemical activity, there has been no formal randomized study of its clinical efficacy. An attempt to remedy this situation has led to a combined German-Danish study (17), which suggested that weekly infusion of human α1-antitrypsin in patients with an initial FEV_1 predicted value of 30%-65% may slow the annual decline of FEV_1. Because this was not a randomized trial, its results are limited by the potential for unknown or unmeasured differences between the treatment groups that could bias the results. A recent study (18) showed that another major proteinase inhibitor, α1-antichymotrypsine, is inactivated in the lungs of patients with chronic bronchitis and emphysema. The conformational transition of α1-antichymotrypsine, from an active to an inactive state within the lung, may play an important role in the pathogenesis of chronic lung disease. The significance of these protein inactivations in progressive lung disease, their relationship to smoking, and the possibilities for prevention by pharmacological treatment are of great interest but require further research.

Pharmacological Therapy to Optimize Lung Function, Symptoms, and Health Status

Pharmacological therapy, including bronchodilator treatments, has been used to optimize lung function, symptoms, and patients' health status.

Are Bronchodilator Treatments Effective in Stable COPD?

Some bronchodilator treatments have proven to be beneficial in treating patients with stable COPD.

Effectiveness of Ipratropium Bromide, Short-Acting B2-Agonist, or a Combination of the Two Drugs Short-acting B2-agonists provide a rapid response, which makes them useful for symptom relief and protection from exercise-induced dyspnea. It is commonly thought that in COPD, anticholinergic drugs are more effective bronchodilators than B2-agonists. Some studies support this premise in stable disease, although other studies have shown similar degree of bronchodilation. In contrast to the use of relative high dose of either salbutamol (800 mcg) and ipratropium bromide (120 mcg) (19), the response to the combination of bronchodilators both at submaximal doses or recommended doses for outpatients is better than either agent studied alone. Due to the high level of prescription of B2-agonist and an anticholinergic, a combination formulation of salbutamol and ipratropium bromide has been developed to afford the convenience of two drug classes in a single inhalation delivery system. Clinical trial studies (20) have established that the fixed combination product provides significant bronchodilator benefit over its individual components.

Long-Term Use of Inhaled Bronchodilators and Sustained Effectiveness In a recent study, effects of extended treatment with bronchodilator therapy in patients with COPD have been assessed by combining results from seven clinical trials (21). Regular treatment with B2-agonist was associated with minimal change in baseline lung function and a decline in acute response to bronchodilator therapy after 90-day administration. In contrast, regular treatment with ipratropium bromide was associated with improvement both in baseline lung function and in acute response to bronchodilator therapy. Shortness of breath assessed by a symptom score was improved significantly ($p < 0.005$) in the exsmokers treated with ipratropium. Quality of life, as measured with a disease-specific instrument, the chronic respiratory questionnaire (CRQ), improved slightly for the entire study population. Ipratropium, in comparison to B2-agonist, resulted in more quality of life improvement among the exsmokers ($p < 0.0003$), although these changes were small (0.35 vs. 0.17 on a seven-point scale), and none exceeded the threshold for a clinically significant change (0.5 or more on a seven-point scale). Interestingly, in the Lung Health Study I (5), an improvement in baseline lung function was also found after initiation of ipratropium therapy, and this effect was sustained as long as the patient was taking the bronchodilator. When inhaler was withheld at the end of the 5-year study, pre-bronchodilator FEV_1 dropped, losing the benefit on baseline lung function.

Effectiveness of Long-Acting Bronchodilators Long-acting bronchodilators have been developed in two classes of drugs, the B2-agonists and the anticholinergics, of which only the B2-agonists are presently available for clinical use. Short-term use of inhaled salmeterol, a long-acting B2-agonist, over 4 hours has been associated with reduction in dyspnea, increased airflow, and reduced hyperinflation in patients with symptomatic COPD who had not taken any inhaled bronchodilator for at least 12 hours or oral bronchodilators for 24 hours (22). Short-term use of salmeterol over 12 hours has been shown to be equally effective improving forced vital capacity (FVC), FEV_1, and forced expiratory flow after 50% of vital capacity (FEF_{50}), but longer-acting than formoterol (23). The effectiveness of the long-acting B2-agonists over a longer interval is only available in salmeterol. In a randomized clinical trial (24), patients received either salmeterol 50 mcg or 100 mcg twice a day or placebo treatment in addition to their existing drug regimen for a period of 16 weeks. The results of the study showed statistically significant improvement in FEV_1, up to 7% in each salmeterol group compared to placebo. There was no difference for the distance walked in 6 min, but patients included in the 50 mcg salmeterol group were significantly less breathless after exertion. There was also significant improvement in daily symptom scores with a corresponding decrease in additional short-acting B2-agonist requirements. The same pattern was seen for nighttime scores, although it didn't reach statistical significance. Compared with placebo, salmeterol 50 mcg taken twice daily was associated with significant improvements in disease-specific quality of life, and St. George's Respiratory Questionnaire (SGRQ) total and impact scores exceeded the threshold for a clinically significant change (25). This was not seen with salmeterol 100 mcg twice daily. Significant quality of life gains confined to those patients receiving salmeterol 50 mcg twice daily may be explained by the better tolerance and fewer adverse events of salmeterol 50 mcg twice daily as compared to 100 mcg twice daily. Other studies comparing salmeterol to other bronchodilator treatments (26) or in addition to concurrent anticholinergic therapy (27) in stable COPD have been presented, but are yet to be published. In one study (26), patients with COPD of all levels of severity responded well to salmeterol and ipratropium. Although patients with more severe disease receiving ipratropium tended to have smaller changes in FEV_1 area under the curve (AUC), the supplemental albuterol use and the overall daytime symptom scores were similar between patients receiving ipratropium and those receiving salmeterol. In another study (27), the addition of salmeterol to anticholinergic treatment improved the FEV_1 from 60 ml at 4 weeks to 30 ml at 24 weeks. The clinical significance of these changes remains to be shown.

Only one compound, tiotropium, has been developed as a long-acting anticholinergic bronchodilator. This compound, not yet available, is a quaternary ammonium structurally related to ipratropium bromide and is known to have an excellent safety profile. Binding studies in humans (28) have confirmed that this is a potent muscarinic antagonist, approximately 10-fold more potent than ipratropium bromide, with receptor subtype selectivity of M3 and M1 over M2. This slow receptor dissociation found its clinical correlate in significant and long-lasting bronchodilation and bronchoprotection in patients with COPD. Clinical studies (29,30) confirm that it is a potent and long-lasting bronchodilator in COPD. Tiotropium achieves very stable long-lasting effects with comparatively low variation of bronchodilation between peak and trough (31). Tiotropium showed a statistically significant improvement in FEV_1 and FVC over ipratropium starting 3 hours postdosing (32), and FEV_1 remained about 12% above baseline over the 13-week duration of the study. International multicenter randomized clinical trials are presently under way in patients with COPD.

Other Novel Inhaled Bronchodilators A novel class of dual D2-receptor and B2-adrenoreceptor agonist activity has been recently developed for the treatment of COPD. Based on the results of animal experimentation, it is postulated that the D2-receptor agonist activity of the first compound AR-C68397AA will inhibit pulmonary neurogenic reflex and result in reduction of bronchoconstriction, cough, mucus production, and, possibly, the perception of dyspnea. Initial studies have been completed in healthy volunteers and in patients with COPD. The clinical development program is continuing with further studies to determine the efficacy and safety of AR-C68397AA administered by inhalation in patients with COPD.

Effectiveness of Theophylline Theophylline prescriptions have decreased significantly over the last 10 years (33). Theophylline may have several potentially useful effects although numerous randomized clinical trials have not been able to consistently show improvement in respiratory symptoms, exercise capacity, and health status. This may be explained by the fact that many studies had a small sample size or were using nonvalidated quality of life indices. Theophylline improved health status in three trials (34,35,36) in which a validated instrument was used and improved exercise capacity in two other trials (35,36). A recent randomized study (37) comparing n of 1 trial to standard practice showed that 21% of 34 patients with COPD improved their dyspnea as measured by the CRQ during theophylline treatment compared with placebo treatment. Thus, there remains a rationale for a trial of theophylline in patients with COPD who remain symptomatic despite inhaled bronchodilators.

Theophylline, a weak and nonselective phosphodiesterase (PDE) inhibitor, has recently been shown to reduce neutrophil counts in sputum in patients with COPD. The PDE4 isoenzyme is the predominant cyclic AMP metabolizing enzyme in inflammatory and immune cells. Several PDE4 inhibitors are presently in clinical development. Second-generation PDE4 inhibitors, such as Ariflo (SB 207499), may have fewer side effects, although it is not yet certain whether these drugs will be useful in patients with COPD.

Are Corticosteroid Treatments Effective in Stable COPD?

Both oral and inhaled corticosteroids have been used to treat patients with stable COPD.

Oral Corticosteroids Before concluding that a patient has benefited from oral corticosteroids, the patient's disease and pulmonary function must be stable and the benefits documented objectively. A recent meta-analysis (38) estimated that the percentage of patients with stable COPD, who improved their FEV_1 by 20% or more with 20 mg of prednisone or more for a treatment period of at least 7 days, was only 10% more (95% confidence interval, 2%-18%) than in the placebo groups. The percentage of patients who benefit from oral corticosteroid therapy appears to be modest, and the potential for adverse effects, when oral corticosteroids are taken regularly, represents a major problem.

Inhaled Corticosteroids Inhaled corticosteroids for stable COPD cannot be viewed simply as a logical extension of their use in the treatment of asthma. In the few short-term studies (39,40) in which small numbers of patients have been selected according to a significant response to oral steroids, the proportion of patients and the size of the effect have been consistently less in patients receiving inhaled corticosteroids than those receiving oral corticosteroids. In the large subgroup of patients who do not improve significantly with an oral corticosteroid, inhaled corticosteroids, even at high doses, failed to show beneficial physiological and functional effects in those with advanced COPD on maximal bronchodilator treatment (41). The results of the long-term EUROSCOP (15) and ISOLDE (16) studies have demonstrated acute, short-term improvements in lung function, and this effect was maintained over the following years. In the ISOLDE study, health status measured with the SGRQ showed a lower health status at each time point for patients in the placebo group compared to those treated with inhaled corticosteroids, and the rates of change against time were continuing to diverge at the end of the study. This effect was achieved with a relatively high dose of fluticasone (1000 mcg per day), a dose potentially associated with a risk of cataracts, glaucoma, and osteoporosis in the elderly population. The effect of a lower dose of inhaled corticosteroids or in combination with maximal bronchodilator treament remains to be determined.

Pharmacological Therapy to Prevent and Treat COPD Exacerbations

COPD exacerbations are difficult to define. It has been estimated that infections play a role in 50% of exacerbations, and, in 30% of these, the infection is of viral, mycoplasmic, or chlamydial origin (42). The role of infection in the pathogenesis of COPD is controversial. However, moderate to severe exacerbations represent an important cause of hospital admissions. Any intervention that could reduce the incidence of acute exacerbations is likely to have impact on morbidity, quality of life, health care services, and resulting costs.

What Pharmacological Approaches Can Prevent Exacerbations in Patients With COPD?

Several pharmacological approaches, including vaccination, immunostimulating agents, and corticosteroid treatments, may be useful in preventing exacerbations of COPD.

Vaccination Patients who are elderly, but do not specifically have COPD, have been shown to have a 70% reduction in mortality from influenza vaccination. Vaccinations are recommended (43) although, for pneumococcal vaccination, no studies specific to COPD have been performed.

Immunostimulating Agents Immunostimulating agents made from bacterial extracts were suggested to lead to potential benefit resulting from the stimulation of the nonspecific components of the immune system. One double-blind, placebo-controlled, randomized clinical trial (44) set out to assess the benefit of OM-85 BV, an immunostimulating extract from eight bacterial species. The risk of having an acute exacerbation of COPD was similar in the treatment and placebo groups. In contrast, the risk of being hospitalized for respiratory problems was 30% lower, and patients treated with OM-85 BV spent an average of 1.5 days in hospital compared with 3.4 days for patients treated with placebo ($p = 0.037$). These results suggest that immunostimulating agents may be beneficial for patients with COPD because they reduce the likelihood of severe respiratory events leading to hospitalization.

Corticosteroid Treatment In patients with mild COPD at risk for acute exacerbation, one recent short-term study (45) showed that fluticasone propionate at a relatively high dose (1000 mcg per day) in comparison to placebo was not associated with a difference in numbers of patients with at least one exacerbation. However, significantly fewer patients had moderate to severe exacerbations during the 6-month treatment with fluticasone propionate. One recent long-term study, ISOLDE (16), showed that fluticasone propionate, again at a relatively high dose (1000 mcg per day), reduced the exacerbation rate by 25% from 1.33 exacerbations per year in the placebo group to 0.99 in the fluticasone group ($p = 0.023$). This will be equivalent to a reduction of one exacerbation for three years of treatment. No reduction of exacerbations was demonstrated in patients with FEV_1 above 1.54 L, and the most important reduction was in patients with FEV_1 below 1.25 L. This may have clinical significance as further data analysis suggests that patients with reduced exacerbation rate also showed reduction in the rate of decline of health status. The EUROSCOP (15) and Copenhagen City Lung (14) studies included patients with mild disease and were likely not empowered to investigate the effects of treatment on exacerbations. Exacerbations were slightly lower in the treated group but the differences did not reach statistical significance. Together, these results provide some indications as to how to deal with individual patients. The widespread use of inhaled corticosteroids is not justified, and the potential but limited benefit of inhaled corticosteroids should be balanced with the risk of adverse systemic effects following a long-term treatment with a relatively high dose of inhaled corticosteroids.

Pharmacological Approaches to Treating an Exacerbation of COPD

Antibiotics, bronchodilator treatments, and corticosteroids have all been used to treat patients with exacerbation of COPD.

Antibiotic Treatments With regard to treatment with antibiotics in exacerbations of COPD, a recent meta-analysis identified only nine randomized, placebo-controlled trials of at least 5 days of antibiotic treatment. The effect score of antibiotic was positive in seven and negative in two (46). Overall, a small benefit in favor of antibiotic treatment was found. It also appears that antibiotic treatment is linked to accelerated recovery from exacerbations in patients with more severe disease (47). Exacerbations of COPD are routinely treated with antibiotics and increasingly treated with newer and more expensive antibiotics even if their superiority over older antibiotics remains to be proven (48,49,50).

Bronchodilator treatments During acute exacerbations of disease, the apparent advantage of ipratropium bromide in COPD becomes less clear than in stable disease. In hospital emergency settings, the addition of nebulized ipratropium bromide to nebulized B2-agonist seems to produce a similar degree of bronchodilation (51,52). It would, therefore, seem that there is no difference in effect and no advantage in combining the two classes of drugs in acute exacerbations of COPD.

Corticosteroid Treatments In the management of exacerbations of airway diseases, corticosteroids are widely prescribed. Published data are now supporting their efficacy in exacerbations of COPD. In the Albert study (53), the group treated with methyl prednisolone 0.5 mg per kg every 6 hours for 72 hours had a greater improvement of pre- and postbronchodilator FEV_1, already detectable after 12 hours of treatment. However, the validity of these results has since been questioned, mainly because of the statistical methods used in the analysis (54). In another study (55), no improvement was demonstrated in lung function within 4 hours following the intravenous injection of 100 mg methylprednisolone compared to placebo. There was also no difference in the rate of hospitalization. More recently, a randomized, double-blind, placebo-controlled study was done to assess the efficacy of 9 days of tapering dose of oral corticosteroids in the treatment of outpatients with COPD exacerbation (56). The results showed that treatment with prednisone accelerated recovery of PaO_2, FEV_1, and PEF; reduced the treatment failure rate; and improved subjective dyspnea. However, the potential for more reversibility in the prednisone treatment group compared to the placebo group could have confounded the treatment effect observed. A more recent study (57), in patients with acute exacerbations randomly assigned to oral prednisolone 30 mg once daily (n = 29) or placebo (n = 27) for 14 days in addition to standard treatment, showed that postbronchodilator FEV_1 increased more rapidly and to a greater extent in the corticosteroid treated group. Up to day five of a hospital stay, FEV_1 increased by 90 ml daily in the intervention group and by 30 ml daily in the placebo group ($p = 0.039$). Hospital stays were shorter in the corticosteroid treated group. The group did not differ at the 6-week follow up. With regard to safety, even on a short-term basis, the use of systemic steroids is not devoid of adverse effects. A double-blind, double-dummy, parallel group comparison study (58), designed to investigate the efficacy of nebulized budesonide and prednisolone in comparison to placebo in the management of exacerbations of COPD requiring hospitalization, has recently been completed in Canada, France, and Belgium. At 72 hours, mean change to postbronchodilator FEV_1 was substantially greater with active treatments than with placebo (95% confidence interval): inhaled steroids versus placebo 0.11 L (0.02-0.19); prednisolone versus placebo 0.16 L (0.08-0.25). Higher incidence of hyperglycemia and minor psychiatric disorders was observed in prednisolone group. Nebulized budesonide may be an alternative to oral prednisolone.

Conclusion

Quitting smoking is the preferred therapeutic approach, but this has proved to be difficult in the majority of patients. Future pharmacotherapy of COPD must include a better understanding of the disease and factors that determine why patients develop COPD. Focusing essentially on reversal of damage is not a realistic goal of treatment in patients with a respiratory disease defined in principle as mainly irreversible. There is a pressing need for the development of new drugs effective in halting the progression of COPD. There is also a need for physiopathological markers that may predict the clinical usefulness of new pharmacological treatment. However, one should not assume disease improvements based only on measurement of physiopathological markers; the patient's functional status and health status should also be measured in a properly designed study. Unfortunately, in the past, these outcomes have often not been assessed, either because of a lack of validated instruments or simply because of the inappropriate assumption that physiopathological changes are associated with a similar change in somatic status, functional capacity, or health status.

References

1. Canadian Thoracic Society Workshop Group. 1992. Guidelines for the assessment and management of chronic obstructive pulmonary disease. *Can Med Assoc J* 147(4):420-428.
2. American Thoracic Society. 1995. Standard for the diagnosis and care of patients with chronic obstructive pulmonary disease. *Am J Respir Crit Care Med* 152:577.
3. Siafatas, N., P. Vermaire, and N. Pride, et al. on behalf of the Task Force European Respiratory Society Consensus Statement. 1995. Optimal assessment and management of COPD. *Eur Respir J* 8:1398-1420.
4. Fletcher, C., and R. Peto. 1977. The natural history of chronic airflow obstruction. *Br Med J* 1:1645-1648.
5. Anthonisen, N., J. Cornett, and J. Kiley, et al. 1994. The Lung Health Study: effects of smoking cessation and the use of an inhaled anticholinergic bronchodilator on the rate of decline of FEV_1. The Lung Health Study. *JAMA* 272:1497-1505.
6. Prochaska, J., and C. Dillemente. 1986. Toward a comprehensive model of change. In *Treating Addictive Behaviors: Process of Change,* ed. W. Miller and N. Heather. New York: Plenum Press.
7. Velicer, W., J. Fava, J. Prochaska, D. Abrams, K. Emmons, and J. Pierce. 1995. Distribution of smokers by stage in three representative samples. *Preventive Med* 24:401-411.
8. Nisell, M., G. Nomikos, and T. Svensson. 1995. Nicotine dependence, midbrain dopamine systems and psychiatric disease. *Pharmacol Toxicol* 76:157-162.
9. Pontieri, F., G. Tanda, F. Orzi, and G. DiChiara. 1996. Effects of nicotine on the nucleus accumbens and similarity to those of addictive drugs. *Nature* 382:255-257.
10. Thompson, G., and D. Hunter. 1998. Nicotine replacement therapy. *Ann Pharmacother* 32:1067-1075.

11. Fiore, M., S. Smith, D. Jorenby, and T. Baker. 1994. The effectiveness of the nicotine patch for smoking cessation. *JAMA* 271(24):1940-1949.

12. Hurt, R., D. Sachs, and E. Glover, et al. 1997. A comparison of sustained release buproprion and placebo for smoking cessation. *N Engl J Med* 337(17):1195-1202.

13. Jorenby, D.E., S.J. Leischow, and M.A. Nides, et al. 1999. A controlled trial of sustained-release bupropion, a nicotine patch, or both for smoking cessation. *N Engl J Med* 340:685-691.

14. Vestbo, J., T. Sorensen, P. Lang, A. Brix, P. Tone, and K. Viskum. 1999. Long-term effect of inhaled budesonide in mild and moderate chronic obstructive pulmonary disease: a randomized controlled trial. *Lancet* 353:1819-1823.

15. Pauwels, R.A., C.G. Lofdahl, L.A. Laitinen, J.P. Schouten, D.S. Postma, N.B. Pride, and S.V. Ohlsson for the European Respiratory Society Study on COPD. 1999. Long-term treatment with inhaled budesonide in persons with mild chronic obstructive pulmonary disease who continue smoking. *N Engl J Med* 340:1948-1953.

16. Calverley, P.M.A., P.S. Burge, P.W. Jones, J.A. Anderson, and T.K. Maslen on behalf of the ISOLDE study group. 1999. Effect of three years' treatment with fluticasone proprionate in patients with moderate to severe COPD. *Am J Respir Crit Care Med* 159:A524.

17. Seersholm, N., M. Wencker, and N. Banik, et al. 1997. Does Alpha1-antitrypsin augmentation therapy slow the annual decline in FEV_1, in patients with severe hereditary Alpha1-antitrypsin deficiency? *Eur Respir J* 10:2260-2263.

18. Chang, W.S., and D. Lomas. 1998. Latent Alpha1-antichymotrypsin: a molecular explanation for the inactivation of Alpha1-antichymotrypsin in chronic bronchitis and emphysema. *J Biol Chem* 273:3695-3701.

19. Easton, P.A., C. Jadue, S. Dhingra, and N.R. Anthonisen. 1986. A comparison of the bronchodilating effects of a beta-2 adrenergic agent (albuterol) and an anticholinergic agent (ipratropium bromide), given by aerosol alone or in sequence. *N Engl J Med* 315(12):735-739.

20. COMBIVENT Inhalation Aerosol Study Group. 1994. In chronic obstructive pulmonary disease, a combination of ipratropium and albuterol is more effective than either agent alone. An 85-day multicenter trial. *Chest* 105(5):1411-1419.

21. Rennard, S., C. Serby, M. Ghabouri, P. Johnson, and M. Friedman. 1996. Extended therapy with ipratropium is associated with improved lung function in COPD: a retrospective analysis of data from seven clinical trials. *Chest* 110:62-70.

22. Ramirez-Venegas, A., J. Ward, T. Lantine, and D. Mahler. 1997. Salmeterol reduces dyspnea and improves lung function in patients with COPD. *Chest* 112:336-340.

23. Cazzola, M., M. Matera, G. Santangelo, A.Vinciguerra, F. Rossi, and G. D'Amato. 1995. Salmeterol and formoterol in partially reversible severe chronic obstructive pulmonary disease: a dose-response study. *Resp Med* 89:357-362.

24. Boyd, G., A. Morice, and J. Pounsford, et al. 1997. An evaluation of salmeterol in the treatment of chronic obstructive pulmonary disease (COPD). *Eur Respir J* 10:1283-1289.

25. Jones, P., and T. Bosh. 1997. Quality of life changes in COPD patients treated with salmeterol. *Am J Respir Crit Care Med* 155:1283-1289.

26. Donahue, J., A. Emmett, K. Richard, and K. Knobil. 1999. Salmeterol is effective bronchodilator therapy for all stages of COPD. *Am J Respir Crit Care Med* 159:A.

27. Chapman, K., M.H. James, A.F. Kuipers, and R. Goldstein. 1999. Addition of salmeterol 50 mcg bid to anticholinergic treatment in COPD. *Am J Respir Crit Care Med* 159:A523.

28. Haddad, E., J. Mak, and P. Barnes. 1994. Characterization of [3H] Ba 679, a slow-dissociating muscarinic receptor antagonist in human lung: radioligand binding and autoradiographic mapping. *Mol Pharmacol* 45:899-907.

29. Maesen, F., J. Smeets, T. Sledsens, F. Wald, and P. Cornelissen. 1995. Tiotroprium bromide, a new long-acting antimuscarinic bronchodilator: a pharmacodynamic study in patients with chronic obstructive pulmonary disease (COPD). *Eur Respir J* 8:1506-1513.

30. Maesen, F., J. Smeets, M. Costongs, F. Wald, and P. Cornelissen. 1993. Br 679 B2, a new long-acting antimuscarinic bronchodilator: a pilot dose-escalation study. *Eur Respir J* 6:1031-1036.

31. Disse, B., G.A. Speck, K. Ludwig Rominger, T.J. Witek, and R. Hammer. 1999. Tiotropium (Spririva): mechanistic considerations and clinical profile in obstructive lung disease. *Life Sci* 64:457-464.

32. Van Noord, J.A., T. Bantje, and M. Eland, et al. 1999. Superior efficacy of tiotropium (TIO) compared to ipratropium (IpBr) as a maintenance bronchodilator in COPD. *Am J Respir Crit Care Med* 159:A525.

33. Van Andel, A.E., C. Reisoner, S.S. Menjoge, and T.J. Witek. 1999. Analysis of inhaled corticosteroid and oral theophylline use among patients with stable COPD from 1987 to 1995. *Chest* 115:703-707.

34. Mahler, D.A., R.A. Matthay, P.E. Snyder, C.K. Wells, and J. Loke. 1985. Sustained-release theophylline reduces dyspnea in nonreversible obstructive airway disease. *Am Rev Respir Dis* 131:22-25.

35. Guyatt, G.H., L.B. Berman, M. Townsend, S.O. Pugsley, and L.W. Chambers. 1987. A measure of quality of life for clinical trials in chronic lung disease. *Thorax* 42:773-778.

36. Kirsten, D., R. Wegner, and R. Jorres, et al. 1993. Effects of theophylline withdrawal in severe chronic obstructive pulmonary disease. *Chest* 104:1101-1107.

37. Mahon, J.L., A. Laupacis, and R.V. Hodder, et al. 1999. Theophylline for irreversable chronic airflow limitation. A randomized study comparing n of 1 trials to standard practice. *Chest* 115:38-48.

38. Callaghan, C.M., R.S. Dittus, and B.P. Katz. 1991. Oral corticosteroid therapy for patients with stable chronic obstructive pulmonary disease. A meta-analysis. *Ann Intern Med* 114(3):216-223.

39. Shim, C.S., and M.H. Williams, Jr. 1985. Aerosol beclomethasone in patients with steroid-responsive chronic obstructive pulmonary disease. *Am J Med* 78:655-658.

40. Bourbeau, J., M. Rouleau, S. Boucher, and M. Krusky. 1993. A double blind randomized study of inhaled budesonide in patients with steroid-responsive COPD. *Am Rev Respir Dis* 147:A317.

41. Bourbeau, J., M. Rouleau, and S. Boucher. 1998. A randomized controlled trial of inhaled corticosteroids in patients with advanced obstructive pulmonary disease. *Thorax* 53:477-482.

42. Ball, P. 1995. Epidemiology and treatment of chronic bronchitis and its exacerbations. *Chest* 108(suppl. 2):43S-52S.

43. Fiebach, N., and W. Beckett. 1994. Prevention of respiratory infections in adults: influenza and pneumococcal vaccines. *Arch Intern Med* 154:2545-2457.

44. Collet, J.P., S. Shapiro, and P. Ernst, et al. 1997. Effects of an immunostimulating agent on acute exacerbations and hospitalizations in patients with chronic obstructive pulmonary disease. *Am J Respir Crit Care Med* 156:1719-1724.

45. Paggiaro, P., R. Dahle, and I. Bakran, et al. 1998. Multicentre randomized placebo controlled trial of inhaled fluticasone propionate in patients with chronic obstructive pulmonary disease. *Lancet* 351:773-780.

46. Saint, S., S. Bent, E. Vittinghoff, and D. Grady. 1995. Antibiotics in chronic obstructive pulmonary disease exacerbations: a meta-analysis. *JAMA* 273:957-960.

47. Pines, A., H. Raafat, K. Plucinski, J. Greenfield, and M. Solari. 1968. Antibiotic regimens in severe and acute purulent exacerbations of chronic bronchitis. *Br Med J* 2:735-738.

48. Cazzola, M., A. Vinciguerra, and G. Beghi, et al. 1995. Comparative evaluation of the clinical and microbiological efficacy of co-amoxiclav vs. cefuxime or ciprofloxacin in bacterial exacerbation of chronic bronchitis. *J Chemother* 7:432-441.

49. Chodosh, S., J. Tuck, K.D. Stottmeier, and D. Pizzuto. 1989. Comparison of ciprofloxacin with ampicillin in acute infectious exacerbations of chronic bronchitis: a double-blind crossover study. *Am J Med* 87:10S-12S.

50. Wollschlager, M., S. Rasof, F. Khan, J. Guarneri, V. Bombardi, and Q. Afzal. 1987. Controlled, comparative study of ciprofloxacin versus ampicillin in treatment of bacterial respiratory tract infections. *Am J Med* 82:164-168.

51. Rebuck, A.S., K.R. Chapman, and R. Abboud, et al. 1987. Nebulized anticholinergic and sympathomimetic treatment of asthma and chronic obstructive airways disease in the emergency room. *Am J Med* 82:59-64.

52. Karpel, J.P. 1991. Bronchodilator responses to anticholinergic and beta-adrenergic agents in acute and stable COPD. *Chest* 99(4):871-876.

53. Albert, R.K., T.R. Martin, and S.W. Lewis. 1980. Controlled clinical trial of methylprednisolone in patients with chronic bronchitis and acute respiratory insufficiency. *Ann Intern Med* 92:753-758.

54. Glenny, R. 1987. Steroids in COPD. *Chest* 91:289-290.

55. Emerman, C.L., A.F. Connors, T.W. Lukens, M.E. May, and D. Effron. 1989. A randomized controlled trial of methylprednisolone in the emergency treatment of acute exacerbations of COPD. *Chest* 95(3):563-567.

56. Thompson, W., D. Christopher, P. Carvalho, N. Charan, and J. Crowley. 1996. Controlled trial of oral prednisone in outpatients with acute COPD exacerbation. *Am J Respir Crit Care Med* 154:407-412.

57. Davis, L., R.M. Angus, and P.M.A. Calverley. 1999. Oral corticosteroids in patients admitted to hospitals with exacerbations of chronic obstructive pulmonary disease: a prospective randomized controlled trial. *Lancet* 354: 456-460.

58. Maltais, F., J. Bourbeau, A. Tonnel, J. Ostinelli, J. Haddon, N. Jacquemet, B. Jennings, and P. Duroux. 1999. Comparison of nebulized budesonide and oral prednisolone with placebo in the treatment of acute exacerbations of COPD. *Eur Respir J* 14(suppl 30):2815.

PART III

Selecting, Recruiting, and Screening Candidates

CHAPTER 5

Selection of Best Candidates for Cardiac Rehabilitation in the Future

William A. Dafoe
University of Ottawa Heart Institute, Ottawa, Canada

From a historical perspective, cardiac rehabilitation (CR) has been defined by prevailing research trials, position statements, and funding sources. The scientific community in the late 1940s (1,2) eventually challenged the dogma of prolonged bed rest following a myocardial infarct. Despite this emerging openness to mobilization and exercise, these recommendations only extended to those with uncomplicated infarcts since this population was the only group that had been studied. By 1964, prevailing research prompted the World Health Organization (WHO) to expand CR indications (3) to include those with rheumatic heart disease, arterial hypertension, chronic cor pulmonale, and congenital heart disease. The rehabilitation services should also include vocational, social, and family counseling interventions. The historical progression toward the recommendations of the present day was neither linear nor lacking controversy. To illustrate, in 1975, a decade after the WHO document, a position statement from Tel Aviv entitled "Critical Evaluation of Cardiac Rehabilitation" still limited the services of CR to postmyocardial infarction (MI) patients and the intervention was primarily exercise therapy. In the 1980s, however, the inclusion criteria for CR were expanded to include coronary artery bypass graft (CABG) patients, those with implantable defibrillators, myoplasty, and heart transplants, and those with congestive heart failure. In 1982, the Third World Congress on Cardiac Rehabilitation in Jerusalem outlined that comprehensive CR should include risk factor modification and exercise training, as well as psychological and vocational counseling. Recent indications would include cardiac patients with almost any underlying pathology as well as high-risk "primary prevention" patients who do not have any obvious manifestation of disease. As a result of expanded services and a greater selection of patients, CR can be considered a scarce medical resource with only a subset of possible patients being enrolled in such programs.

Several studies, including recent national surveys in Canada and the United States, estimate that only 20%-50% of eligible candidates receive CR (4-8). These surveys consistently reveal lower rates of participation among women, older individuals, those with less education, and the unemployed. A multivariate logistic regression analysis showed that for patients with a myocardial infarction, the strongest predictor of utilization was age, with younger patients more likely to enroll in CR than older patients. For patients with angina, the strongest predictor of enrollment was CABG surgery (4).

Allocation of Scarce Medical Resources

It is unlikely that there will be an adequate expansion of formal programs to accommodate all potentially acceptable candidates. Thus, efforts should be made to develop criteria for the selection of best candidates. The present intake processes are heterogeneous and are often dependent on the referring physician's biases and subjective criteria with regard to which patients should be referred to CR. It is proposed that a more objective referral process be developed that would include consistent criteria for the evaluation of referred patients. As an initial template, the criteria used from the Council on Ethical and Judicial Affairs from the American Medical Association for the allocation of scarce medical resources would include the following categories:

1. Likelihood of benefit
2. Change in quality of life
3. Duration of benefit
4. Urgency of need
5. Efficiency of resources (13)

Likelihood of Benefit

Assigning priorities according to likelihood of benefit for a given intervention should maximize the number of lives saved as well as the quality of life. The primary difficulty with this criterion is the degree of uncertainty that exists for various predictors. Large differences in outcome are necessary to apply this criterion ethically. Although it is generally accepted that CR can decrease subsequent mortality by up to 25%, it is not possible to predict which individuals will benefit. Other limitations include the heterogeneity of programs and variable efficacy that may be affected by ethnicity and gender. For example, Romeo and Saccucci (9), using the Sickness Impact Profile (SIP), surveyed the perceived health status of three ethnic groups—Jews, Italian-Americans, and Blacks—during and after CR. Their results demonstrated that while Jews and Italian-Americans showed improvement in self-assessed perceived health status, Black men showed only slight improvement. The perceived health status of Black women actually deteriorated.

Another study by Loose and Fernhall, although it did not measure the perceived health status prior to CR, found that women participating in CR experienced a poorer quality of life than men participating in CR (10). The Council on Ethical and Judicial Affairs felt that as long as patients have some chance of benefiting, to whatever degree, their exclusion cannot be justified.

Minimal Anticipated Benefit There are patients in CR who may have little chance of further benefit. Possibilities include individuals with serious comorbidities that dictate the health of the individual with cardiac disease. An individual with significant cancer, for example, may be a more appropriate candidate for cancer rehabilitation or palliative care. The other extreme would include patients who already have demonstrated an excellent recovery, have a low risk of subsequent events, and who have minimal psychosocial problems.

Nonmedical Factors That May Present Obstacles to Treatment It is possible that a patient's life circumstances may impede the success of medical treatment. Certain obstacles such as difficulties in communication and transportation, as well as physical difficulties, may be overcome with appropriate intervention. If a patient's personality traits or behaviors are perceived to lessen the likelihood of benefit, then efforts must be made to overcome these obstacles before the patient is deemed ineligible. An example encountered in CR is the patient with a drug dependency problem. In our experience, such patients do poorly according to standardized expectations. These patients, however, should not be automatically denied access to CR services. It is reasonable to contract with such patients that acceptance into CR be contingent on the successful completion of an appropriate treatment program. Such factors may prejudice a decision maker's judgment of a particular patient's likelihood of benefit from a given intervention. Such nonmedical factors should be cautiously used, if used at all, when assigning priorities due to the risk of "arbitrariness and overgeneralization." The committee expressed concern regarding the danger of allocating a lower priority to such patients, who could benefit greatly from a given intervention, with some extra support.

Change in Quality of Life

If resources are limited and the likelihood of benefit similar, then treatment should be provided to those patients who are anticipated to derive the greatest improvement in quality of life. The difficulty with this criterion relates to the inherent variability in the assessment of quality of life. The Council suggested that in the absence of a recognized quality of life tool, a suitable proxy would be functional status because it is the most objective measure. Using functional status as an objective tool has serious limitations. For example, a sedentary individual with significant left ventricular dysfunction may be pleased with a peak achieved capacity of

5 metabolic equivalents (METs), while a professional athlete correctly surmises that this dictates the end to participation in professional sports.

Prevention of Extremely Poor Outcome If functional status is used as a proxy for quality of life, then the Council suggested that prevention of an extremely poor outcome should be considered the first priority. In CR, extremely poor outcomes occur infrequently, but one example to consider is the patient immobilized by the fear of subsequent cardiac events. This could be the fear of a recurrent myocardial infarction or the firing of an implantable defibrillator. Since these situations have the potential for significant deterioration in the patient and family, early intervention is required.

Differences in Magnitude of Change If functional status is a proxy for quality of life, then a higher priority should be assigned to individuals with a greater anticipated magnitude of change. In CR, the improvement in quality of life is greater for those individuals with a low score at program entry. Using exercise capacity as an example, the largest increment occurs in individuals with low initial functional capacities.

Discrimination Against the Disabled Population The disabled population may be discriminated against if it were perceived that their disabilities would impair their improvement in quality of life following treatment. Allocation decisions should not be based on the absolute functional status of a patient before treatment, but by how much the patient's functioning might benefit from treatment. A disabled patient might receive a lower priority only if that patient's preexisting disabilities substantially limit potential improvement relative to that of another patient, despite any reasonable adaptations that the program might attempt. For example, a proposed CR participant might present with both cardiac and neurological impairment (say from a stroke with significant hemiparesis). The anticipated aerobic improvement might be limited by balance problems, thus initial efforts should be directed toward neuromuscular rehabilitation. If these are successful, then a trial of CR could be considered.

Duration of Benefit

The length of time a patient will benefit from a treatment can influence that patient's overall gain and may be an appropriate consideration for some allocation decisions. In medicine, this criterion has been applied most appropriately to treatments such as organ grafts. There is considerable uncertainty regarding the prediction of a patient's life span or of the longevity of an organ graft. Also, this criterion has the inherent danger of prejudicing against the elderly. It would be difficult to use the duration of benefit criteria for the selection of patients for CR, unless there were a well-accepted predictive model for ongoing adherence. Those with life-threatening illnesses would by definition have limited duration of benefit.

Urgency of Need

In medicine, "urgency of need" usually refers to life-threatening situations such as those requiring ICU beds or organ transplants for patient survival. It is somewhat related to the "prevention of extremely poor outcome" concept discussed previously. In the cardiovascular domain, an example might include the patient, incapacitated and suicidal due to fear of another cardiac event, who requires an immediate psychiatric intervention. In CR, a participant might present with unstable angina or heart failure. The first rehabilitation need is to arrange appropriate cardiac stabilization by way of the treating cardiovascular physicians. Another possible circumstance is a situation in which a family is near collapse from stresses inherent in the patient's illness. In this case, arranging early admission in a program with appropriate psychosocial supports might avoid the rapid, inexorable decline of patient and family.

Efficiency of Resources

Using a utilitarian argument, a higher priority is given to those who require less of a limited resource. This would enable more patients to benefit from the remaining resources. The Council stressed that this criterion should only be applied when all other criteria are equal. An example in transplant medicine would include assigning a higher priority to a patient requiring only a heart transplant as opposed to a patient requiring both a heart and lung transplant. This way, two lives may be saved instead of one. At this point in time for CR, it is difficult to quantify the resources required for different types of patients. Nevertheless, CR practitioners do appreciate that certain medical conditions (e.g., unstable angina) require more staff supervision and that patients with multiple psychosocial problems predating the cardiac event tend to consume more resources over a longer period of time. In practice however, this "efficiency factor" may be counterbalanced by other criteria. A patient that requires minimal staff intervention (i.e., a "high-efficiency patient") may show minimal net gain if the initial starting indices are high. Conversely, a patient requiring intense staff resources may also show large incremental gains.

Factors That Should Be Used Cautiously or Not Used at All

Some factors are ethically questionable and should either be applied very cautiously, or not at all, when determining how health care resources should be allocated.

Social Worth Evaluation of an individual's contribution to society, or social worth, has been used to justify denial of medical services for those who are judged to fail to make a positive contribution to society. Such social worth arguments have been used against providing medical treatment for the elderly, the economically disadvantaged, criminals, and those with substance addictions. Although this criterion may be advocated by those who idealize attempts to maximize the return on the societal investment for medical resources, the Council on Ethical and Judicial Affairs is against its use as a factor for allocation decisions. Similarly, CR practitioners should not use judgments of prospective patients' social worth to influence entry criteria. Not only do such analyses deflect the traditional focus of the medical profession from a patient-centered approach, but also any single definition of social worth is rarely based on objective criteria and ultimately devalues cultural diversity.

Patient Contribution to Disease In many fields of medicine, a lower priority is assigned to patients whose past behaviors have contributed significantly to their present need for scarce medical resources or costly interventions. Should cardiovascular surgeons, for example, refuse to operate on patients whose smoking or eating habits may have contributed to their heart disease? The arguments justifying this position are often tenuous at best. Not only is it not always clear which elements contribute most to a disease, but factors with negative stigmas associated with them tend to be most singled out. An obese patient or a patient who smokes is more likely to be denied treatment than a patient in a high-ranking profession whose work-related stress may have contributed to his or her cardiac condition. Most often these judgments are couched in less offensive terms that emphasize the impact of these behaviors on a poor medical outcome. Yet, these judgments are frequently sociomoral rather than empirical evaluations. In the context of CR, they are not relevant because it is not only the morbidity of cardiovascular disease that is targeted, but also the very behaviors that contributed to it as well. Furthermore, it often happens that those patients with the "worst behaviors" may display the greatest gain.

Past Use of Resources Patients should be evaluated for their suitability for a particular medical intervention according to their current needs. It is possible that past use of the resource contributes to that patient's current likelihood of benefit or expected improvement in quality of life. For instance, there is often a poorer likelihood that subsequent organ grafts will succeed in a transplant candidate, if previous ones have already failed. Similarly, patients who have previously had a course of CR with minimal improvement are unlikely to make any significant gains.

Application to Practice

Once some general criteria are established to evaluate prospective patients, it is necessary to design a method by which these criteria are applied.

Use of These Criteria

The Council (13) recommends that all patients initially be assessed according to the five previously mentioned criteria, but because of the uncertainty involved in assessment measures and outcome predictions, these criteria should only be used to discriminate between patients when substantial differences exist. If it is not possible to discriminate on the basis of these ethical criteria, then a first come, first served philosophy should be used. When patients are evaluated by any standards, three groups of patients are usually identified: those who are clearly good candidates for treatment, those who are clearly poor candidates, and those who fall somewhere in the middle. Some CR programs have a preset number of patients that can be admitted to a program at any one time. Therefore, patients who will derive littlc benefit from rehabilitation may not be admitted. Other approaches attempt to maximize the number of patients who are accepted. Once those candidates who meet a minimal standard are identified, individuals are triaged so that resources can be optimally allocated. For example, it may be appropriate to provide some patients who are already doing well with a one-time assessment; others who require more intervention may benefit from a home-based program; and still others may require a more intensive and complete CR program. Whichever method is used, allocation of placements into a CR program and provision of other scarce medical resources should be guided by the mandate to prioritize patients such that preventing an extremely poor outcome of one patient should take precedence over a general improvement in quality of life in another. For example, preference might be given to a patient immobilized with fear of any activity, as compared with a patient who wishes to improve his maximum oxygen uptake from 105% to 115% of that predicted for age and gender.

Decision Makers

Once criteria and methods for establishing priorities are established, someone must be responsible for making the actual decisions. The American Medical Association Council on Ethical and Judicial affairs notes that physicians of patients competing for resources are poorly positioned to make impartial decisions (13). The traditional model of CR involves the treating physician deciding whether a patient is a suitable candidate. As mentioned previously, referral decisions by physicians reflect underlying biases about particular patients and about the benefits and limitations of CR. If all patients are referred to CR programs, the staff must then become the decision makers with respect to appropriate access to program services. Once a patient begins an intake process, however brief, expectations for program participation are generated. An alternative model would involve the establishment of a centralized formula, which would generate the most consistent decisions. Any process for the allocations of scarce resources, from kidney transplants to placements into a cardiac rehabilitation service, must use allocation mechanisms that, in addition to being consistent, are perceived to be objective and flexible. The limitation of centralized mechanisms is the lack of flexibility. Furthermore, the so-called objective point values given during the prioritization process may disguise ethical decisions regarding the importance of the different factors.

Legal Considerations

In our litigious society, the legal implications of any discussion on the allocation of scarce medical resources concern physicians in both the Canadian system and in managed care organizations of the United States. Although a comprehensive analysis of the legal issues and precedents exceeds the scope of this paper, certain issues must be raised. As noted by Alice Gosfield, there remains a "temporal parallax" in case law, where precedent does not keep pace with the market changes that constrain physicians to make allocation decisions (11). Among the litigation that has been brought to court, the conclusions have tended to be the same:

- Treating physicians are legally accountable for the treatment they provide.
- It is not sufficient for a physician to argue as a defense that the failure to provide the standard of care was based on financial constraints imposed on the health care provider (11,12).

The American Medical Association has confirmed patient welfare as the first consideration for all physicians working within health maintenance organizations (13). According to the Supreme Court of Canada (1971), physicians are only held responsible to provide a reasonable standard of care. Specifically, that they use "that reasonable degree of learning and skill ordinarily possessed by practitioners in similar communities in similar cases." This Canadian ruling provides little guidance regarding allocation of scarce resources.

Conclusion

The evolution of CR over the last four decades has been remarkable in terms of the types of patients who may benefit, as well as the number of potential candidates. Despite the strong evidence for its efficacy and the position statements advocating its common use, the percentage of patients accessing such programs remains low. An ideal scenario would see the provision of CR services to all that require it. A more realistic scenario is the realization that CR should be viewed as a scarce medical resource. Using criteria developed by the Council on Ethical and Judicial Affairs from the American Medical Association, the categories of (a) likelihood of benefit, (b) change in quality of life, (c) duration of benefit, (d) urgency of need, and (e) efficiency of resources can be modified to develop criteria for the selection of the best candidates for CR. Equal attention will be required for the use of these criteria, guidelines for decision makers, and resulting ethical and legal considerations with the application of such criteria.

References

1. Levine, S.A. 1944. Some harmful effects of recumbency in the treatment of heart disease. *JAMA* 126:80-84.
2. Taylor, H., A. Henschel, and J. Brozek. 1949. Effects of bedrest on cardiovascular function and work performance. *J Appl Physiol* 2:223-224.
3. WHO Committee. 1964. Rehabilitation with cardiovascular diseases: report of a WHO expert committee. *World Health Org Tech Rep Ser* 270.
4. Evenson, K.R., W.D. Rosamond, and R.V. Luepker. 1998. Predictors of outpatient cardiac rehabilitation utilization: the Minnesota Heart Surgery Registry. *J Cardiopulm Rehabil* 18:192-198.
5. Ades, P., M. Waldmann, D. Polk, and J. Coflesky. 1992. Referral patterns and exercise response in the rehabilitation of female coronary patients aged >62 years. *Am J Cardiol* 69:1422-1425.
6. Ades, P., M. Waldmann, W. McCann, and S. Weaver. 1992. Predictors of cardiac rehabilitation participation in older coronary patients. *Arch Intern Med* 152:1033-1035.
7. Armstrong, K.L., L.A. Wolfe, and M.C. Amey. 1994. Cardiovascular rehabilitation in Canada: a national survey. *J Cardiopulm Rehabil* 14:262-272.
8. Thomas, R.J., N.H. Miller, and C. Lamendola, et al. 1996. National survey on gender differences in cardiac rehabilitation programs. Patient characteristics and enrollment patterns. *J Cardiopulm Rehabil* 16(6):402-412.
9. Romeo, K.C., and M.S. Saccucci. 1991. Ethnic and gender differences in cardiac rehabilitation. *J Cardiopulm Rehabil* 11:214-220.
10. Loose, M.S., and B. Fernhall. 1995. Differences in quality of life among male and female cardiac rehabilitation participants. *J Cardiopulm Rehabil* 15(3):225-231.
11. Gosfield, A. 1995. The legal subtext of the managed care environment: a practitioner's perspective. *J Law Med Ethics* 23(3):230-235.
12. Capen, K. 1997. Resource allocation and physician liability. *Can Med Assoc J* 156(3):393-395.
13. Council on Ethical and Judicial Affairs, American Medical Association. 1995. Ethical considerations in the allocation of organs and other scarce medical resources among patients. *Arch Intern Med* 155(1):29-40.

CHAPTER 6

Evaluation of Cardiac Patients With Standard Exercise ECG Testing

Victor Froelicher

Cardiology Division, Palo Alto Veterans Affairs Health Care Systems, Palo Alto, California, USA

Motivated by recent studies describing new diagnostic modalities and techniques and a renewed interest in applying them as screening tests, it would seem wise to review lessons learned from past mistakes. Therefore, we examined experiences from the early studies of the standard exercise test. Four major mistakes that have been made by researchers when evaluating the exercise test's diagnostic characteristics are

1. choosing patients for study that provide a limited challenge to the diagnostic performance of the test,
2. not limiting the amount of workup bias in identifying patients for study,
3. considering soft end points instead of hard end points, and
4. using surrogates instead of a gold standard.

We will examine each of these errors and provide illustrations for each.

Limited Challenge

Limited challenge means that rather than studying the test in consecutive patients, a group of healthy or least-diseased patients is compared to patients who have severe disease. This is only appropriate as the first step in evaluating a new test or measurement and is not appropriate for evaluating or demonstrating true test characteristics (figure 6.1). Actual test characteristics are only defined in consecutive patients with the complaint that requires testing (i.e., chest pain). Such patients are the only patients who should be included in a study to determine test discriminating characteristics. When the healthy or least diseased are studied the specificity of the test should be very high, usually greater than 90%. When the most diseased are studied, the sensitivity should be very high, often 90% or more (figure 6.2). Even when ROC curves are calculated from results from these two disparate groups, a relatively large area will be obtained. It is only when the test or measurement is applied in consecutive patients with a complaint that requires testing that we see the actual test characteristics. Usually the sensitivity and specificity are much lower.

An argument could be made that limited challenge does not matter if only certain measurements are being compared. However, limited challenge can cause differences in other factors that cause the measurements to be different. For instance, heart rate, SBP, and exercise capacity are markedly different in healthy normal subjects compared to those with severe disease (figure 6.3). The discriminatory capacity of any ST measurement divided by heart rate (HR) (i.e., ST/HR index) is exaggerated when compared in samples with limited challenge.

Workup Bias

Another problem with most of the studies evaluating the diagnostic characteristics of the exercise test has been failure to limit workup bias. Consider figure 6.4: patients with chest pain being seen in the office are in the upper left circle. Normal clinical practice then results in an exercise test being done and in only certain patients being selected for further workup. Cardiac catheterization would be chosen particularly for those with a low exercise capacity and an abnormal ST response. Others will be catheterized but the population will be selected to favor these responses. Patients excluded from cardiac catheterization after the exercise test will be those with a high exercise capacity and a normal ST response. Others will also be excluded, but in the majority, these characteristics will predominate. Figure 6.5 shows the results. Most of the studies that have examined the characteristics of the exercise test, using the gold standard of cardiac catheterization, had workup bias. Sensitivity usually is about 70% and specificity is about 70% in such populations. What is unknown is how the test functions in the population of patients who present to the office, depicted in the upper left circle of the figure. In the few studies that have limited workup bias by protocol or that have had a lower degree of workup bias because of clinical practice (where the exercise test is largely ignored) and that showed different test characteristics, the sensitivity is roughly 45% and the specificity is 85%. These are the characteristics of test performance in the typical office setting.

A meta-analysis of 50 studies that have performed tests with angiographic correlates has been reanalyzed considering the percentage of patients with abnormal exercise-induced ST-segment depression in each study (see figures 6.6 and 6.7) (1). One assumes that there is less workup bias in the studies with the lower percentage of patients with an abnormal exercise test and more workup bias in those with a higher percentage of patients with abnormal exercise tests. Clearly there is a high

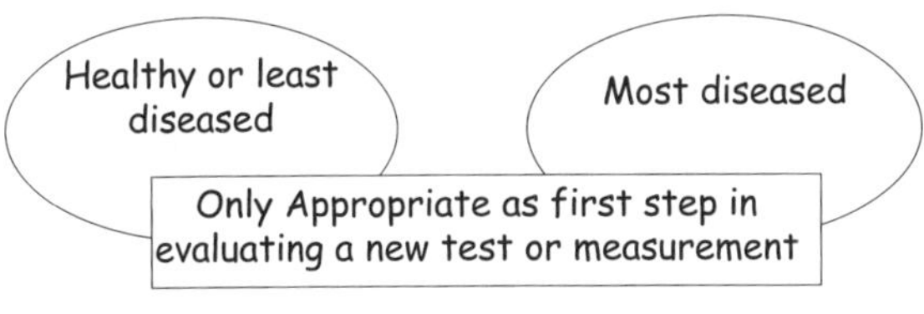

Consecutive Patients with the complaint which requires testing

should be studied to determine test or measurement characteristics

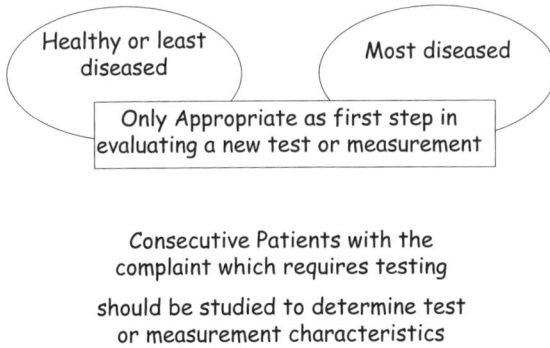

Figure 6.1 Illustration of limited challenge.

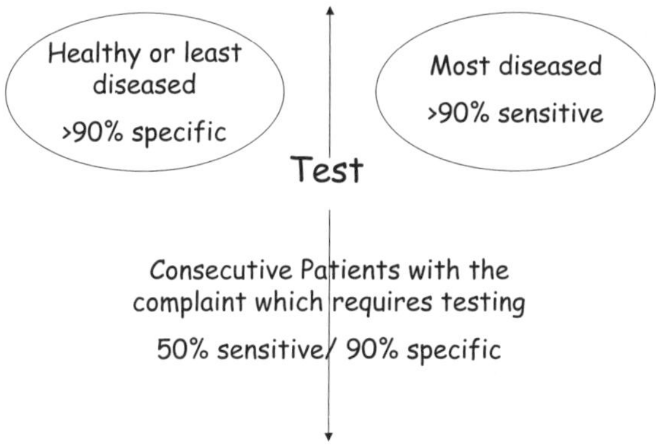

Figure 6.2 Exercise test characteristics in studies with and without limited challenge.

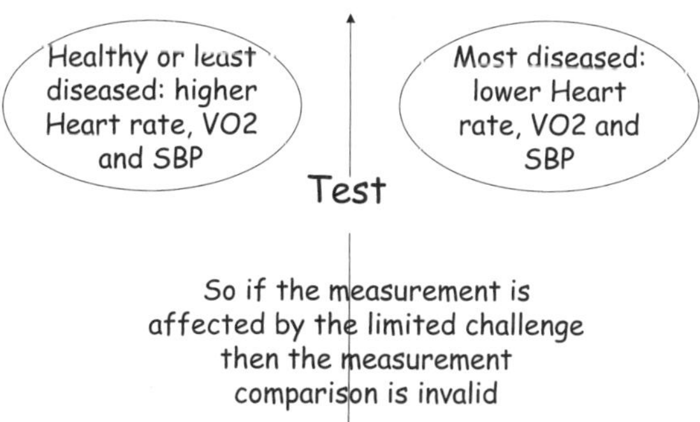

Figure 6.3 The effect of limited challenge on the hemodynamic responses.

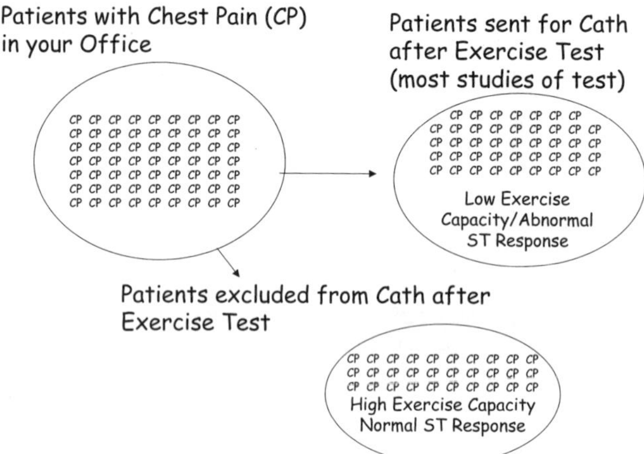

Figure 6.4 An illustration of work up bias.

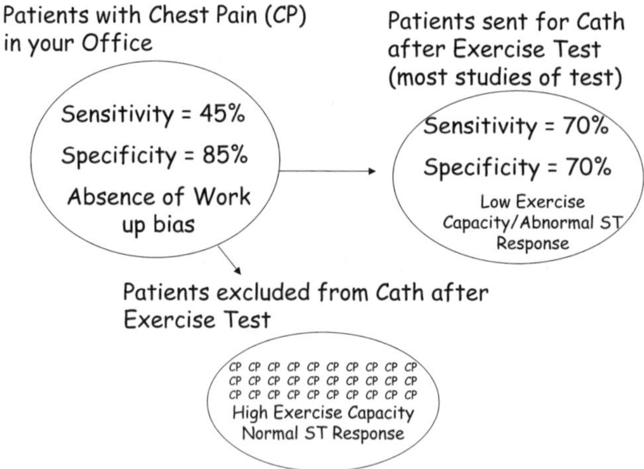

Figure 6.5 The effects of workup bias on test diagnostic characteristics.

correlation between the percentage of abnormal tests and specificity and sensitivity. Specificity is higher with less workup bias and sensitivity is lower. This is consistent with the studies that have removed workup bias by study design.

In summary, workup bias results from the fact that not all patients seen with chest pain and undergoing exercise tests also receive a cardiac catheterization. Excluded by workup bias are those with high exercise capacity and normal ST responses. Patients with low exercise capacity and abnormal ST responses are selected for further study. Though this is not always the case in any of the studies, tendencies toward this pattern vary from study to study, and that is why different test performance characteristics have been obtained with the exercise test. In the studies that have removed workup bias

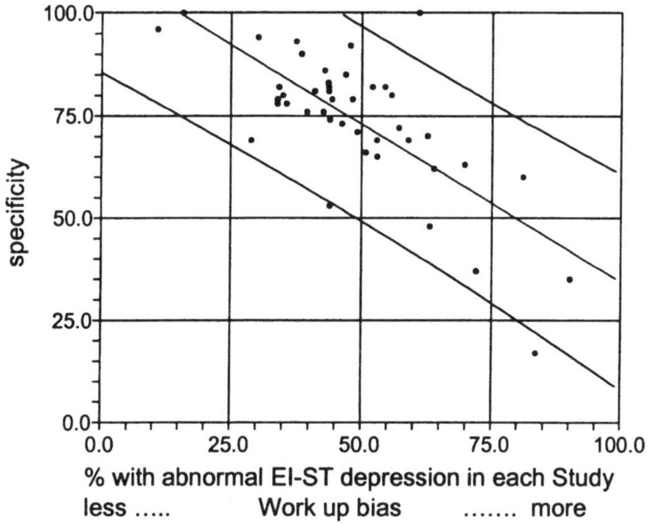

Figure 6.6 Plot of the 50 exercise studies diagnosing any angiographic CAD excluding patients with a history of MI.

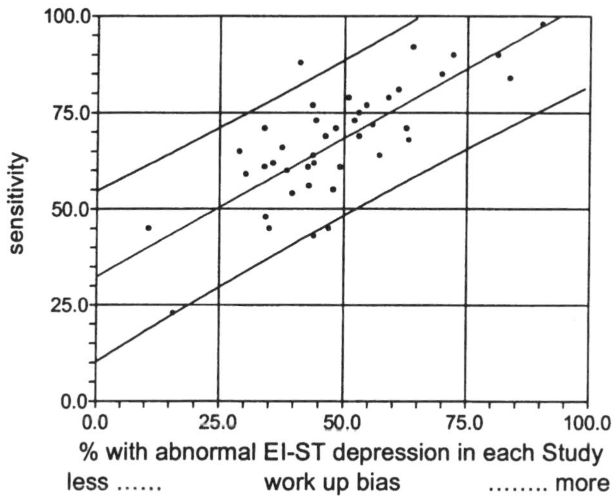

Figure 6.7 Plot of the 50 exercise studies diagnosing any angiographic CAD excluding patients with a history of MI.

by study design, these differences are very clearly seen. As shown in table 6.1, approximately 12,000 patients have been included in the 58 studies with varying degrees of workup bias. The mean sensitivity has been 67% and mean specificity 72%. The two studies that have removed workup bias by protocol have included 2000 patients and have considerably different test characteristics (2,3).

Table 6.1 Angiographic Correlative Studies for Diagnosis of Any CAD

Studies	No. of patients	Sensitivity	Specificity
58 with workup bias	12,000	67%	72%
2 without workup bias	2,000	45%	90%

An argument could be made that the clinician does not want to conduct a cardiac catheterization on everyone. That is not the point. To determine the discriminatory characteristics of a test, a study protocol must be strictly followed to catheterize and exercise test all patients presenting with chest pain. Then the practicing physician can tell from the study how effective the exercise test is in office practice and make better decisions regarding which patients need further evaluation.

Hard Versus Soft End Points

The best example of the problem of using soft end points instead of hard end points comes from screening studies. Twelve studies have used the exercise test to screen asymptomatic individuals for cardiac disease (table 6.2). Patients have been screened for silent heart disease using the exercise test and have been followed for 5 to 10 years for cardiac events. Considerably different results have been obtained in these studies according to the end points considered. When angina is included as an end point, nonspecific symptoms in a subject with an abnormal test are more likely to be called coronary disease during the follow-up period. Hard end points, such as death or myocardial infarction, are more appropriately used in such studies because of this lack of clarity. The first screening studies included angina as an end point; the last four have used only hard end points. Table 6.2 shows that the first studies tested 5526 subjects in all and ranged in size from 100-1390 individuals. Sensitivity was 50%, specificity was 90%, risk ratio was nine times (meaning that those with an abnormal ST depression were nine times more likely to have a cardiac event than those with a normal response), and the predictive value of a positive response was 25%. That means that one out of four patients with abnormal tests went on to have a cardiac event. Remember that some of these events were angina, which was probably not truly due to cardiac disease and may not have truly been angina. The last four studies have been larger in size and have included only hard end points. The sensitivity of the test has been about 25%, specificity about 90%, risk ratio four times (i.e., those with an abnormal ST depression were four times more likely to have a cardiac even than those with a normal response), and the predictive value of a positive response was only 5%. This means that only 1 out of 20 people with an abnormal test truly went on to a cardiac event.

Table 6.2 The Twelve Screening Studies

Study	No. of patients	Sensitivity	Specificity	RR	PV+
First 8 (soft end points)	5526 (100–1390)	50%	90%	9×	25%
Last 4 (hard end points)	12,212	25%	90%	4×	5%

Because of this very limited predictive value, in any asymptomatic population, screening has not been recommended. It can cause more harm than good and can lead to unnecessary tests. Several studies have even tried to raise the pretest probability by considering risk factors and have not been able to do so to a level that limits the false-positives and improves the predicted value.

The argument could be made that we should be able to predict which patients are going to develop milder forms of coronary disease than death or myocardial infarction, such as angina. Certainly we would like to do this but the problem is that the test result is creating end points. Thus, using soft end points exaggerates the sensitivity and predictive value of the test. This could be avoided by blinding all parties to the test result, but this is considered unethical. Because some of the asymptomatic individuals developing chest pain really have angina resulting from coronary disease, the sensitivity probably lies between the 25% and 50% obtained in the studies that used hard or soft end points.

Misleading Surrogates

Using surrogates for various measurements and outcomes has invalidated a number of studies. One method of using surrogates involves using the same criteria for computer measurement of the ST segments as are used for visual analysis. A misleading surrogate is applying strict 1-mm and horizontal slope criteria with a computer. This results in a totally different classification of abnormal ST responses than when the analysis is done visually. As it turns out, truly horizontal slopes are rare with a computer, whereas the human eye flattens things routinely in reading the ST segment. In addition, 1 mm by computer includes visual measurements to approximately 0.75 mm. Fewer patients are classified as abnormal using standard criteria if a computer does classification, in comparison to a physician visually using classic criteria. If comparing computer and visual analysis, one has to adjust for this fuzz factor inherent in the visual analysis.

A problematic surrogate is using nuclear imaging instead of angiography as a gold standard. It is well known that nuclear imaging has test limitations and cannot be used to replace angiography. Even though angiography has limitations, it is the best standard we have for obstructive coronary disease.

Another misleading surrogate is using interventions as definitions of cardiac events. Numerous studies have found that with modern treatment, there are few cardiovascular deaths and infarctions in most populations studied. This is particularly the case when patients with congestive heart failure are excluded. In order to have enough end points, follow-up studies have included bypass surgery or PTCA as an end point. This creates problems because the test results often determine who gets these procedures, and so it is not really valid to include them as events predicted by the test. A built-in bias favors the test predicting the result.

Screening

The American Heart Association and other organizations have expressed renewed interest in applying screening tests to asymptomatic individuals because of the data showing the ability of the statins to lower cholesterol and decrease cardiac events. The thought is that a marker of atherosclerosis could help to decide who should or should not be started on a statin rather than simply relying on a risk factor score or threshold. Because of the association of radiographically imaged calcification with atherosclerotic plaque burden, the new technology of electron beam computed tomography (EBCT) has been proposed as such a screening test. Unfortunately, studies avoiding the previously mentioned problems have not been performed with EBCT, and its test characteristics are still unknown. An obvious result of some of the screening studies of EBCT is that a finding of calcium leads to catheterization and surgical intervention in asymptomatic individuals (4). Unfortunately, this creates end points and exaggerates the discriminatory power of the test. Other tests considered for screening include carotid ultrasound, the ankle-brachial index, the resting ECG, and the standard exercise test.

Exercise test guidelines have not recommended using the standard exercise test for screening because of the problem with false-positives (5). Given its test characteristics, in a low-prevalence population, roughly 9 out of 10 individuals with an abnormal test will be falsely positive; that is, they will not have coronary disease. This can lead to insurance and employment problems and can even start a healthy person through the cardiologist's diagnostic cascade. If the results of a screening test were reported as a probability (for instance, as a treadmill or calcium score) rather than a pure negative or positive and only used to tailor the preventive treatment, then any screening test could be helpful. However even this approach remains a hypothesis until the following study is performed: an asymptomatic population is identified and then randomized to either receiving the screening test and a standardized strategy of response, or not. Such a study has been accomplished for mammography but is unlikely to be conducted for coronary disease due to the cost.

Considering Bayes Theorem we would like to increase the pretest probability of detecting disease before applying a screening test by using risk factors to identify asymptomatic individuals with a higher prevalence of coronary disease. Although this seems reasonable, the only study to attempt this did not document a better predictive value. The Lipid Research Clinics Coronary Primary Prevention Trial investigators attempted to predict coronary heart disease morbidity and mortality in men with hypercholesterolemia from an exercise test (6). To study whether the test was more predictive for men with hypercholesterolemia (i.e., thus increasing the pretest probability for disease), data from 3806 asymptomatic men with hypercholesterolemia were analyzed. The prevalence of an abnormal test was 8.3%. During a mean four-year follow-up, the mortality rate from coronary heart disease was 6.7% (21 of 315) in men with an abnormal test and 1.3% (46 of 3460) in men with a negative test (7). The age-adjusted rate ratio for an abnormal test, compared with a negative test, was nearly seven times in the placebo group and five times in the cholestyramine group. These results are comparable to the Lipid Research Clinics screening results in asymptomatic individuals without hypercholesterolemia.

Scores

Rather than rely on the ST segments and the simple cut point of 1 mm of depression, better test characteristics can be obtained by using more information obtained from the test (7). For instance, the DUKE treadmill score that includes METs and symptoms during the test along with ST depression can improve the predictive accuracy of the test (8). This is analogous to a calcium measurement with EBCT, an echo wall motion score, or a thallium reperfusion score.

Comparison of Diagnostic Tests for Coronary Artery Disease

It is appropriate to compare the newer diagnostic modalities with the standard exercise test because it is a mature, established technology. The equipment and personnel for performing it are readily available. Exercise testing equipment is relatively inexpensive, so replacement or updating is not a major limitation. The test can be performed in the doctor's office and does not require injections or exposure to radiation. It can be an extension of the medical history and physical exam, providing more than simply diagnostic information. Furthermore, it can determine the degree of disability and impairment to quality of life as well and can also be the first step in rehabilitation and altering a major risk factor (physical inactivity).

Some of the newer add-ons or substitutes for the exercise test have the advantage of being able to localize ischemia as well as diagnose coronary disease when the baseline ECG negates ST analysis (more than 1 mm ST depression, left bundle branch block, WPW). Also, although the newer technologies appear to have better diagnostic characteristics, this is not always the case, particularly when more than the ST segments from the exercise test are used in scores.

Test evaluation has been advanced by the writings of Reid and Feinstein (9) and Guyatt (10) and so we are now in a better position to evaluate studies of test characteristics. A number of researchers have applied these guidelines along with meta-analysis to come to consensus on the diagnostic characteristics of the available tests for angiographic coronary artery disease (11,12). Table 6.3 presents some of the results from meta-analyses and from multicenter studies. Because sensitivity and specificity are inversely related and altered by the chosen cut point for normal versus abnormal, the predictive accuracy (percentage of patients correctly classified as normal and abnormal) is a convenient way to compare tests. For instance, although the sensitivity and specificity for exercise testing and EBCT are nearly opposite, the predictive accuracies of the tests are similar. This means altering their cut points (i.e., lowering the amount of ST segment depression or raising the calcium score) would result in similar sensitivities and specificities. Because predictive accuracy can be thought of as the number of individuals correctly classified out of

Table 6.3 Comparison of Exercise Testing and Add-Ons or Other Test Modalities

Grouping	No. of studies	Total # patients	Sensitivity	Specificity	Predictive accuracy
Meta-analysis of standard exercise ECG	147	24,047	68%	77%	73%
• Excluding MI patients	41	11,691	67%	72%	69%
• Limiting workup bias	2	>1000	50%	90%	69%
Meta-analysis of exercise test scores	24	11,788			80%
Thallium scintigraphy	59	6,038	85%	85%	85%
SPECT w/o MI	27	2136	86%	62%	74%
Exercise ECHO	58	5000	84%	75%	80%
Exercise ECHO excluding MI patients	24	2109	87%	84%	85%
Nonexercise stress tests					
• Persantine thallium	11	<1000	85%	91%	87%
• Dobutamine ECHO	5	<1000	88%	84%	86%
Cardiokymography (CKG)	1	617	71%	88%	79%
Electron beam computed tomography (EBCT)	4	1631	90%	45%	68%

100 tested, simply subtracting predictive accuracies provides an estimate of how many more patients are classified by substituting one test for another test.

Although the nonexercise stress tests are very useful, the results shown previously are probably better than their actual performance because of the effects of patient selection. The results of the cardokymography (CKG) multicenter study are included because of its excellent design (13). For studies of diagnostic characteristics, patients with a prior myocardial infarction should be excluded since diagnosis of coronary disease is not an issue in them.

The Exercise ECG Test

Gianrossi et al. investigated the variability of the reported diagnostic accuracy of the exercise ECG by applying meta-analysis (14). One hundred forty-seven consecutively published reports, involving 24,074 patients who underwent both coronary angiography and exercise testing, were summarized and the results entered into a computer spreadsheet. Wide variability in sensitivity and specificity was found (the mean sensitivity was 68% with a range of 23%-100% and a standard deviation of 16%; the mean specificity was 77% with a range of 17%-100% and a standard deviation of 17%). The median predictive accuracy (percentage of total true calls) is approximately 73%.

To more accurately portray the performance of the exercise test, only the results in 41 studies out of the original 147 were reanalyzed. These 41 studies excluded patients with a prior myocardial infarction, fulfilling one of the criteria for evaluating a diagnostic test, and provided all of the numbers for calculating test performance. These 41 studies, including nearly 10,000 patients, demonstrated a lower mean sensitivity of 68% and a lower mean specificity of 74%; this means that there was also a lower predictive accuracy (69% rather than 73%). Notice that the predictive accuracy has the least variation. In several studies in which workup bias was lessened, fulfilling the other major criteria, the sensitivity was approximately 50% and the specificity 90% with the predictive accuracy staying at 70% (2,3). Workup bias has not been removed in any of the other studies of diagnostic tests.

Nuclear Perfusion and Echocardiography

Investigators from the University of California in San Francisco reviewed the contemporary literature to compare the diagnostic performance of exercise echocardiography (ECHO) and exercise nuclear perfusion scanning (NUC) in the diagnosis of coronary artery disease (15). Studies published between January 1990 and October 1997 identified from MEDLINE search, bibliographies of reviews and original articles, and suggestions from experts in each area were reviewed. Articles were included if they discussed exercise ECHO and/or exercise NUC imaging with thallium or sestamibi for detection and/or evaluation of coronary artery disease; if data on coronary angiography were presented as the reference test; and if the absolute numbers of true-positive, false-negative, true-negative, and false-positive observations were available or derivable from the data presented. Studies performed exclusively in patients after myocardial infarction, after percutaneous transluminal coronary angioplasty, after coronary artery bypass grafting, or with recent unstable coronary syndromes were excluded. Two reviewers used a standardized spreadsheet to independently extract clinical variables, technical factors, and test performance. Discrepancies were resolved by consensus. Forty-four articles met inclusion criteria: 24 reported exercise ECHO results in 2637 patients with a weighted mean age of 59 years. Sixty-nine percent were men, 66% had CAD, and 20% had prior myocardial infarction. Twenty-seven studies reported exercise single proton emission computed tomography (SPECT) at first use in 3237 patients, 70% of whom were men, 78% had CAD, and 33% had prior myocardial infarction. In pooled data weighted by the sample size of each study, exercise ECHO had a sensitivity of 85% (95% CI, 83%-87%) with a specificity of 77% (95% CI, 74%-80%). Exercise NUC yielded a similar sensitivity of 87% (95% CI, 86%-88%) but a lower specificity of 64% (95% CI, 60%-68%). Comparing exercise ECHO performance to exercise NUC, exercise ECHO was associated with significantly better discriminatory power when adjusted for age, publication year, and a setting including known coronary artery disease for NUC studies. In models comparing the discriminatory abilities of exercise ECHO and exercise NUC versus exercise testing without imaging, both ECHO and NUC performed significantly better than the exercise ECG.

It appears that exercise ECHO (specificity of 84%) has better specificity than SPECT (specificity of 62%) but not than the exercise ECG (specificity of 90%). The earlier meta-analysis of thallium perfusion imaging suggested better test characteristics with planar imaging than the currently used SPECT.

CKG

A multicenter study has demonstrated the diagnostic accuracy of CKG recorded 2-3 minutes after exercise in 617 patients undergoing cardiac catheterization (13). Twelve participating centers used a standardized protocol. Adequate CKG tracings, which were obtained in 82% of patients, were dependent on the skill of the operator and on certain patient characteristics. Of the 327 patients without prior myocardial infarction who had technically adequate CKG and ECG tracings, 166 (51%) had coronary disease. Both the sensitivity and specificity of CKG (71 and 88%, respectively) were significantly greater than the values for the exercise ECG (61 and 76%, respectively). The CKG is a simple, inexpensive add-on to the standard exercise test.

Electron Beam Computed Tomography

One hundred sixty men and women with coronary disease (45-62 years), of whom 138 had obstructive coronary artery disease and 22 had normal coronary arteries, and 56 age-matched healthy control subjects, underwent double-helix computed tomography (16). Sensitivity in detecting obstructive coronary artery disease was high (91%); however, specificity was low (52%) because of calcification in nonobstructive lesions. A multicenter study evaluated patients referred for angiography (17). Four hundred ninety-one symptomatic patients underwent coronary angiography and electron beam computed tomography at five different centers between 1989 and 1993. The area under the ROC curve was 0.75 for the coronary calcium score, indicating moderate discriminatory power for this score for predicting angiographic findings. In this group, sensitivity of any detectable calcification by EBCT as an indicator of significant stenosis (greater than 50% narrowing) was 92% and specificity 43%. When these computed tomography images were reinterpreted in a blinded and standardized manner, however, specificity was only 31%. In another multicenter study (18) of 710 enrolled patients, 427 had significant angiographic disease, and coronary calcification was detected in 404, yielding a sensitivity of 95%. Of the 283 patients without angiographically significant disease, 124 had negative EBCT studies for a specificity of 44%.

Conclusion

The lessons from exercise testing are pertinent today particularly as we investigate new diagnostic technologies. It is interesting to note the evolution of test evaluation that has occurred over the history of exercise testing. Certainly the clinical exercise test investigators, some of whom made some of the mistakes noted above, can feel at least partially responsible for these advances.

References

1. Gianrossi, R., R. Detrano, K. Lehmann, P. Dubach, A. Colombo, and V.F. Froelicher. 1989. Exercise-induced ST depression in the diagnosis of CAD. A meta-analysis. *Circulation* 80:87-98.
2. Morise, A., and G.A. Diamond. 1995. Comparison of the sensitivity and specificity of exercise electrocardiography in biased and unbiased populations of men and women. *Am Heart J* 130(4):741-747.

3. Froelicher, V.F., K.G. Lehmann, R. Thomas, S. Goldman, D. Morrison, J. Myers, C. Dennis, R. Shabetai, D. Do, and J. Froning. 1998. The electrocardiographic exercise test in a population with reduced workup bias: diagnostic performance, computerized interpretation, and multivariable prediction. Veterans Affairs Cooperative Study in Health Services #016 (QUEXTA) Study Group. Quantitative Exercise Testing and Angiography. *Ann Intern Med* 128(12, pt. 1):965-974.

4. Arad, Y., L.A. Spadaro, K. Goodman, A. Lledo-Perez, S. Sherman, G. Lerner, and A.D. Guerci. 1996. Predictive value of electron beam CT of the coronary arteries: 19-month follow-up of 1173 asymptomatic subjects. *Circulation* 93:1951-1953.

5. Gibbons, R.J., G.J. Balady, J.W. Beasley, J.T. Bricker, W.F. Duvernoy, V.F. Froelicher, D.B. Mark, T.H. Marwick, B.D. McCallister, P.D. Thompson, Jr., W.L. Winters, and F.G. Yanowitz. 1997. ACC/AHA Guidelines for Exercise Testing. A report of the American College of Cardiology/American Heart Association Task Force on Practice Guidelines (Committee on Exercise Testing). *J Am Coll Cardiol* 30(1):260-311.

6. Ekelund, L.G., C.M. Suchindran, R.P. McMahon, G. Heiss, A.S. Leon, D.W. Romhilt, C.L. Rubenstein, J.L. Probstfield, and R.F Ruwitch. 1989. Coronary heart disease morbidity and mortality in hypercholesterolemic men predicted from an exercise test: the Lipid Research Clinics Coronary Primary Prevention Trial. *J Am Coll Cardiol* 14:556-563.

7. Yamada, H., D. Do, A. Morise, and V. Froelicher. 1997. Review of studies utilizing multi-variable analysis of clinical and exercise test data to predict angiographic coronary artery disease. *Progr Cardiovasc Dis* 39:457-481.

8. Shaw, L.J., E.D. Peterson, L.K. Shaw, K.L. Kesler, E.R. DeLong, F.E. Harrell, Jr., L.H. Muhlbaier, and D.B. Mark. 1998. Use of a prognostic treadmill score in identifying diagnostic coronary disease subgroups. *Circulation* 98(16):1622-1630.

9. Reid, M., M. Lachs, and A. Feinstein. 1995. Use of methodological standards in diagnostic test research. *JAMA* 274:645-651.

10. Guyatt, G.H. 1991. Readers' guide for articles evaluating diagnostic tests: what ACP Journal Club does for you and what you must do yourself. *ACP J Club* 115:A-16.

11. Gianrossi, R., R. Detrano, A. Columbo, and V.F. Froelicher. 1990. Cardiac fluoroscopy for the diagnosis of coronary artery disease: a meta-analytic review. *Am Heart J* 120(5):1179-1188.

12. Detrano, R., A. Janosi, G. Marcondes, N. Abbassi, K. Lyons, and V.F. Froelicher. 1988. Factors affecting sensitivity and specificity of a diagnostic test: the exercise thallium scintigram. *Am J Med* 84:699-710.

13. Weiner, D.A. 1985. Accuracy of cardiokymography during exercise testing: results of a multicenter study. *J Am Coll Cardiol* 6:502-509.

14. Gianrossi, R., R. Detrano, D. Mulvihill, K. Lehmann, P. Dubach, A. Colombo, D. McArthur, and V.F. Froelicher. 1989. Exercise-induced ST depression in the diagnosis of coronary artery disease: a meta-analysis. *Circulation* 80:87-98.

15. Fleischmann, K.E., M.G. Hunink, K.M. Kuntz, and P.S. Douglas. 1998. Exercise echocardiography or exercise SPECT imaging? A meta-analysis of diagnostic test performance. *JAMA* 280(10):913-920.

16. Shemesh, J., S. Apter, J. Rozenman, A. Lusky, S. Rath, Y. Itzchak, and M. Motro. 1995. Calcification of coronary arteries: detection and quantification with double-helix CT. *Radiology* 197(3):779-783.

17. Detrano, R., T. Hsiai, S. Wang, G. Puentes, J. Fallavollita, P. Shields, W. Stanford, C. Wolfkiel, D. Georgiou, M. Budoff, and J. Reed. 1996. Prognostic value of coronary calcification and angiographic stenoses in patients undergoing coronary angiography. *J Am Coll Cardiol* 27(2):285-290.

18. Budhoff, M.J., D. Georgiou, A. Brody, A.S. Agatston, J. Kennedy, C. Wolfkiel, W. Stanford, P. Shields, R.J. Lewis, W.R. Janowitz, S. Rich, and B.H. Brundage. 1996. Ultrafast computed tomography as a diagnostic modality in the detection of coronary artery disease: a multicenter study. *Circulation* 93:898-904.

19. Shemesh, J.S., Apter, J. Rozenman, A. Lusky, S. Rath, Y. Itzchak, M. Motro. 1995. Calcification of coronary arteries: detection and quantification with double-helix CT. *Radiology* 197(3):779-783.

20. Detrano, R.T., Hsiai, S. Wang, G. Puentes, J. Fallavollita, P. Shields, W. Stanford, C. Wolfkiel, D. Georgiou, M. Budoff, J. Reed. 1996. Prognostic value of coronary calcification and angiographic stenoses in patients undergoing coronary angiography. *J Am Coll Cardiol* 27(2):285-290.

21. Budhoff, M.J., D. Georgiou, A. Brody, A.S. Agatston, J. Kennedy, C. Wolfkiel, W. Stanford, P. Shields, R.J. Lewis, W.R. Janowitz, S. Rich, and B.H. Brundage. 1996. Ultrafast computed tomography as a diagnostic modality in the detection of coronary artery disease: a multicenter study. *Circulation* 93:898-904.

CHAPTER 7

Can Women Benefit From Exercise Cardiac Rehabilitation?

T. Kavanagh[1,2,3], L.F. Hamm[1], R.J. Shephard[1,3,4], D.J. Mertens[1], J. Kennedy[1], and J. Beyene[4]

[1]Toronto Rehabilitation Centre, Cardiac Rehabilitation and Secondary Prevention Program, Toronto, Ontario, Canada

[2]Department of Medicine, University of Toronto, Toronto, Ontario, Canada

[3]Faculty of Physical Education and Health, University of Toronto, Toronto, Ontario, Canada

[4]Department of Public Health Sciences, University of Toronto, Toronto, Ontario, Canada

Cardiovascular disease is the leading cause of death among women in North America. Despite this, women who survive a coronary event are less likely to be referred for cardiac rehabilitation than men. Previous reports suggest that this is because they are older and, consequently, more likely to fatigue easily and suffer from concurrent medical conditions such as arthritis, diabetes, obesity, hypertension, vision difficulties, and neurological problems. They are also less likely to own or drive a car and more likely to have a dependent spouse at home. All of these factors may persuade the physician that referral for rehabilitation is unrealistic (1-4).

Younger women, on the other hand, tend to return to their previous work too soon following myocardial infarction. They underestimate the energy required when they rejoin the workforce or attempt routine household chores, tire quickly, and as a consequence become discouraged and depressed (5). They are thus less receptive to joining a structured exercise program.

A number of previous reports have suggested that women respond less favorably than men to exercise-centered programs of cardiac rehabilitation (6-8). Suggested reasons for the poorer response (9) include a failure of women to identify with male-oriented exercise programs (10) and differences in physical and psychosocial needs (11), as well as a greater level of anxiety and lesser sense of self-efficacy (12). However, the supposed difference in response is not well established. It could reflect no more than a gender-linked age variation in those recruited, or the adoption of a less vigorous program for women because more class time was devoted to discussion of women's issues (11), or because exercise leaders held the mistaken belief that women would be less willing than their male peers to accept pain or tiredness (13). In contrast, a number of recent studies have demonstrated that both compliance and training responses can match that of male patients (1,14-17).

Accordingly, we compared the response of large samples of age-matched male and female patients who had participated faithfully in a 12-month conditioning program that began 3-4 months following a coronary event. The response to rehabilitation was assessed in terms of changes in anthropometric and physiological variables.

Methods

Our research methods are discussed below.

Patients

The patients were 547 women and 547 men matched for age (age 61.4 ± 8.1 years, range 40-79 years) with a diagnosis of fully documented myocardial infarction (n = 278, 278); coronary bypass graft surgery (n = 225, 225); or angioplasty (n = 44, 44). All had been referred to the Toronto Rehabilitation Centre's Cardiac Rehabilitation and Secondary Prevention Programme under conditions approved by the Institutional Committee on Human Experimentation.

Patients were recruited 3-4 months after the primary episode; none had undergone any formal exercise training subsequent to the event. Although the majority of the group had been advised by their personal physician to begin walking after discharge from hospital, many had been afraid to do so.

Exercise Program

This has been described in previous publications (18, 19, 20), but in essence consists of a walking/jogging regimen, the pace of the walk being determined from the results of a cardiopulmonary exercise test, taking 70% of measured peak oxygen intake, and/or the ventilatory threshold, and/or a perceived exertion of 13-14 on the original Borg scale (21). The average initial prescription calls for a distance of 1.6 km, five times weekly, the aim being to increase this to 4.8 km for a total of 24 km per week over a period of 1 year. In the absence of complications, attendance at the centre is once a week, with four other exercise sessions carried out away from the centre and monitored by an exercise log that is returned on a weekly basis. Men and women exercise together at the centre, and the supervisory staff comprises both men and women. Other aspects of the program include lectures on cardiovascular conditioning and exercise physiology; advice on participation in other types of sports activities; and discussions on smoking cessation, diet, weight control, stress reduction, effects and side effects of medications, and return to work. The Toronto program has operated since 1968 and presently accepts some 1600 new referrals annually. The current dropout rate over a 1-year interval is 28%-33% for women and 25%-31% for men. All patients included in this trial necessarily remained compliant throughout the 12-month period: attendance averaged 78.6 ± 13.4% of prescribed sessions.

Anthropometric Measurements

Height and body mass were determined by standard clinical scales. Skinfold readings were taken at three standard sites (triceps, subscapular, and suprailiac) using John Bull calipers, and the percentage of body fat was calculated according to the formulas of Durnin and Womersley (22). Lean body mass was estimated from total body mass and percent body fat.

Cardiopulmonary Exercise Testing

The peak work rate and peak oxygen intake were determined by a progressive cycle ergometer test. The work rate was increased stepwise by increments of 16.7 watts every minute to subjective exhaustion, a Borg rating of perceived exertion between 18 and 20, the attainment of an oxygen intake plateau, or the appearance of symptoms or clinical or electrocardiographic signs requiring halting of the test (23).

The electrocardiogram (leads V_1, CM_5, III) was monitored continuously, blood pressure was measured in the last 15 seconds of every second minute of testing, and patients reported their overall rating of perceived exertion at 1-minute intervals.

Patients breathed through a mouthpiece and low-resistance (Hans Rudolph) valve connected to a Sensor-Medics/Horizon Metabolic Cart calibrated against cylinder gas mixtures. Respiratory rate, respiratory minute volume, and oxygen intake were recorded every 15 seconds.

Measurements of anthropometric characteristics, peak work rate, and peak oxygen intake were completed on entry and at the end of 12 months of conditioning.

Statistical Analysis

Two-way analysis of variance (ANOVA) was used to determine the effect of age (categorized in four age-decade groups: 40-49, 50-59, 60-69, 70-79) and gender on selected physiological variables at baseline and in changes from baseline measured after 1 year of training. Whether or not the effect of gender depended on the age decade was assessed from the age-gender interaction term in the model. When the interaction term was statistically significant at the 5% level, simple effects were tested at fixed levels of age decade.

Results

The results of our analysis are given below in terms of training regimen, initial status, and response of the patients.

Training Regimen

When first seen, since the men had a higher initial fitness level, they were prescribed a somewhat longer walking/jogging distance than the women and they covered this at a faster pace. In both genders, the pace decreased progressively with age group.

The increase in prescribed distance over the year also diminished with age group, but was slightly larger for men than for women throughout. Likewise, the men showed a somewhat greater increase of pace than the women did over the year of rehabilitation.

Initial Status

Pretraining body composition and cardiorespiratory status were assessed for both men and women.

Body Composition When first seen, the men were substantially heavier than the women, but this was due in part to body size. The average body mass index was closely similar for men and women, tending to decrease in the older age categories. There was also an age-related decrease in lean body mass in both men and women. On average, both sexes were somewhat above the ideal body mass for their height. Men had a substantially lower percentage of body fat than the women, which is normal even among highly trained athletes (table 7.1).

Cardiorespiratory Status In the women the average values for peak oxygen intake were marginal for independent living. ANOVA showed that the resting heart rate was somewhat lower in men than in women ($p < 0.0041$), and in both sexes values tended to decrease with age group ($p < 0.0045$); however, there was no significant gender/age interaction. The peak respiratory gas exchange (R) values

Table 7.1 Comparison of Initial Anthropometric Status Between Women (W) and Men (M), Grouped by Age Decade

Variable	40-49 years 54W, 54M	50-59 years 176W, 176M	60-69 years 231W, 231M	70-79 years 86W, 86M
Initial body mass (kg)*				
W	72.6 ± 15.1	68.3 ± 12.1	66.2 ± 11.6	63.5 ± 10.7
M	87.8 ± 17.8	80.8 ± 11.8	79.8 ± 11.3	77.1 ± 10.7
Initial BMI (kg/m^2)				
W	28.0 ± 5.8†	26.7 ± 4.5†	26.1 ± 4.5	25.9 ± 4.2
M	28.5 ± 5.1	27.1 ± 3.3	26.8 ± 3.5	26.1 ± 3.1
Initial body fat (%)*				
W	35.6 ± 4.6	34.7 ± 4.3	33.2 ± 4.5	31.8 ± 4.1
M	23.9 ± 4.4	22.5 ± 3.6	21.6 ± 3.9	20.1 ± 3.8
Initial lean body mass (kg)*				
W	46.6 ± 7.3	44.2 ± 6.0	43.8 ± 5.8	43.0 ± 5.5
M	66.3 ± 11.1	62.4 ± 7.7	62.3 ± 7.0	61.4 ± 7.3

Gender differences significant by two-way ANOVA (age-decade vs. gender) are marked by *; age/gender interactions by †.

and the peak Borg ratings suggest that all participants made a good peak effort; the peak R was lower in women than in men ($p < 0.0071$) and also declined significantly with age group ($p < 0.0015$). The peak work rate showed the expected gender effect ($p < 0.001$) and a significant age-group effect ($p < 0.0001$); equally the peak oxygen intake was less in women ($p < 0.0001$) and declined with age ($p < 0.0001$) (table 7.2).

Training Responses

Changes in body composition and cardiorespiratory status in response to training were assessed (see table 7.3).

Body Composition Patients in all age groups tended to increase body mass over the year of training; the younger women responded more than the younger men in this regard. The increase in body mass index showed a significant age-group effect for women only ($p = 0.0044$), with a significant age/gender interaction ($p = 0.0367$) and a significant gender difference for those aged 40-49 and 50-59 years only ($p = 0.0093, 0.0324$, respectively).

Body fat showed decreases in the men aged up to 69 only. ANOVA indicated a gender effect ($p = 0.0084$), but no age-group or age/gender interaction.

Table 7.2 Comparison of Initial Response to Progressive Exercise Test Between Women (W) and Men (M), Grouped by Age Decade

Variable	40-49 years 54W, 54M	50-59 years 176W, 176M	60-69 years 231W, 231M	70-79 years 86W, 86M
Resting heart rate (b/min)*				
W	74.6 ± 11.8	70.8 ± 13.7	69.8 ± 14.8	68.0 ± 13.6
M	69.3 ± 15.2	68.9 ± 15.1	67.9 ± 14.6	63.5 ± 11.5
Peak respiratory gas exchange ratio*				
W	1.19 ± 0.14	1.14 ± 0.12	1.11 ± 0.12	1.07 ± 0.12
M	1.16 ± 0.13	1.15 ± 0.09	1.13 ± 0.09	1.15 ± 0.10
Peak Borg rating (units)				
W	18.9 ± 1.5	18.7 ± 1.7	18.6 ± 1.7	18.6 ± 1.9
M	18.9 ± 1.4	18.8 ± 1.5	18.7 ± 1.8	18.7 ± 1.5
Peak work rate (watts)*				
W	100 ± 23	87 ± 23	80 ± 20	67 ± 21
M	151 ± 42	132 ± 32	122 ± 30	104 ± 24
Peak oxygen intake (ml/[kg • min])*				
W	17.3 ± 3.1	14.7 ± 3.0	14.7 ± 3.0	13.4 ± 2.4
M	22.2 ± 6.0	18.9 ± 4.4	18.9 ± 4.4	16.4 ± 3.4

Gender differences significant by two-way ANOVA (age-decade vs. gender) are marked by *; age/gender interactions by †.

Lean body mass tended to increase in all age categories. There were no gender or gender/age group effects.

Cardiorespiratory Status Resting heart rate showed decreases over the year of training, with the largest changes in younger women. ANOVA by age group and gender showed a significant gender difference ($p = 0.0426$).

Peak work rate increased significantly with training, with larger responses in the men than in the women. Both gender ($p = 0.0057$) and age group ($p = 0.0019$) exerted significant effects.

Peak oxygen intake showed consistent increases with training, the response throughout being larger in men than in women. There were highly significant differences in training response with gender ($p = 0.0001$) and age group ($p = 0.0003$).

Discussion

Findings regarding participants' initial status, compliance, and training response are generally in agreement with those of previous authors.

Table 7.3 Responses to Training, Differences Expressed as Percent of Initial Measure

Variable	40-49 years 54W, 54M	50-59 years 176W, 176M	60-69 years 231W, 231M	70-79 years 86W, 86M
Body mass				
W	3.2*	2.1*	0.4	0.3
M	0.2	0.6	0.7	0.6
BMI†				
W	2.8*	2.2*	0.4	0.3
M	0.6	1.3	1.2	0.3
Body fat*				
W	0.34	–0.32	–0.87	–0.3
M	–3.3	–2.6	–2.2	–0.2
LBM				
W	2.8	2.3	0.9	0.2
M	0.9	1.3	1.1	0.7
HR_{rest}*				
W	–5.9	–4.9	–4.3	–4.9
M	0.3	–2.6	–5.7	–1.3
WR_{max}*				
W	22.0	16.0	13.7	17.9
M	15.2	13.6	13.1	16.3
$\dot{V}O_2max$*				
W	8.6	10.8	9.5	9.7
M	16.6	14.5	11.6	10.9

Gender differences significant by two-way ANOVA (age-decade vs. gender) are marked by *; age/gender interactions by †.

Initial Status

Our findings are in agreement with those of previous authors who determined that older women who have sustained a coronary event enter a rehabilitation program with a poorer peak oxygen intake than their male counterparts (1,5). Indeed, many female members of our sample fell below the level at which difficulty is first encountered with the tasks of everyday living (24). In the younger women at least, (40-59 years), markers of the extent of peak effort (peak heart rate, peak respiratory gas exchange ratio, and peak Borg rating) all suggest that the difference in peak oxygen intake between men and women is real, rather than an expression of a poorer peak effort in the women. At least part of the female disadvantage is attributable to a low lean body mass and a higher percentage of body fat than that found in male subjects.

The loss of lean mass begins at an earlier age for untrained men and women than what we have seen in masters athletes who sustain their training (25), and the loss of lean tissue could play a role in limiting both peak aerobic performance and the response to training. This highlights the need to include an element of resistance training in a well-designed coronary rehabilitation program (26).

Compliance

All of the present group of patients were selected on the basis that they had remained compliant throughout the 12-month trial. Nevertheless, we would agree with a number of recent authors in finding that compliance does not differ substantially between men and women (1,14,15,17). The extensive experience of the Toronto Rehabilitation Centre shows that some 69%-75% of men and 67%-72% of women will attend a progressive training program faithfully for a 12-month period.

Problems of female compliance may have arisen in some earlier studies because no allowance was made for gender differences in initial condition or rate of response to training. Patients quickly become discouraged if the required program is beyond their capacity. Failure to customize the baseline exercise prescription and the rate of progression of prescriptions could well explain the poor compliance of women noted in previous reports.

With regard to this present study, because women entered with a poorer aerobic fitness level, it was necessary to prescribe a shorter initial training distance and a slower initial training pace than for the typical male patient, and this contributed to a smaller training response. There was also some evidence of a slower progression of the exercise prescription in the women.

Training Response

Our current data show clearly that women cardiac patients respond to a progressive training program, making substantial gains in various measures of endurance fitness over a 12-month progressive exercise program. In some respects (increases in body mass index and decreases in resting heart rate), the younger women (40-59 years) show significantly larger changes than their male counterparts. This increase in body mass index reflects in large part an increase in lean tissue mass; the women begin the program with much weaker skeletal muscles than the men and have a correspondingly greater potential to enhance their strength; this in turn reduces cardiac afterloading and makes an important contribution to aerobic performance.

The men made significantly larger gains of aerobic function than the women over the 12-month program. This may be a consequence of the lower training intensity (i.e., walking pace) achieved by the women. Alternatively, it may be that training enabled the men to push themselves to a higher peak heart rate and a higher systolic pressure. It remains unclear how far this change in response reflects a true physiological gain (a strengthening of the myocardium or an increase in chronotropic and inotropic responses) and how far it merely reflects a willingness to make a greater peak effort after 1 year of contact with centre staff. However, there was no significant increase of peak respiratory gas exchange ratio value except in the oldest age category and no significant change in Borg rating at any age, so it seems reasonable to propose that an enhanced physiological response accounts for much of the observed gains. In the women, in whom initial aerobic function was poor, the average gain in measured peak oxygen intake, although less than in the men, nevertheless may have been enough to allow independent living for several more years than would have been the case if no rehabilitation had been undertaken.

Conclusion

We conclude that middle-aged and older women suffering from ischemic heart disease compare favorably with men in their compliance record and physiological responses to a rehabilitation exercise training regimen, provided that it is tailored to their specific needs. Physicians should be encouraged to refer them to such programs.

Acknowledgments

The authors wish to thank Meenakshi Bhagi and Janet Will of the Toronto Rehabilitation Centre for their help with data collection and manuscript preparation, respectively.

References

1. Ades, P.A., M.L. Waldmann, D.M. Polk, and J.T. Coflesky. 1992. Referral patterns and exercise response in the rehabilitation of female coronary patients aged greater than or equal to 62 years. *Am J Cardiol* 69:1422-1425.
2. Harlan, W.R., S.A. Sandler, K.L. Lee, L.C. Lam, and D.B. Mark. 1995. Importance of baseline functional and socio-economic factors for participation in cardiac rehabilitation. *Am J Cardiol* 76:36-39.
3. Lavie, C.J., and R.V. Milani. 1997. Benefits of cardiac rehabilitation and exercise training in elderly women. *Am J Cardiol* 79:664-666.
4. Thomas, R.J., N.H. Miller, and C. Lamendola, et al. 1996. National survey on gender differences in cardiac rehabilitation programs. Patient characteristics and enrollment patterns. *J Cardiopulm Rehabil* 6:402-412.

5. Boogard, M.A.K. 1984. Rehabilitation of the female patient after myocardial infarction. *Nurs Clin N Am* 19:433-439.
6. Brezinka, V., and F. Kittel. 1996. Psychosocial factors of coronary heart disease in women: a review. *Soc Sci Med* 42:1351-1365.
7. Hamilton, G.A. 1990. Recovery from acute myocardial infarction in women. *Cardiology* 77 (suppl. 2):58-70.
8. O'Callahan, W.G., K.K. Teo, and J. O'Riordan, et al. 1984. Comparative response of male and female patients with coronary artery disease to exercise rehabilitation. *Eur Heart J* 5:649-651.
9. Ginzel, A.R. 1996. Women's compliance with cardiac rehabilitation programs. *Progr Cardiovasc Nurs* 11:30-35.
10. Moore, S.M. 1996. Women's views on cardiac rehabilitation programs. *J Cardiopulm Rehabil* 16:123-129.
11. Arnold, E. 1997. The stress connection. Women and coronary heart disease. *Crit Care Nurs Clin N Am* 9:565-575.
12. Shuster, P.M., and J. Waldron. 1991. Gender differences in cardiac rehabilitation patients. *Rehabil Nurs* 16:248-253.
13. Moore, S.M., and F.M. Kramer. 1996. Women's and men's preferences for cardiac rehabilitation program features. *J Cardiopulm Rehabil* 16:163-168.
14. Cannistra, L.B., G.J. Balady, C.J. O'Malley, D.A. Weiner, and T.J. Ryan. 1992. Comparison of the clinical profile and outcome of women and men in cardiac rehabilitation. *Am J Cardiol* 69:1274-1279.
15. Balady, G.J., D. Jette, J. Scheer, and J. Downing. 1996. Changes in exercise capacity following cardiac rehabilitation in patients stratified according to age and gender. Results of the Massachusetts Association of Cardiovascular and Pulmonary Rehabilitation Multicenter Database. *J Cardiopulm Rehabil* 16:38-46.
16. Lavie, C.J., and R.V. Milani. 1995. Effects of cardiac rehabilitation and exercise training on exercise capacity, coronary risk factors, behavioural characteristics, and quality of life in women. *Am J Cardiol* 75:340-343.
17. Warncr, J.G., Jr., P.H. Brubacker, and Y. Zhu, et al. 1995. Long-term (5-year) changes in HDL cholesterol in cardiac rehabilitation patients. Do sex differences exist? *Circulation* 92:773-777.
18. Kavanagh, T., M.H. Yacoub, D.J. Mertens, J. Kennedy, R.B. Campbell, and P. Sawyer. 1988. Cardio-respiratory responses to exercise training after orthotopic cardiac transplantation. *Circulation* 1:162-171.
19. Kavanagh, T., M.G. Myers, R.S. Baigrie, D.J. Mertens, P. Sawyer, and R.J. Shephard. 1996. Quality of life and cardiorespiratory function in chronic heart failure: effects of 12 months' aerobic training. *Heart* 76:42-49.
20. Kavanagh. T. 1998. *Take Heart!* Toronto, ON: Key Porter Books Ltd.

21. Borg, G.A.V. 1962. *Physical Performance and Perceived Exertion.* Lund, Sweden: Gleerup.

22. Durnin, J.V.G.A., and J.A. Womersley. 1974. Body fat assessed from total body density and its estimation from skinfold thickness: measurements on 481 men and women aged from 16 to 72 years. *Br J Nutr* 32:77-97.

23. American College of Sports Medicine. 1991. *Guidelines for Graded Exercise Testing and Exercise Prescription*, 4th ed. Philadelphia: Lea & Febiger, 1991.

24. Morey, M.C., C.F. Pieper, and J. Coroni-Huntley. 1998. Is there a threshold between peak oxygen uptake and self-reported physical functioning in older patients. *Med Sci Sports Exerc* 30:1223-1229.

25. Kavanagh, T., L.J. Lindley, R.J. Shephard, and R. Campbell. 1988. Health and socio-demographic characteristics of the masters competitor. *Ann Sports Med* 4(2):55-64.

26. Beniamini, Y., J.J. Rubenstein, L.D. Zaichkowsky, and M.C. Crim. 1997. Effects of high-intensity strength training on quality-of-life parameters in cardiac rehabilitation patients. *Am J Cardiol* 80:841-846.

PART IV

Peripheral Components of Exercise Intolerance: Implications for Cardiopulmonary Rehabilitation

CHAPTER 8

Peripheral Muscle Limitations to Exercise in Patients With Congestive Heart Failure: Implications For Rehabilitation

Jean Jobin and Jean-François Doyon
Hôpital Laval, Institut Universitaire de Cardiologie et de Pneumologie de l'Université Laval, Québec, Canada

In postindustrial civilizations, chronic heart failure (CHF) is a very important health problem. Its prevalence is estimated to be between 3 and 20 per 1000 people (1). These numbers increase to 30 to 130 per 1000 for people aged 65 and above. Each year, the incidence of new patients diagnosed with heart failure is at least 0.5% in the United States and in Europe (2,3). Because reduced work capacity is a well-known characteristic of heart failure patients compared to age-matched healthy subjects (4-7), and because most functional class III-IV patients are disabled (8), heart failure is becoming a growing liability for industrial countries. Therefore, potential causes of limitations of work capacity have been largely investigated in the last decade. Furthermore, the recent introduction of the muscle hypothesis (9) among the six main models of progression of heart failure (2) leads to a considerable amount of new research oriented toward the study of skeletal muscle in CHF. Recent review articles have considered peripheral factors in exercise intolerance and symptomatology in CHF (10-12). This chapter reviews studies relating skeletal muscle anomalies to exercise intolerance in patients with CHF. Findings on the effect of exercise training on these anomalies and their implications for rehabilitation in the treatment of CHF are also discussed.

Skeletal Muscle Alterations and Exercise Intolerance in CHF

Exercise tolerance in heart failure patients is reduced to about 50% of that of healthy subjects of the same age and sex (13). Interestingly, the exercise intolerance is more important if the etiology of CHF is ischemic disease (14). Contrary to common belief, however, exercise intolerance does not seem to result merely from a failure in cardiac function, since studies found a very weak correlation between cardiac function measurements such as left ventricular ejection fraction and exercise tolerance (7,15-17). More recently, Gulec et al. (18) found no significant relationship between resting indices of systolic and diastolic dysfunction determined by echo Doppler and exercise tolerance in patients with dilated cardiomyopathy. Moreover, it seems that peak $\dot{V}O_2$ is a better single predictor of mortality and morbidity than left ventricular ejection fraction for patients with CHF (7,19-21). Furthermore, during submaximal exercise at any given workload, patients with CHF have similar oxygen uptake and cardiac output but greater anaerobiosis and increased fatigue when compared to healthy subjects (22). Thus if we consider that work capacity (peak $\dot{V}O_2$) is determined by a central component, cardiac output, and a peripheral one, arteriovenous oxygen difference, according to the Fick principle, then the study of the skeletal muscle function, one of the peripheral components, becomes of paramount importance.

Muscle Mass

Earlier researchers determined that muscle atrophy was part of the CHF syndrome (23-25). Mancini et al. (26) concluded that severe muscle atrophy occurred in 68% of 76 patients with CHF. Furthermore, Minotti et al. (27) reported that the decrease in skeletal muscle mass was correlated with the decrease in peak $\dot{V}O_2$ in CHF.

Muscle Function

Because it is noninvasive and easily performed, an assessment of muscular strength is one the most currently used measurements of overall muscular function. Muscular strength studies reported a significant decrease in isokinetic and isometric absolute strength for patients with CHF compared to healthy subjects (28-30). However, relative strength for these patients with CHF, the ratio of muscle strength per muscle cross-sectional area, was not significantly different from that in healthy subjects. This leads to the conclusion that the decrease in muscle strength resulted from the decreased muscle cross-sectional area and not to a defect in contractile mechanism per se. However, Harrington et al. (31) found that isokinetic muscle strength remained lower in patients compared to healthy subjects even after normalization for muscle cross-sectional area, leading them to suggest that the changes in skeletal muscles of patients with CHF were not only quantitative but also qualitative in nature. The relationship of muscle strength to peak $\dot{V}O_2$ in CHF remains controversial: two studies found no significant correlation between these two variables (15,27), whereas three others reported a significant correlation (28,29,31).

A different method of studying skeletal muscle function consists of measuring time to reach fatigue during maximal or submaximal contractions either dynamic or isometric: muscle endurance. Studies on muscle endurance of patients with CHF reported interesting results. First, these studies demonstrated that endurance of the quadriceps femoris muscles was decreased in patients with CHF compared to healthy subjects (15,27,29,30,32). Harrington et al. (31) obtained similar results with isokinetic contractions. Furthermore, electromyographic studies carried out on patients with CHF objectively demonstrated early development of muscle fatigue (33). Decreased muscle endurance correlates with decreased peak $\dot{V}O_2$ in patients with CHF (27,29), indicating that muscle endurance must be considered with muscle strength as potential determinants of exercise intolerance in CHF. Minotti et al. (15, 32) tried to determine whether muscle bulk, muscular failure, or failure of neuromuscular transmission was responsible for fatigue of skeletal muscle. In one study, they found that failure of neuromuscular transmission was not responsible for the failure of muscle to maintain the physical load (32). They had previously studied the effect of muscle mass reduction on skeletal muscle endurance (15). They concluded that, contrary to the earlier reported important effect of decreased muscle cross-sectional area on muscle strength, the decrease in muscle cross-sectional area did not entirely explain the decrease in muscle endurance, as Harrington et al. (31). They further concluded that muscle alterations in CHF were not only quantitative, but also qualitative in nature.

One of the difficulties in studying skeletal muscle anomalies in cardiac or pulmonary patients is that it is always difficult to isolate the skeletal muscle factor from cardiovascular ones in studies using dynamic exercise, unless one uses a very small muscle mass such as the forearm or a single finger flexor. Obviously, large muscle mass such as the quadriceps femoris cannot be exercised dynamically at any significant intensity without some cardiovascular and respiratory involvement. However, when performing sustained isometric contractions of a relatively high intensity such as 60% of maximum voluntary contraction (MVC) or more, it is possible to conclude that the cardiorespiratory systems were not involved in any significant manner. This is so, first, because above 60% of MVC, blood flow is almost totally stopped in the contracting muscle (34). And second, the exercise duration is so short that it can be done without any additional contribution from the cardiovascular or respiratory systems. Thus, isometric testing allows the researcher to study the muscle function as an isolated organ, independent from significant solicitation of the cardiovascular and respiratory systems.

Skeletal Muscle Metabolism

In the past 10 to 15 years, researchers have extensively studied skeletal muscle metabolism in an effort to better understand the role of muscle function in exercise intolerance in patients with CHF. One of the first interesting findings on skeletal muscle metabolism in exercising patients with CHF was high blood lactate concentration (4,35-39). Furthermore, this increased concentration of blood lactate appeared prematurely, at submaximal workloads (39).

Skeletal muscle metabolism can also be studied noninvasively with nuclear magnetic resonance (^{31}P-NMR). These studies found a decrease of intramuscular pH, a decrease in phosphocreatine levels, and an increase in inorganic phosphate during muscle contractions in patients with CHF compared to healthy subjects (5, 40,41). These changes in muscle metabolism are linked to an increased glycolytic metabolism that results in premature intramuscular acidosis and decreased metabolic efficiency to do physical work (12). Furthermore, a recent study by Van der Ent et al. (42) found these metabolic anomalies to be present even in very small finger flexor muscles and at workloads below significant pH changes. Thus they must have happened independently from any significant cardiopulmonary involvement.

These results on muscle metabolism are supported by invasive interventions: enzymatic activity analyses on muscle samples from transcutaneous needle biopsy studies. Such studies reported a decrease in mitochondrial enzyme activities in patients with CHF compared to healthy subjects (43-45). The free fatty acid pathway was also shown to be affected as demonstrated by a decreased activity of the β-oxidation enzymes (5,44). However, glycolytic enzymes were not found to be altered (5,43-45), this being consistent with an alteration of the skeletal muscle cell oxidative metabolism in patients with CHF compared to healthy subjects. In a study on acid-base balance and some blood metabolites during exercise at low workloads, Opasich et al. (46) concluded recently that these important cellular metabolic alterations, which are present at rest, must at least partially affect daily physical activities.

Skeletal Muscle Ultrastructure

Not surprisingly, alterations in the skeletal muscle function and metabolism of patients with CHF are also accompanied by modifications in the ultrastructure of the cell. First, some studies demonstrated that patients with CHF had an increase in type II muscle fiber proportion compared to healthy subjects (28,43-45), and that this was specific to type IIb muscle fiber proportion (5,44). In addition to this increase in the proportion of fast-twitch muscle fibers, investigators have found evidence of atrophy in some types of muscle fiber compared to healthy subjects. However, results are not always consistent among studies. Some studies reported that the reduction of muscle fiber cross-sectional area occurs in all fiber types (28,47), whereas other studies concluded that the atrophy was present only in type II fibers (5), or only in type IIb fibers (44).

The inconsistencies reported on muscle fiber capillarity in CHF may be related to the poor power of most studies. Two studies demonstrated a decrease in the number of capillaries per muscle fiber (43,44), whereas another study did not show any significant difference in the capillary-to-fiber ratio compared to healthy subjects (5). Some studies quantified the number of capillaries per fiber cross-sectional surface area, but results are inconsistent. Some studies reported a decrease in the capillary number per surface area in patients with CHF compared to healthy subjects (43,45); other studies did not show any significant difference between patients with CHF and healthy subjects (28,44); and another study found an increase in the number of capillaries per surface area for patients with CHF (5). Consistent with the decreased oxidative metabolism, Drexler et al. (45) found that patients with CHF had a reduction of the mitochondrial density and a reduction of the mitochondrial mass compared to healthy subjects.

These results on muscle ultrastructure combined with other results on muscle metabolism and muscle endurance help us better understand how skeletal muscle may contribute to exercise intolerance during physical work in patients with CHF. These patients overuse the glycolytic metabolic pathway preferentially over oxidative metabolism, which results in premature skeletal muscle fatigue even during submaximal exercise.

Despite the fact that there is still no direct evidence (other than the increase in $\dot{V}O_2$max without changes in maximum cardiac output following exercise training reported by some [6]) that skeletal muscle alterations cause exercise intolerance in patients with CHF, research during the past two decades has helped us to better understand that exercise intolerance is much more complex than it was once believed to be. It is a multifactorial phenomenon that includes peripheral limitations, and skeletal muscle is an important component (12,48).

We still do not know what are the causes of skeletal muscle alterations in CHF. The following sections discuss some potential causes of skeletal muscle alterations in CHF, followed by a consideration of some intervention practices, such as exercise training, as potential means to restore skeletal muscle function in patients with CHF, and therefore to decrease the impact of disability on them.

Potential Causes of Skeletal Muscle Alterations in Patients With CHF

Some studies have suggested potential causes for skeletal muscle alterations in CHF. However, very few have identified the mechanism of action that would produce the observed alterations.

Physical Inactivity or Disuse Hypothesis

One of the most cited cause to explain exercise intolerance in patients with CHF is physical inactivity, often called "detraining" or "disuse." The similarities between changes occurring in patients with CHF and those observed in otherwise healthy subjects submitted to a long period of physical inactivity or drastically reduced activity are numerous (49-52). Furthermore, it is well known that patients with CHF rapidly become less and less active, first at the appearance of the first symptoms, and second after confirmation of the diagnosis, a time when decreased physical activity was the most common recommendation until a few years ago (53). Furthermore, a review by McKelvie et al. (54) on the effect of exercise training on patients with CHF revealed that it can improve exercise tolerance, increase skeletal muscle oxidative capacity, and partially restore fiber type proportions as well as muscle function. Thus, many authors concluded that if increased activity reversed muscle alterations, they were probably initiated by decreased physical activity. However, this is a long way from considering physical inactivity the only culprit of skeletal muscle dysfunction. Recent studies revealed that some alterations observed in patients with CHF were different from those observed following disuse or sedentarism. Changes reported by Sullivan et al. (55) on myosin heavy chain gene expression in CHF skeletal muscle are usually not seen with detraining or disuse. These results were confirmed in animal studies in the absence of a decreased level of physical activity (56). Furthermore, Vescovo et al. (57) brought evidence that prolonged bed rest in stroke patients did not decrease type I muscle fiber proportion, and concomitantly increase type II fiber proportion, as much as it did in patients with CHF. Thus one must conclude that physical inactivity is only one of many factors involved in skeletal muscle alterations in CHF.

The Hemodynamic Hypothesis

Logically, it makes sense that a decreased left ventricular function will affect central and peripheral hemodynamics (58), decreasing blood flow and consequently oxygen supply to the skeletal muscle. Leg blood flow has been reported to be decreased in patients with CHF during exercise (4,59,60). However, some studies on leg blood flow of patients with CHF found that leg blood flow can be maintained near normal in some patients with CHF compared to healthy subjects (61,62). Despite this controversy, it is of interest to compare skeletal muscle characteristics of patients with CHF to those of healthy subjects submitted to hypoxia. Some studies brought evidence that exposure to hypoxia decreases skeletal muscle oxidative enzyme activities, causes skeletal muscle atrophy, and brings about a shift in the proportion of type II fibers at the expense of type I fibers (63,64). Furthermore, studies using near-infrared spectroscopy to evaluate skeletal muscle oxygenation during exercise concluded that the decreased skeletal muscle oxygen supply might be related to problems in the muscle fiber itself and not entirely to decreased blood flow in CHF (65,66).

Other Probable Causes Some other factors have been identified as possible causes for skeletal muscle changes in patients with CHF. Malnutrition is one of them (12). However, dietary supplementation in patients with CHF failed to improve muscle abnormalities and exercise tolerance (67). It is important to note that although muscle mass is related to muscular strength in patients with CHF, it is not significantly related to muscle endurance (27).

Increased sympathetic activity has been suggested as a potential mechanism responsible for the skeletal muscle alterations observed in CHF (58). Hara and

Floras (68) observed a higher muscle sympathetic nerve activity at rest in young patients with dilated cardiomyopathy. However, even using exercise as a potent source of increased sympathetic activity failed to show any aftereffect of submaximal exercise at an intensity of 70% heart rate reserve on muscle sympathetic nerve activity of patients with CHF compared to healthy subjects. This does not rule out the potential effect of increased sympathetic neurohormonal activity on muscle metabolism and ultrastructure alterations found in patients with CHF, but indicates that changes observed in muscle metabolism during exercise are not likely to be related to exercise or postexercise sympathetic hyperactivity in this type of patient with CHF. On the other hand, studies on ACE (enalapril and losartan) treatment of patients with CHF reported an improvement in functional class, an improvement in exercise capacity, and a shift in skeletal muscle fiber toward slow myosin heavy chain, indicating that normalization in the neurohormonal activity may be responsible for the restoration of some metabolic and ultrastructure parameters (69,70).

Furthermore, the change in myosin heavy chain correlates with the net change in peak $\dot{V}O_2$ (71). However, the shift observed in fiber type proportions was not accompanied by significant changes in oxidative enzyme activities with enalapril (70). Effects of the neurohormonal system on skeletal muscle alterations are also suggested by the results of Sabbah et al. (72) on the fiber type distribution of the leg muscle of dogs with CHF. One month after induction of heart failure, the decrease in exercise duration for these dogs was associated with the decrease in type I muscle fiber surface area. However, these changes appeared before any significant change in cardiac output was observed, indicating that changes in left ventricle (LV) geometry might be sufficient to trigger some skeletal muscle changes very early in the evolution of CHF (72). Some pharmacological treatments of CHF may also be involved in the skeletal muscle alterations observed in patients as suggested by the results obtained by Schaufelberger et al. (73) with digoxin.

Implications for Future Rehabilitation in the Treatment of Skeletal Muscle Alterations Do skeletal muscle alterations reported here have any meaning for rehabilitation specialists? The obvious answer is yes, of course. In the 1970s and early 1980s, CHF was considered a contraindication to exercise (53). This conduct was dictated by fear that exercise would put patients at risk by increasing cardiovascular and especially LV stress and accelerate the natural evolution of the disease. Since then many studies have shown that if correctly prescribed, exercise, far from being deleterious, was beneficial to a great majority of patients with LV dysfunction (30,54,71,74,75). Despite these findings, many clinicians are still reluctant to enroll patients with advanced CHF (functional class III and IV) in rehabilitation programs. This is mainly a result of lack of knowledge of recent studies on exercise training, as well as the weaknesses of some of these early studies in which there was no control group. Furthermore, the cardiovascular and LV stress of exercise is still feared by many, despite the fact that even severe LV dysfunction patients (LVEF ≤30%) are not harmed by exercise programs (75,76). This is why some recent findings may help, especially those relating skeletal muscle anomalies to functional capacity and those indicating that these anomalies may be partially reversed by exercise training programs. Recent studies have shown that it is now possible to induce training effects in skeletal muscle metabolism and function, with consequent improvement in functional capacity and quality of life (77,78), without overstressing the cardiovascular system or the LV. This can be done through localized skeletal muscle training, either through strength or endurance exercises or a combination of both types of training regimens (78-80). Furthermore, recent studies using electrical stimulation provide evidence that skeletal muscle metabolism, structure, and function, as well as functional capacity, can be improved with minimal cardiovascular stress (81-83). This opens new possibilities for patients with very low work capacities such as those in class IV, especially in the light of the muscle hypothesis in CHF, which would imply that reversal of skeletal muscle anomalies may have a positive effect on the progression of the CHF syndrome (9). Furthermore it is possible to obtain very interesting improvement in functional exercise capacity with training regimens inducing minimal LV wall stress (84).

Conclusion

We can say that the future should witness the adoption of cardiac rehabilitation as an important component in the treatment of CHF, and especially in the treatment of the peripheral factors involved in diminished functional capacity, and in consequence decrease the disability burden of this disease as implied by recent reviews on this topic (85-87). This will even be more so if the so-called muscle hypothesis (9,88) is verified and proved to be a significant factor in the evolution of the disease, exercise training having the potential to restore muscle metabolism and ultrastructure (54,74,89). Therefore, exercise training—and especially rehabilitation because it is a multifactorial intervention (90) integrating biopsychosocial aspects of living with heart disease—will become important factors in the control of disability, morbidity, and mortality in patients with CHF through its impact on cardiovascular function, on skeletal muscle function, and last but not least: the patient's overall quality of life.

Finally, new noninvasive investigative techniques such as near-infrared spectroscopy (65,66) and surface electromyography (EMG) will allow researchers to better monitor the effects of different types of exercise training regimens, including skeletal muscle electrical stimulation, on skeletal muscle blood flow, oxygenation, and function. Therefore, this new knowledge should improve understanding of how training regimens work, as well as their interaction with pharmacological treatments and with psychosocial interventions. Furthermore, noninvasive techniques, through serial measurements, will help us to understand the time course of skeletal muscle alterations and their relationship with the time course of the left ventricular function and the CHF syndrome as a whole. Thus, integrative medicine will be an important factor in the future treatment of patients with CHF.

References

1. Delahaye, F., and G. Gevigney. 1997. Épidémiologie et histoire naturelle de l'insuffisance cardiaque. *Rev Prat* 47:2114-2117.

2. Poole-Wilson, P.A. 1997. History, definition, and classification of heart failure. In *Heart Failure: Scientific Principles and Clinical Practice*, ed. P.A. Poole-Wilson, W.S. Colucci, B.M. Massie, K. Chatterjee, and A.J.S. Coats. New York: Churchill Livingstone.

3. Sutton, G.C., and M.R. Cowie. 1997. Epidemiology of heart failure in the United States. In *Heart Failure: Scientific Principles and Clinical Practice*, ed. P.A. Poole-Wilson, W.S. Colucci, B.M. Massie, K. Chatterjee, and A.J.S. Coats. New York: Churchill Livingstone.

4. Wilson, J.R., J.L. Martin, D. Schartz, and N. Ferraro. 1984. Exercise intolerance in patients with chronic heart failure: role of impaired nutritive flow to skeletal muscle. *Circulation* 69:1079-1087.

5. Mancini, D.M., E. Coyle, and A. Coggan, et al. 1989. Contribution of intrinsic skeletal muscle changes to 31P NMR skeletal muscle abnormalities in patients with chronic heart failure. *Circulation* 80:1338-1346.

6. Sullivan, M.J., M.B. Higginbotham, and F.R. Cobb. 1989. Exercise training in patients with chronic heart failure delays ventilatory anaerobic threshold and improves submaximal exercise performance. *Circulation* 80:1338-1346.

7. Cohn, J.N., G.R. Johnson, and R. Shabetai, et al. 1993. Ejection fraction, peak exercise oxygen consumption, cardiothoracic ratio, ventricular arrhythmias, and plasma norepinephrine as determinants of prognosis in heart failure. *Circulation* 87(suppl. VI):VI5-VI16.

8. Sullivan, M.J., and M.H. Hawthorne. 1997. Nonpharmacologic interventions. In *Heart Failure: Scientific Principles and Clinical Practice*, ed. P.A. Poole-Wilson, W.S. Colucci, B.M. Massie, K. Chatterjee, and A.J.S. Coats. New York: Churchill Livingstone.

9. Coats, A.J.S., A.L. Clarck, M. Piepoli, M. Volterrani, and P.A. Poole-Wilson. 1994. Symptoms and quality of life in heart failure: the muscle hypothesis. *Br Heart J* 72(suppl.):S36-39.

10. Clark, A.L., P.A. Poole-Wilson, and A.J.S. Coats. 1996. Exercise limitation in chronic heart failure: central role of the periphery. *JACC* 28:1092-1102.

11. Stassijins, G., R. Lysens, and M. Decramer. 1996. Peripheral and respiratory muscles in chronic heart failure. *Eur Respir J* 9:2161-2167.

12. Harrington, D., and A.J.S. Coats. 1997. Skeletal muscle abnormalities and evidence for their role in symptom generation in chronic heart failure. *Eur Heart J* 18:1865-1872.

13. Weber, K., G. Kinasewitz, J. Janicki, and A. Fishman. 1982. Oxygen utilization and ventilation during exercise in patients with chronic heart failure. *Circulation* 65:1213-1223.

14. Clark, A.L., D. Harrington, T.P. Chua, and A.J.S. Coats. 1997. Exercise capacity in chronic heart failure is related to the aetiology of heart disease. *Heart* 78:569-571.

15. Minotti, J.R., I. Christoph, R. Oka, M.W. Weiner, L. Wells, and B.M. Massie. 1991. Impaired skeletal muscle function in patient with congestive heart failure. Relationship to systemic exercise performance. *J Clin Invest* 88:2077-2082.

16. Volterrani, M., A.L. Clark, and P.F. Ludman, et al. 1994. Predictors of exercise capacity in chronic heart failure. *Eur Heart J* 15:801-809.

17. Wilson, J.R., G. Rayos, T.K. Yeoh, P. Gothard, and K. Bak. 1995. Dissociation between exertional symptoms and circulatory function in patients with heart failure. *Circulation* 92:47-53.

18. Gulec, S., F. Ertas, and E. Tutar, et al. 1998. Exercise performance in patients with dilated cardiomyopathy: relationship to resting left ventricular function. *Int J Cardiol* 65:247-253.

19. Likoff, M.J., S.L. Chandler, and H.R. Kay. 1987. Clinical determinants of mortality in chronic congestive heart failure secondary to idiopathic dilated or to ischemic cardiopathy. *Am J Cardiol* 59:634-638.

20. Goldman, S., G. Johnson, J.N. Cohn, G. Cintron, R. Smith, and G. Francis. 1993. Mechanism of death in heart failure. *Circulation* 87(suppl. VI):VI24-VI31.

21. Smith, R.F., G. Johnson, S. Ziesche, G. Bhat, K. Blankenship, and J.N. Cohn. 1993. Functional capacity in heart failure: comparison of methods for assessment and their relation to other indexes of heart failure. *Circulation* 87(suppl. VI):VI88-VI93.

22. Steele I.C., A. Moore, A.M. Nugent, M.S Riley, N.P.S. Campbell, and D.P. Nicholls. 1997. Noninvasive measurement of cardiac output and ventricular ejection fractions in chronic cardiac failure: relationship to impaired exercise tolerance. *Clin Science* 93:195-203.

23. Katz, A.M., and P.B. Katz. 1962. Diseases of the heart in works of Hippocrates. *Br Heart J* 24:257-264.

24. Aronson, J.K. 1985. *An Account of the Foxglove and its Medical Uses.* London: Oxford University Press.

25. Morley-Davies, A., and J. Nolan. 1996. Heart failure: a historical context. In *Heart Failure in Clinical Practice,* ed. J.V.V. McMurray and J.G.F. Cleland. London: Martin Dunitz.

26. Mancini, D.M., G. Walter, and N. Reichnek, et al. 1992. Contribution of skeletal muscle atrophy to exercise intolerance and altered muscle metabolism in heart failure. *Circulation* 85:1364-1373.

27. Minotti, J., P. Pillay, R. Oka, L. Wells, I. Christoph, and B.M. Massie. 1993. Skeletal muscle size: relationship to muscle function in heart failure. *J Appl Physiol* 75:373-381.

28. Lipkin, D., D. Jones, J. Round, and P. Poole-Wilson. 1988. Abnormalities of skeletal muscle in patients with chronic heart failure. *Int J Cardiol* 18:187-195.

29. Buller, N.P., D. Jones, and P.A. Poole-Wilson. 1991. Direct measurements of skeletal muscle fatigue in patients with chronic heart failure. *Br Heart J* 65:20-24.

30. Magnusson, G., B. Isberg, K. Karlberg, and C. Sylven. 1994. Skeletal muscle strength and endurance in chronic congestive heart failure secondary to idiopathic dilated cardiomyopathy. *Am J Cardiol* 73:307-309.

31. Harrington, D., S.D. Anker, and T.P. Chua, et al. 1997. Skeletal muscle function and its relationship to exercise tolerance in chronic heart failure. *J Am Coll Cardiol* 30:1758-1764.

32. Minotti, J.R., P. Pillay, L. Chang, L. Wells, and B.M. Massie. 1992. Neurophysiological assessment of skeletal muscle fatigue in patients with congestive heart failure. *Circulation* 86:903-908.

33. Buonocore, M., Opasich, C., and R. Casale. 1998. Early development of EMG localized muscle fatigue in hand muscles of patients with chronic heart failure. *Arch Phys Med Rehab* 79:41-45.

34. Sadamoto, T., F. Bonde-Petersen, and Y. Suzuki. 1983. Skeletal muscle tension, flow pressure, and EMG during sustained isometric contractions in humans. *Eur J Appl Physiol* 51:395-408.

35. Meakins, J., and C.N.H. Lang. 1927. Oxygen consumption, oxygen debt and lactic acid in circulatory failure. *J Clin Invest* 4:273-293.

36. Huckabee, W.K., and W.E. Judson. 1958. The role of anaerobic metabolism in the performance of mild muscular work. I. Relationship to oxygen consumption and cardiac output and the effect of congestive heart failure. *J Clin Invest* 37:1577-1592.

37. Donald, K.W., J. Gloster, E.A. Harris, J. Reeves, and P. Harris. 1961. The production of lactic acid during exercise in normal subjects and patients with rheumatic heart disease. *Am Heart J* 62:494-510.

38. Weber, K.T., and J.S. Janicki. 1985. Lactate production during maximal and submaximal exercise in patients with chronic heart failure. *J Am Coll Cardiol* 6:717-724.

39. Sullivan, M.J., M.B. Higginbotham, and F.R. Cobb. 1988. Increased exercise ventilation in patients with chronic heart failure: intact ventilatory control despite hemodynamic and pulmonary abnormalities. *Circulation* 77:552-559.

40. Wilson, J.R., L. Fink, and J. Maris, et al. 1985. Evaluation of energy metabolism in skeletal muscle of patients with heart failure with gated phosphorus-31 nuclear magnetic resonance. *Circulation* 71:57-62.

41. Massie, B.M., M. Conway, and R. Yonge, et al. 1987. 31-P nuclear magnetic resonance evidence of abnormal skeletal muscle metabolism in patients with congestive heart failure. *Am J Cardiol* 60:309-315.

42. Van der Ent, M., J.A.L. Jeneson, W.J. Remme, R. Berger, R. Ciampricotti, and F. Visser. 1998. A noninvasive selective assessment of type I fibre mitochondrial function using ^{31}P-NMR spectroscopy. *Eur Heart J* 19:124-131.

43. Yancy, C.W., Jr., D. Parsons, L. Lane, M. Carry, B.G. Firth, and C.G. Blomqvist. 1989. Capillary density, fiber type and enzyme composition of skeletal muscle in congestive heart failure. *J Am Coll Cardiol* 13(suppl.):38A.

44. Sullivan, M.J., H.J. Green, and F.R. Cobb. 1990. Skeletal muscle biochemistry and histology in ambulatory patients with long-term heart failure. *Circulation* 81:518-527.

45. Drexler, H., U. Riede, T. Munzel, H. Knigt, E. Funke, and H. Just. 1992. Alteration of skeletal muscle in chronic heart failure. *Circulation* 85:1751-1759.

46. Opasich, C., E. Pasini, and R. Aquilani, et al. 1997. Skeletal muscle function at low work level as a model for daily activities in patients with chronic heart failure. *Eur Heart J* 18:1626-1631.

47. Belardinelli, R., D. Georgiou, V. Scocco, T.J. Barstow, and A. Puracaro. 1995. Low intensity exercise training in patients with chronic heart failure. *J Am Coll Cardiol* 26:975-982.

48. Brubaker, P.H. 1997. Exercise intolerance in congestive heart failure: a lesson in exercise physiology. *J Cardiopulm Rehabil* 17:217-221.

49. Refenberick, D.H., J.G. Gamble, and S.R. Max. 1973. Responses of mitochondrial enzymes to decreased muscular activity. *Am J Physiol* 225:1295-1299.

50. Holloszy, J.O. 1976. Adaptations of muscular tissue to training. *Prog Cardiovasc Dis* 18:445-458.

51. MacDougall, J.D., G.R. Ward, D.G. Sale, and J.R. Sutton. 1977. Biochemical adaptation of human skeletal muscle to heavy resistance training and immobilization. *J Appl Physiol* 43:700-703.

52. Edwards, R.H.T. 1981. Human muscle function and fatigue. In *Human Muscle Fatigue: Physiological Mechanisms,* ed. R. Porter and J. Whelan. London: Pitman Medical.

53. American College of Sports Medicine. 1995. Common medications. In *ACSM Guidelines for Exercise Testing and Prescription,* 5th ed. New York: Williams and Wilkins.

54. McKelvie, R.S., K.K. Teo, N. McCartney, D. Humen, T. Montague, and S. Yusuf. 1995. Effects of exercise training in patients with congestive heart failure: a critical review. *J Am Coll Cardiol* 25:789-796.

55. Sullivan, M.J., B.D. Duscha, H. Klitgaard, W.E. Kraus, F.R. Cobb, and B. Saltin. 1997. Altered expression of myosin heavy chain in human skeletal muscle in chronic heart failure. *Med Sci Sports Exerc* 29:860-866.

56. Simonini, A., C.S. Long, G.A. Dudley, P. Yue, J. McElhinny, and B.M. Massie. 1996. Heart failure in rats causes changes in skeletal muscle phenotype and gene expression unrelated to locomotor activity. *Circulation* 79:128-136.

57. Vescovo, G., L. Facchin, and P. Tenderini, et al. 1995. A new micro-method for assessing myosin heavy chain composition in skeletal muscle needle biopsies. Differences between chronic heart failure and diffuse muscle atrophy. *Eur Heart J* 16(Suppl):357.

58. Sullivan, M.J., and Cobb F.R. 1992. Central hemodynamic response to exercise in patients with chronic heart failure. *Chest* 101(suppl. 5):340S-346S.

59. Sullivan, M.J., J.D. Knight, M.B. Higginbotham, and F.R. Cobb. 1989. Relation between central and peripheral hemodynamics during exercise in patients with chronic heart failure. Muscle blood flow is reduced with maintenance of arterial perfusion pressure. *Circulation* 80:769-781.

60. Weiner, D.H., L.I. Fink, J. Maris, R.A. Jones, B. Chance, and J.R. Wilson. 1986. Abnormal skeletal muscle bioenergetics during exercise in patients with heart failure: role of reduced muscle blood flow. *Circulation* 73:1127-1136.

61. Massie, B.M., M. Conway, and R. Yonge, et al. 1987. Skeletal muscle metabolism in patients with congestive heart failure: relation to clinical severity and blood flow. *Circulation* 76:1009-1019.

62. Howald, H., D. Pette, J.A. Simoneau, A. Uber, H. Hoppeler, and P. Cerretelli. 1990. Effects of chronic hypoxia on muscle enzyme activities. *Int J Sports Med* 11(suppl.):S10-S14.

63. Hilderbrand, I.L., C. Sylvén, M. Esbjornsson, K. Hellstrom, and E. Jansson. 1991. Does chronic hypoxaemia induce transformations of fibre types? *Act Physiol Scand* 141:435-439.

64. Hoppeler, H., and D. Desplanches. 1992. Muscle structural modifications in hypoxia. *Int J Sports Med* 13(suppl. 1):S166-S168.

65. Wilson, J.R., D.M. Mancini, K. McCully, N. Ferraro, N. Lanoce, and B. Chance. 1989. Noninvasive detection of skeletal muscle underperfusion with near-infrared spectroscopy in patients with heart failure. *Circulation* 80:1668-1674.

66. Matsui, S., N. Tamura, T. Hirakawa, S. Kobayashi, N. Takekoshi, and E. Murakami. 1995. Assessment of working skeletal muscle oxygenation in patients with chronic heart failure. *Am Heart J* 129:690-695.

67. Broquist M., H. Arnquist, U. Dahlstrom, J. Larsson, E. Nylander, and J. Permert. 1994. Nutritional assessment and muscle energy metabolism in

severe chronic heart failure—effects of long term dietary supplementation. *Eur Heart J* 15:1641-1650.

68. Hara, K., and J.S. Floras. 1998. Resting muscle sympathic nerve activity does not predict duration of symptom-limited submaximal exercise in young patients with dilated cardiomyopathy. *Can J Cardiol* 14:689-694.

69. Schaufelberger, M., G. Andersson, B.O. Eriksson, G. Grimby, P. Held, and K. Swedberg. 1996. Skeletal muscle changes in patients with chronic heart failure before and after treatment with enalapril. *Eur Heart J* 17:1678-1685.

70. Vescovo, G., L. Dalla Libera, and F. Serafini, et al. 1998. Improved exercise tolerance after losartan and enalapril in heart failure: correlation with changes in skeletal muscle myosin heavy chain composition. *Circulation* 98:1742-1749.

71. Hambrecht, R., J. Niebauer, and E. Fiehn, et al. 1995. Physical training in patients with stable chronic heart failure: effects on cardiopulmonary fitness and ultrastructural abnormalities of leg muscles. *J Am Coll Cardiol* 25:1239-1249.

72. Sabbah, H.N., F. Hansen-Smith, and V.G. Sharov, et al. 1993. Decreased proportion of type I myofibers in skeletal muscle of dogs with chronic heart failure. *Circulation* 87:1729-1737.

73. Schaufelberger, M., B.O. Eriksson, G. Grimby, P. Held, and K. Swedberg. 1997. Skeletal muscle alterations in patients with chronic heart failure. *Eur Heart J* 18:971-980.

74. Giannuzzi, P., P.L. Temporelli, U. Corrà, M. Gattone, A. Giordano, and L. Tavazzi. 1997. Attenuation of unfavorable remodeling by exercise training in postinfarction patients with left ventricular dysfunction: results of the exercise in left ventricular dysfunction (ELVD) trial. *Circulation* 96:1790-1797.

75. Digenio, A.G., A. Cantor, T.D. Noakes, L. Cloete, D. Mavunda, and J.D. Esser. 1996. Is severe left-ventricular dysfunction a contraindication to participation in an exercise rehabilitation program. *S Afric Med J* 86:1106-1109.

76. Keteyian, S.J., A.B. Levine, and C.A Brawner, et al. 1996. Exercise training in patients with heart failure: a randomized controlled trial. *Ann Intern Med* 124:1051-1057.

77. Kavanagh, T., M.G. Myers, R.S. Baigrie, D.J. Mertens, P. Sawyer, and R.J. Shephard. 1996. Quality-of-life and cardiorespiratory function in chronic-heart-failure—effects of 12 month aerobic training. *Heart* 76:42-49.

78. Magnusson, G., A. Gordon, and L. Kaijser, et al. 1996. High-intensity knee extensor training in patients with chronic heart-failure—major skeletal muscle improvement. *Eur Heart J* 17:1048-1055.

79. Meyer, K., L. Samek, and M. Schwaibold, et al. 1996. Physical responses to different modes of interval exercise in patients with chronic heart-failure—application to exercise training. *Eur Heart J* 17:1040-1047.

80. Gordon, A., R. Tyni-Lenné, H. Persson, L. Kaijser, E. Hultman, and C. Sylvén. 1996. Markedly improved skeletal muscle function with local muscle patients with chronic heart failure. *Clin Cardiol* 19:568-574.

81. Pette, D., and G. Vrbova. 1992. Adaptation of mammalian skeletal muscle fibers to chronic electrical stimulation. *Rev Physiol Biochem Pharmacol* 120:115-202.

82. Kraus, W.E., C.E. Torgan, and D.A. Taylor. 1994. Skeletal muscle adaptation to chronic low-frequency motor nerve stimulation. *Exerc Sports Sci Rev* 22:313-360.

83. Maillefert, J.F., J.C. Eicher, and P. Walker, et al. 1998. Effects of low-frequency electrical stimulation of quadriceps and calf muscles in patients with chronic heart failure. *J Cardiopulm Rehabil* 18:277-282.

84. Demopoulos, L., R. Bijou, I. Fergus, M. Jones, J. Strom, and T. LeJemtel. 1997. Exercise training in patients with severe congestive heart failure: enhancing peak aerobic capacity while minimizing the increase in ventricular wall stress. *J Am Coll Cardiol* 29:597-603.

85. Balady, G.J. 1998. Exercise training in the treatment of heart failure: what is achieved and how? *Ann Med* 30(suppl. 1):61-65.

86. Braith, R.W. 1998. Exercise training in patients with CHF and heart transplant recipients. *Med Sci Sports Exerc* 30(suppl.):S367-S378.

87. Clark, J.R., and C. Sherman. 1998. Congestive heart failure—training for a better life. *Phys Sports Med* 26:53-56.

88. Gordon, A., and L.M. Voipiopulkki. 1997. Crosstalk of the heart and periphery: skeletal and cardiac muscles as therapeutic targets in heart failure. *Ann Med* 29:327-331.

89. Hambrecht, R., E. Fiehn, and J. Yu , et al. 1997. Effects of endurance training on mitochondrial ultrastructure and fiber type distribution in skeletal muscle in patients with stable chronic heart failure. *JACC* 29:1067-1073.

90. American Association of Cardiovascular and Pulmonary Rehabilitation. 1999. *Guidelines for Cardiac Rehabilitation and Secondary Prevention Programs,* 3rd ed. Champaign, IL: Human Kinetics.

CHAPTER 9

Peripheral Muscle Dysfunction in Patients With Chronic Obstructive Pulmonary Disease

François Maltais[1], Jean Jobin[1], and Pierre LeBlanc[1,2]
[1]Institut Universitaire de Cardiologie et de Pneumologie de l'Université Laval, Québec, Canada
[2]Unité de Recherche, Centre de Pneumologie de l' Hôpital Laval Sainte-Foy, Québec, Canada

Despite optimal bronchodilator therapy, many patients with chronic obstructive pulmonary disease (COPD) have a poor functional status and are unable to perform normal daily activities. Simple clinical observations indicate that factors other than impairment in lung function contribute to exercise intolerance in these individuals. It is well known that, while there is a relationship between forced expiratory volume in 1 second (FEV_1) and peak exercise capacity, there is also a wide range of exercise performance for any given degree of airflow obstruction (1). Perhaps the most striking clinical evidence pointing to a peripheral factor in exercise limitation in COPD comes from lung transplant recipients in whom exercise tolerance remains low despite normalization of their lung function (2,3). These observations have generated renewed interest in the evaluation of peripheral muscle function in patients with COPD. In this chapter, the evidence for and the possible etiologies of peripheral muscle dysfunction in patients with COPD are reviewed. The term "muscle dysfunction" is used to signify structural or functional muscle changes with no implication as to whether or not these changes result from a specific muscular pathological process. The possible influence of peripheral muscle dysfunction on exercise tolerance as well as the diagnostic and therapeutic approaches to this problem are also addressed.

Evidences of Peripheral Muscle Dysfunction in COPD

Peripheral muscle abnormalities described in patients with COPD include reduction in muscle mass, weakness, alteration in fiber type distribution, and decreased metabolic capacity (table 9.1). The quadriceps is the most commonly studied peripheral muscle, not only because it is readily accessible, but also because it is a primary effector

Table 9.1 Evidence of Peripheral Muscle Dysfunction in Patients With COPD

Muscle atrophy (Schols et al. 1993 [4])

Weakness (Gosselink, Troosters, and Decramer 1996 [11]; Hamilton et al. 1995 [12])

Morphological changes

- ↓ proportion of type I fibers (Jakobsson, Jorfeldt, and Brundin 1990 [24]; Hildebrand et al. 1991 [25]; Whittom et al. 1998 [26]; Maltais et al. 1999 [27])
- ↑ proportion of type IIb fibers (Whittom et al. 1998 [26]; Hildebrand et al. 1991 [25])
- atrophy of type I and IIa fibers (Whittom et al. 1998 [26])
- ↓ capillarization (Whittom et al. 1998 [26])

Altered metabolic capacity

- ↓ intramuscular pH (Fiaccadori et al. 1987 [32])
- ↓ ATP concentration (Gertz et al. 1977 [31]; Fiaccadori et al. 1987 [32])
- ↑ muscle lactate concentration (Gertz et al. 1977 [31]; Fiaccadori et al. 1987 [32])
- ↑ ionosine monophosphate (Pouw et al. 1998 [33])
- ↓ mitochondrial enzyme activities (Jakobsson et al. 1995 [28]; Maltais et al. 1996 [29])

muscle of ambulation. Because most studies have included patients with moderate to severe disease, muscle changes reported herein pertain to this patient population.

Muscle Wasting and Weakness

Peripheral muscle wasting is an important consequence of advanced COPD, and its prevalence increases with the degree of airflow obstruction (4,5). Using computed tomography to directly measure muscle mass, we found that the thigh muscle cross-sectional area is reduced by approximately 30% in patients with moderate to severe COPD (6). The reduction in muscle mass is clinically relevant because it is associated with impaired muscle strength and exercise capacity (4,7-10) independent of the degree of airflow obstruction (9,10).

Although to a different extent, the strength of both upper and lower limb muscles is commonly reduced in patients with COPD (11,12). In general, the reduction in upper limb muscle strength is of smaller magnitude than that of the lower limb (6,11-14). Peripheral muscle weakness seems to primarily result from muscle atrophy, as suggested by the proportional reduction in muscle mass and strength (6). However, in patients exposed to systemic corticosteroids, the loss in strength may be out of proportion to the loss in total body muscle mass (6,15). This is in keeping with previous animal studies showing that corticosteroids may alter muscle function without causing muscle atrophy (16).

Muscle Fiber Type, Size, and Capillarization

Human skeletal muscle fibers can be grouped into separate categories based on their physiological and metabolic characteristics; type I fibers are characterized by slow contractile velocity and high oxidative capacity, which accounts for their relative resistance to fatigue, whereas type IIb fibers have a fast contractile velocity and a lower oxidative capacity and therefore are more prone to fatigue (17). Type IIa fibers are intermediate between I and IIb (17). Although the evaluation of the skeletal muscle contractile protein profile has shown that the different types of fibers should be seen as a continuum rather than as distinct categories (18), it is still convenient to study the fiber type profile because it is an important determinant of the muscle metabolic capacity both at rest and during exercise (19-21).

The fiber type distribution of the vastus lateralis muscle has been assessed in patients with COPD either using classical histochemical fiber typing or by evaluating the expression of myosin heavy chain isoforms. In patients with mild to moderate airflow obstruction, the proportion of type I fiber is preserved (22,23). In patients with more advanced airflow obstruction, there is a reduction in the proportion of type I fibers with a reciprocal increase in type IIb fibers (24-27). In these individuals, type I and IIa fibers are also atrophic compared to those in age-matched normal subjects (26). Muscle capillarization, another important determinant of skeletal muscle aerobic capacity, is reduced in patients with COPD with a lower number of capillaries in contact with type I and IIa fibers in comparison to normal subjects (26).

Muscle Metabolic Capacity

The activity of citrate synthase (28,29) and 3-hydroxyacyl CoA dehydrogenase (29), two mitochondrial enzymes involved in the citric acid cycle and in the β-oxidation of fatty acids, respectively, is reduced in patients with COPD (figure 9.1), whereas a paradoxical increase in the activity of cytochrome oxidase, an enzyme of the electron-chain transport, has been found in these individuals (30). Apparently, glycolytic enzyme activity is not modified in COPD (29). Altogether these enzymatic changes indicate that the oxidative capacity of the vastus lateralis muscle is reduced in patients with COPD compared to normal subjects and that a discoordinate expression of the skeletal muscle mitochondrial enzyme activities may be present in COPD.

Peripheral Muscle Metabolism at Rest and During Exercise

In keeping with the morphological and enzymatic muscle changes, muscle energy metabolism is modified at rest and during exercise in patients with COPD. Low intracellular pH, reduced phosphocreatine (Pcr) and adenosinetriphosphate (ATP)

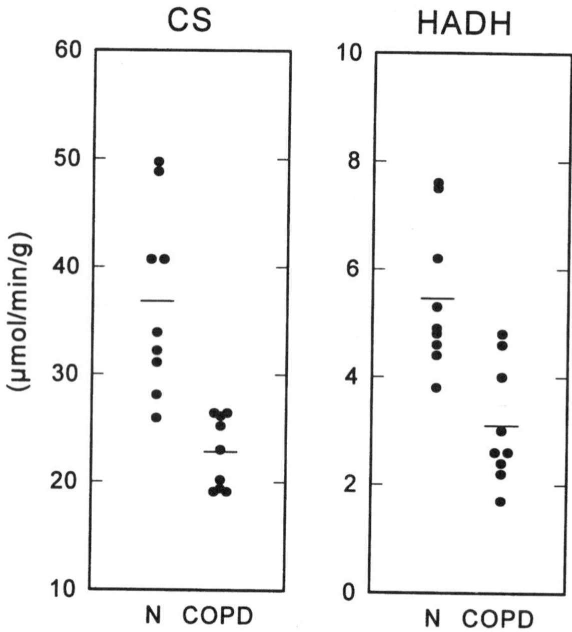

Figure 9.1 The activity of two mitochondrial enzymes, citrate synthase (CS) and 3-hydroxyacyl CoA dehydrogenase (HADH) in normal subjects and in patients with COPD. The activity of the two enzymes was markedly reduced in COPD. From Maltais et al. 1996 (29).

contents, and increased lactate and ionosine monophosphate concentrations have been found in the vastus lateralis muscle (25,31-33). Using nuclear magnetic resonance spectroscopy (^{31}P-NMR) to study the oxidative metabolism of skeletal muscle during exercise, a greater decline in muscle intracellular pH and in phosphocreatine/inorganic phosphate (Pcr/(Pcr + Pi) ratio during exercise occurs in patients with COPD compared to normal subjects (13,34-37). These findings are indicative of impaired oxidative phosphorylation and ATP resynthesis with early activation of anaerobic glycolysis within the contracting muscles (13,34-37). Peripheral muscle metabolic abnormalities during exercise are worsened by hypoxemia and can be partially reversed with oxygen supplementation, indicating more dependency of energy metabolism on anaerobic ATP production during hypoxemia (36-38).

We recently measured leg blood flow, arterial and femoral venous pH, and lactate during leg cycling exercise in eight patients with severe COPD (39). In agreement with the ^{31}P-NMR studies, we found a faster decline in femoral venous pH and an increase in lactate release from the lower limb during exercise in COPD patients compared to normal subjects. These findings could not be explained by differences in peripheral oxygen transport, suggesting that altered muscle metabolism during exercise is related to a poor peripheral muscle oxidative capacity or to abnormal muscle metabolic regulation (40). This contention is further supported by the negative correlation between the increase in arterial lactate during exercise and aerobic enzyme activities in normal subjects (17) and in patients with COPD (29).

Exercise Tolerance and Peripheral Muscle Dysfunction in COPD

Altered peripheral muscle function may affect exercise tolerance through several mechanisms. Two groups of investigators have clearly shown that weakness of the quadriceps strength has a negative impact on exercise tolerance independent of lung impairment (11,12). These effects can be explained by the influence of muscle strength on the perception of leg effort during exercise, the main limiting symptoms in 40%-45% of patients with COPD (12,41,42). A stronger quadriceps should decrease the intensity of leg effort for a given exercise level (12), and this may have important implications in exercise tolerance. Patients are likely to have a better exercise tolerance if they feel less discomfort in the exercising muscles. Reduced endurance of the vastus lateralis muscle, another consequence of COPD, has also been associated with low functional status (43).

Altered muscle metabolism may also influence exercise tolerance. Increased lactic acidosis for a given exercise work rate, which is a common finding in COPD (44-47), enhances the ventilatory needs by increasing nonaerobic CO_2 production (46,48,49). This places an additional burden on respiratory muscles already facing an increased impedance to breathing. In addition, the resulting acidemia may act directly as a breathing stimulus. Last, premature muscle acidosis, a contributory factor to muscle fatigue and early exercise termination in normal subjects (50-52), may be an important mechanism contributing to exercise intolerance in COPD (39).

Other possible consequences of poor peripheral muscle function in COPD include reduction in quality of life (53), greater use of health care resources (54), and poor survival (55).

Etiology of Skeletal Muscle Dysfunction in COPD

The etiology of skeletal muscle dysfunction in patients with COPD has not been elucidated. Several potential mechanisms may contribute to the problem (table 9.2), and their relative importance is likely to vary between patients. A unique mechanism explaining peripheral muscle dysfunction in all patients is unlikely.

Aging

Muscle changes associated with the aging process include a decrease in muscle mass and strength, atrophy of type II fibers with preservation of type I fibers, and

Table 9.2 Possible Etiologies of Skeletal Muscle Dysfunction in Patients With COPD

Chronic inactivity and disuse atrophy
Nutritional imbalance
Systemic corticosteroid
Hypoxemia
Electrolyte disturbances
Generalized myopathy
Systemic inflammation

lower oxidative capacity (56). When compared to age-matched normal subjects, peripheral muscle mass, strength, fiber type characteristics, and metabolic capacity are clearly abnormal in many patients with COPD, therefore, peripheral muscle dysfunction cannot be accounted for by the aging process alone.

Chronic Inactivity and Disuse Atrophy

Because in most studies, control subjects and patients with COPD were not matched for their functional status, differences in the level of activity are a potentially important variable explaining the muscle changes in COPD. Chronic inactivity results in physiological changes in the skeletal muscles that are often referred to as muscle deconditioning (57). Reduction in oxidative enzyme activity and the atrophy of type I fibers seen in the quadriceps of patients with COPD are also characteristics of muscle changes found in chronic inactivity (57-59). In contrast, the extreme reduction in the proportion of type I fibers also found in patients with COPD is usually not demonstrated in studies evaluating the effects of a few weeks of inactivity (60,61). This is possibly related to the short duration of these studies because prolonged reduction in physical activity level clearly has the potential to alter the proportion of the different types of fibers (62). Improvement in skeletal muscle oxidative capacity observed after training also supports the role of deconditioning (63).

Although chronic inactivity and muscle deconditioning may well be the primary mechanisms of the development of poor peripheral muscle function in COPD, the potential role of other mechanisms should not be overlooked. In a recent study, important modifications in the myosin heavy chain profile were found in patients with COPD compared to normal subjects, despite modest differences in peak exercise capacity between the two groups, suggesting that other potential factors alone or in conjunction with inactivity may be involved in peripheral muscle dysfunction in COPD.

Nutritional Imbalance

Increased total daily and resting energy expenditure is common in patients with COPD and could contribute to body weight and muscle loss (9,64). In many patients, the greater energy expenditure is compensated by increasing the caloric intake so that body weight is maintained. However, this adaptation is progressively lost in patients with severe COPD as indicated by Schols and colleagues (9) who reported a decrease in caloric intake with increasing severity of airflow obstruction. Although nutritional imbalance may play a role in muscle wasting in some patients, the absent or modest improvement in peripheral muscle function associated with nutritional supplementation suggests that a negative energetic balance is not the primary mechanism of muscle wasting in most cases.

Hypoxemia

In normal subjects, chronic hypoxemia decreases the muscle mass, lowers the oxidative capacity of the skeletal muscle, and reduces the area of type I fibers (65,66). In keeping with this, a positive correlation between PaO_2 and percentage of type I fibers in the vastus lateralis muscle has been reported in patients with COPD (24,25). Although such a relationship should be interpreted with caution because hypoxemia only occurs in patients with advanced disease and severe functional impairment, it raises the possibility that chronic hypoxemia may play a role in patients with low resting PaO_2 or in those with repeated O_2 desaturation occurring during sleep and/or exercise (67,68).

Corticosteroids

Steroid-induced myopathy is characterized by muscle wasting and weakness and affects preferentially type IIb fibers (69). The potential role of corticosteroid in the development of muscle weakness should not be overlooked in some individuals submitted to chronic or even intermittent systemic corticosteroid treatment (15,70). In patients with COPD, muscle weakness may appear with low doses of corticosteroids (<10 mg/day), perhaps because of a greater susceptibility to developing corticosteroid-induced myopathy (15).

Electrolyte Disturbances

Hypokalemia, hypomagnesemia, and hypophosphatemia may be present in patients with COPD and may impair skeletal muscle function. In these patients, hypophosphatemia may be related to a defect in renal phosphate reabsorption and may be worsened by the use of furosemide, theophylline, and corticosteroid (71). Accordingly, electrolyte disturbances should be looked for when evaluating patients with COPD and muscle weakness (72).

Systemic Inflammatory Response

A systemic inflammatory response appears to be an important mechanism of muscle wasting in chronic disorders such as AIDS (73), cancer (74), and chronic heart failure (75). In these conditions, increased levels of inflammatory cytokines such as IL-6, IL-8, and TNFα may contribute to muscle wasting by promoting muscle protein degradation (76). This might also be the case in patients with COPD in whom increased levels of TNFα, IL-8, and acute phase protein have also been found (77-79). The possibility that a systemic inflammatory process triggers muscle wasting in COPD needs to be further explored.

Specific Generalized Myopathy

The possibility of a specific generalized myopathic process has been raised because the function of several muscle groups including the respiratory muscles may be affected in COPD. Although the occurrence of such a process cannot be ruled out, several observations appear to refute it. For instance, the observation that upper limb strength is better preserved than that of the lower limbs (11,14) is more suggestive of reduced muscle activation as the cause of muscle dysfunction. In contrast to the vastus lateralis muscle, a greater proportion of type I fiber has been found in the diaphragm of patients with severe COPD compared to the diaphragm of healthy subjects (80,81). This differential adaptation of the diaphragm and the peripheral muscle could be related to the difference in the level of activation and physical workload between the two muscle groups (80). The chronic increase in work of breathing faced by the diaphragm in emphysema is, in fact, a continuous training stimulus. As in any other skeletal muscle, the increased proportion in type I fiber in the emphysematous diaphragm is likely to represent an adaptation to training. This reinforces the role of muscle deconditioning in peripheral muscle dysfunction in these individuals (80) and indicates that a generalized myopathy is unlikely.

In summary, the mechanisms conducting to poor peripheral muscle in COPD remains unclear. Several conditions such as chronic inactivity, hypoxia, the use of systemic corticosteroids, nutritional imbalance, and possibly a state of systemic inflammation may be involved.

Clinical Diagnostic of Peripheral Muscle Dysfunction in COPD

To date, there have been no clinical trials looking at the effects of correcting peripheral muscle dysfunction on exercise tolerance and quality of life in patients with COPD. Only empiric recommendations can therefore be made regarding the clinical approach to this problem. Because peripheral muscle dysfunction can be recognized with simple tools, may contribute to poor functional status, and may be improved with simple therapeutic interventions, it seems advisable to incorporate the evaluation of peripheral muscle function in the overall assessment of patients with severe COPD.

Underweight patients and those having specific muscle symptoms or showing a reduction in exercise tolerance out of proportion to their impairment in lung function should be suspected of having impaired peripheral muscle function (1). Patients on long-term systemic corticosteroids are also at particular risk of developing this complication (15,70). In these individuals, evaluation of peripheral muscle function may disclose specific problems such as atrophy or weakness that can be at least be partly corrected by appropriate therapeutic interventions.

Although muscle waste is easy to recognize by physical examination in advanced COPD, loss of muscle mass may be more subtle in the early stage of the disease. With simple anthropometric data such as skinfold thickness and limb circumference measurements, several indices of muscle mass can be referenced to normal predicted values, and a loss of muscle mass not evident from measurement of body weight may be identified (4, 82). Bioelectrical impedance analysis may provide a more accurate estimate of fat-free mass (FFM) than anthropometry and is both easy to perform and reproducible (83). Measurements of albumin, prealbumin, and transferrin levels are not useful to identify loss of muscle mass (4). Several simple devices can be used to measure the maximal voluntary strength. The assessment of handgrip and quadriceps strength can be easily incorporated into the clinical evaluation and provides useful information on the status of peripheral muscle function and distribution of muscle weakness (11,12). Muscle biopsy with morphological and enzymatic analysis remains a research tool in the investigation of the mechanisms of peripheral muscle dysfunction.

Peripheral muscle dysfunction can also be suspected from the results of a progressive symptom limited exercise test. The relationship between FEV_1 and maximal exercise capacity has been evaluated in patients with COPD (1). When the reduction in maximal exercise capacity is disproportionate to disease severity, the presence of another factor such as peripheral muscle dysfunction, which may contribute to exercise limitation, should be suspected. During the exercise test, it may also become obvious that the main symptom limiting exercise is leg fatigue rather than dyspnea. In these individuals, early sensation of peripheral muscle fatigue during exercise may indicate the presence of peripheral muscle weakness (12). A disproportionate increase in arterial lactic acid for a given exercise work rate in the absence of oxygen desaturation may finally point to a poor skeletal muscle oxidative capacity (17,21,29).

Improving Peripheral Muscle Function in COPD

Because the cause of peripheral muscle dysfunction remains unclear, treatment of this condition is difficult and is likely to remain suboptimal as long as our understanding of this problem is not improved. The current therapeutic approach consists of correcting all possible conditions involved with poor peripheral muscle function. Because the etiology of peripheral muscle dysfunction in COPD appears to be multifactorial, one isolated therapeutic strategy is unlikely to completely resolve the problem. A global approach with correction of all possible contributing factors should be used and will ultimately have a better chance of success.

Exercise Training

Because chronic inactivity may explain several of the muscle changes recognized in COPD, exercise training is an important therapeutic option. In young as well as in older normal subjects, the peripheral adaptation in skeletal muscle occurring with endurance training is characterized by an increase in mitochondrial oxidative capacity and muscle capillarization and a transformation of type IIb to type IIa muscle fibers that have a greater oxidative potential (17,19,56). These muscle changes are associated with smaller increases in muscle and blood lactic acid concentrations during exercise (17,19,84,85). The general principles of exercise training in normal subjects also apply to patients with COPD. Physiological adaptation to training is limited to the muscles recruited during training, and the characteristics of muscle adaptation depend on the training strategy used: endurance training improves performance during submaximal exercise such as long distance running, whereas strength training improves the ability to perform explosive tasks such as weightlifting (86).

Although several excellent studies have documented that exercise tolerance can be improved with exercise training in patients with COPD (46,53,87-91), only some have looked at the effect of exercise training on peripheral skeletal muscle function in these individuals (26,53,63,92-94). The training strategies most commonly used are walking, treadmill, and leg-cycling exercise. Proposed mechanisms of improvement include better motivation, desensitization to dyspnea, and improved technique and performance (95). Until recently, skeletal muscle adaptation to training was not believed to occur in COPD (92,96). It was thought that these patients could not achieve a sufficiently high training intensity to achieve a physiological training effect. However, Casaburi and other investigators (111) observed a significant reduction in exercise lactic acidosis, CO_2 production, and ventilation after endurance training in patients with COPD, strongly suggesting the development of physiological adaptation to training in these patients (47,97,98). Studies done in our laboratory also indicated that patients with severe COPD can sustain the necessary training intensity and duration for a skeletal muscle adaptation to training to occur (26,63). After 12 weeks of leg-cycling exercise, improvement in the activity of two mitochondrial enzymes (figure 9.2), an increase in type I fiber size of the vastus lateralis muscle, and a reduction in arterial lactic acid concentration for a given level of exercise were found (26,63). After training, the level of skeletal muscle oxidative activity and the proportion of each fiber type

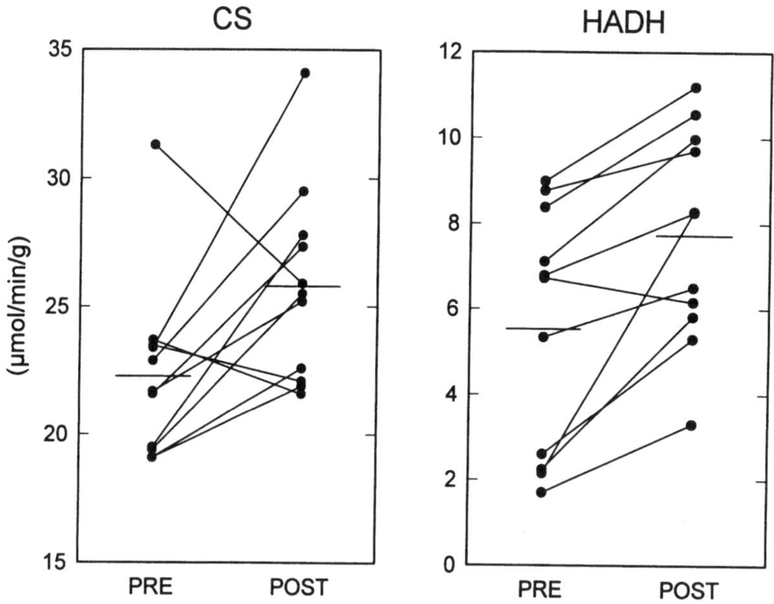

Figure 9.2 The activity of citrate synthase (CS) and 3-hydroxyacyl CoA dehydrogenase (HADH) in 11 patients with COPD before and after a 12-week endurance training program. The activity of the two enzymes increased significantly with training. From Maltais et al. 1996 (63).

were still abnormal, suggesting that the training program was too short or that irreversible muscle changes had taken place. Other investigators have reported increased quadriceps endurance during voluntary contractions after 3 weeks of endurance training (94).

Strength training appears to be an interesting strategy in patients with COPD (53) as this type of training is more effective in improving muscle mass and strength than aerobic training. In addition, strength training causes less dyspnea during the exercise period, making it easier to tolerate than aerobic training for patients with severe COPD (53). Simpson and colleagues (53) studied 34 patients with severe COPD randomized to a control group or to 8 weeks of strength training consisting of three different exercises (one for the arms, two for the legs). Muscle strength increased by 16%-40% depending on the muscle group evaluated, and this was associated with an improvement in the endurance time to submaximal exercise. Notably, improvement in muscle strength after training does not necessarily imply muscle physiological adaptation since it may be due to a more efficient neuromuscular coupling. Low-intensity muscle exercise improves upper and lower limb muscle endurance (93).

Whether strength training is a useful adjunct to aerobic training has been addressed recently (99). In this study, the effects of aerobic training alone or in combination with strength training on peripheral muscle function were evaluated in 36 patients with severe COPD. The combination of aerobic and strength training was associated with greater improvement in peripheral muscle strength and in thigh muscle cross-sectional area (MCSA) than aerobic training alone. Thus, this study confirmed that the peripheral muscles may show structural adaptation with an appropriate training regimen despite severe ventilatory impairment. This observation is important given the potential adverse effects of peripheral muscle dysfunction on exercise tolerance and quality of life in patients with COPD.

Nutritional Intervention

Nutritional support has been used with the hope that restoring nutritional balance would increase body weight, muscle mass, and ultimately functional status. Comparison between studies is difficult because of the variety of nutritional interventions. With oral or enteral nutritional supplementation for 2-12 weeks, weight gain can be achieved (100-103), although the results are often modest and inconsistent (104-107). Typically, the increase in body weight resulting from nutritional supplementation resulted from an increase in fat with little or no improvement in FFM (107,108). It is therefore not surprising that the magnitude of improvement in muscle strength and functional status following nutritional supplementation is rather small (104-107). There are also important limitations to aggressive nutritional intervention in patients with severe COPD. Gastrointestinal symptoms such as bloating, early satiety, meal-related O_2 desaturation, and postprandial dyspnea are common side effects (109). Despite the lack of strong evidence showing beneficial effects of nutritional intervention on muscle function, it is nevertheless advisable to restore a positive energetic balance for patients with low body weight. In most cases, this should be achievable with simple dietetic counseling (109).

Anabolic Drugs and Exercise Training

The efficacy of anabolic steroids to improve muscle mass, especially when combined with exercise training, has been confirmed in normal men (110). Given the positive relationship between quadriceps strength and exercise tolerance in patients with COPD (11,12), the possibility of increasing muscle mass with the use of anabolic drugs appears to be an interesting therapeutic option. A profound reduction in blood testosterone and insulin-like growth factor-1 (IGF-1) levels has been reported in patients with COPD and may provide further rationale for the use of anabolic drugs in these patients (111). The use of anabolic steroids with nutritional support and exercise training increases muscle mass with small or absent improvement in peripheral muscle function (108,112). Similarly, 1 to 8 weeks of exercise training combined with the administration of growth hormone induces gain in muscle mass but does not provide any additional improvement in muscle strength or exercise tolerance (113,114). In summary, modest increase in muscle mass occurs when the administration of anabolic steroids or growth hormone is combined with a training program in patients with COPD. Whether it will be possible to achieve greater improvement in muscle function that could translate into clinically significant gains with the combination of exercise and anabolic drugs is uncertain.

Oxygen Therapy

Although short-term oxygen therapy improves the oxidative metabolism during exercise in hypoxemic patients with COPD (36,38), little is known about the effects of long-term home oxygen supplementation on muscle function. Six to nine months of home oxygen therapy may facilitate the formation of muscle ATP but does not appear to improve skeletal muscle enzyme activity (28,115). It also seems unlikely that long-term oxygen supplementation will significantly improve muscle function although there may be a benefit because oxygen therapy might increase the patient's level of activity.

Conclusion

Peripheral muscle dysfunction is commonly found in patients with moderate to severe COPD and may contribute to exercise intolerance in people with this disease. Simple clinical tools are available to identify this problem, and therapeutic interventions, such as exercise training alone or supplemented by nutritional intervention and anabolic drugs, may improve peripheral muscle function in COPD. Further studies are needed to clarify the mechanisms of peripheral muscle dysfunction and to develop more effective therapeutic interventions. Hopefully, this research will improve our understanding of exercise intolerance and help us develop innovative therapeutic strategies to improve functional status and quality of life in patients with COPD.

Acknowledgments

The authors wish to thank Marthe Bélanger, Sarah Bernard, Marie-Josée Breton, Richard Debigaré, Jean-François Doyon, and François Whittom for their contributions to their research and Dr. Yvon Cormier, Dr. Jean Deslauriers, and Yves Lacasse for helpful suggestions regarding the manuscript. This work was supported in part by the Fonds de la recherche en santé du Québec and by La fondation JD Bégin, Université Laval.

References

1. Jones, N.L., and K.J. Killian. 1991. Limitation of exercise in chronic airway obstruction. In *Chronic Obstructive Pulmonary Disease,* ed. N.S. Cherniack. Philadelphia: W.B. Saunders.
2. Williams, T.J., G.A. Patterson, P.A. McClean, N. Zamel, and J.R Maurer. 1992. Maximal exercise testing in single and double lung transplant recipients. *Am Rev Respir Dis* 145:101-105.
3. Evans, A.B., A.J. Al-Himyary, and M.I. Hrova, et al. 1997. Abnormal skeletal muscle oxidative capacity after lung transplantation by ^{31}P-MRS. *Am J Respir Crit Care Med* 155: 615-621.
4. Schols, A.M.W.J., P.B. Soeters, M.C. Dingemans, R. Mostert, P.J. Frantzen, and E.F.M. Wouters. 1993. Prevalence and characteristics of nutritional depletion in patients with stable COPD eligible for pulmonary rehabilitation. *Am Rev Respir Dis* 147:1151-1156.
5. Schols, A.M.W.J., R. Mostert, P.B. Soeters, W.H.M. Saris, E.F.M. Wouters. 1991. Energy balance in patients with chronic obstructive pulmonary disease. *Am Rev Respir Dis* 143:1248-1252.
6. Bernard, S., P. Leblanc, and F. Whittom, et al. 1998. Peripheral muscle weakness in patients with chronic obstructive pulmonary disease. *Am J Respir Crit Care Med* 158:629-634.
7. Engelen, M.P.K.J., A.M.W.J. Schols, W.C.Baken, G.J. Wesseling, and E.F.M. Wouters. 1994. Nutritional depletion in relation to respiratory and peripheral skeletal muscle function in out-patients with COPD. *Eur Respir J* 7:1793-1797.
8. Schols, A.M.W.J., R. Mostert, P.B. Soeters, L.H. Greve, and E.F.M. Wouters. 1989. Nutritional state and exercise performance in patients with chronic obstructive lung disease. *Thorax* 44:937-941.
9. Schols, A.M.W.J., R. Mostert, P.B. Soeters, and E.F.M. Wouters. 1991. Body composition and exercise performance in patients with chronic obstructive pulmonary disease. *Thorax* 46:695-699.
10. Palange, P., S. Forte, A. Felli, P. Galassetti, P. Serra, and S. Carlone. 1995. Nutritional state and exercise tolerance in patients with COPD. *Chest* 107:1206-1212.
11. Gosselink, R., T. Troosters, and M. Decramer. 1996. Peripheral muscle weakness contributes to exercise limitation in COPD. *Am J Respir Crit Care Med* 153:976-980.
12. Hamilton, A.L., K.J. Killian, E. Summers, and N.L. Jones. 1995. Muscle strength, symptom intensity and exercise capacity in patients with cardiorespiratory disorders. *Am J Respir Crit Care Med* 152:2021-2031.

13. Kutsuzawa, T., S. Shioya, D. Kurita, M. Haida, Y. Ohta, and H. Yamabayashi. 1992. ^{31}P-NMR study of skeletal muscle metabolism in patients with chronic respiratory impairment. *Am Rev Respir Dis* 146:1019-1024.

14. Newell, S.Z., D.K. McKenzie, and S.C. Gandevia. 1989. Inspiratory and skeletal muscle strength and endurance and diaphragmatic activation in patients with chronic airflow limitation. *Thorax* 44:903-912.

15. Decramer, M., L.M. Lacquet, R. Fagard, and P. Rogiers. 1994. Corticosteroids contribute to muscle weakness in chronic airflow obstruction. *Am Rev Respir Dis* 150:11-16.

16. Dekhuijzen, P.N.R., G. Gayan-Ramirez, R. Dom, V. de Bock, and M. Decramer. 1993. Triamcinolone and prednisolone affect contractile properties and histopathology of rat diaphragm differently. *J Clin Invest* 92:1534-1542.

17. Saltin, B., and P.D. Gollnick. 1982. Skeletal muscle adaptability: significance for metabolism and performance. In *The Handbook of Physiology: The Skeletal Muscle System,* ed. L.D. Peachey. Bethesda, MD: American Physiological Society.

18. Staron, R.S., and P. Johnson. 1993. Myosin polymorphism and differential expression in adult human skeletal muscle. *Comp Biochem Physiol* 106:463-475.

19. Holloszy, J.O., and E.F. Coyle. 1984. Adaptations of skeletal muscle to endurance exercise and their metabolic consequences. *J Appl Physiol* 56:831-838.

20. Sullivan, M.J., H.J. Green, F.R. Cobb. 1991. Altered skeletal muscle metabolic response to exercise in chronic heart failure. Relation to skeletal muscle aerobic enzyme activity. *Circulation* 84:1597-1607.

21. Ivy, J.L., R.T. Withers, P.J. Van Handel, D.H. Elger, and D.L. Costill. 1980. Muscle respiratory capacity and fiber type as determinants of the lactate threshold. *J Appl Physiol* 48:523-527.

22. Hughes, R.L., H. Katz, V. Sahgal, J.A. Campbell, R. Hartz, and T.W. Shields. 1983. Fiber size and energy metabolites in five separate muscles from patients with chronic obstructive lung disease. *Respiration* 44:321-328.

23. Satta, A., G.B. Migliori, and A. Spanevello, et al. 1997. Fibre types in skeletal muscles of chronic obstructive pulmonary disease patients related to respiratory function and exercise tolerance. *Eur Respir J* 10:2853-2860.

24. Jakobsson, P., L. Jorfeldt, and A. Brundin. 1990. Skeletal muscle metabolites and fibre types in patients with advanced chronic obstructive pulmonary disease (COPD), with and without chronic respiratory failure. *Eur Respir J* 3:192-196.

25. Hildebrand, I.L., C. Sylvén, M. Esbjornsson, K. Hellstrom, and E. Jansson. 1991. Does hypoxaemia induce transformations of fiber types? *Acta Physiol Scand* 141:435-439.

26. Whittom, F., J. Jobin, and P.M. Simard, et al. 1998. Histochemical and morphological characteristics of the vastus lateralis muscle in COPD patients. Comparison with normal subjects and effects of exercise training. *Med Sci Sports Exerc* 30:1467-1474.

27. Maltais, F., M.J. Sullivan, and P. Leblanc, et al. 1999. Altered expression of myosin heavy chain in the vastus lateralis muscle in patients with COPD. *Eur Respir J* 13:850-854.

28. Jakobsson, P., L. Jorfeldt, and J. Henriksson. 1995. Metabolic enzyme activity in the quadriceps femoris muscle in patients with severe chronic obstructive pulmonary disease. *Am J Respir Crit Care Med* 151:374-377.

29. Maltais, F., A.A. Simard, C. Simard, J. Jobin, P. Desgagnés, and P. Leblanc. 1996. Oxidative capacity of the skeletal muscle and lactic acid kinetics during exercise in normal subjects and in patients with COPD. *Am J Respir Crit Care Med* 153:288-293.

30. Sauleda, J., F. García-Palmer, and R.J. Wiesner, et al. 1998. Cytochrome oxidase activity and mitochondrial gene expression in skeletal muscle of patients with chronic obstructive pulmonary disease. *Am J Respir Crit Care Med* 157:1413-1417.

31. Gertz, I., G. Hedenstierna, G. Hellers, and J. Wahren. 1977. Muscle metabolism in patients with chronic obstructive lung disease and acute respiratory failure. *Clin Sci Mol Med* 52:395-403.

32. Fiaccadori, E., S. Del Canale, P. Vitali, E. Coffrini, N. Ronda, and A. Guariglia. 1997. Skeletal muscle energetics, acid-base equilibrium and lactate metabolism in patients with severe hypercapnia and hypoxia. *Chest* 92:883-887.

33. Pouw, E.M., A.M.W.J. Schols, G.J. van der Vusse, and E.F.M. Wouters. 1998. Elevated inosine monophosphate levels in resting muscle of patients with stable chronic obstructive pulmonary disease. *Am J Respir Crit Care Med* 157:453-457.

34. Wuyam, B., J.F. Payen, and P. Levy, et al. 1992. Metabolism and aerobic capacity of skeletal muscle in chronic respiratory failure related to chronic obstructive pulmonary disease. *Eur Respir J* 5:157-162.

35. Tada, H., H. Kato, and T. Misawa, et al. 1992. ^{31}P-nuclear magnetic resonance evidence of abnormal skeletal muscle metabolism in patients with chronic lung disease and congestive heart failure. *Eur Respir J* 5:163-169.

36. Payen, J.F., B. Wuyam, and P. Levy, et al. 1993. Muscular metabolism during oxygen supplementation in patients with chronic hypoxia. *Am Rev Respir Dis* 147:592-598.

37. Lévy, P., B. Wuyam, J.L. Pépin, H. Reutenauer, and J.F. Payen. 1996. Anomalies des muscles squelettiques des BPCO en insuffisance respiratoire. Apport de la spectroscopie RMN ^{31}P. *Rev Mal Respir* 13:183-191.

38. Mannix, E.T., M.D. Boska, P. Galassetti, G. Burton, F. Manfredi, and M.O. Farber. 1995. Modulation of ATP production by oxygen in obstructive lung disease as assessed by ^{31}P-MRS. *J Appl Physiol* 78:2218-2227.

39. Maltais, F., J. Jobin, and M.J. Sullivan, et al. 1998. Metabolic and hemodynamic responses of the lower limb during exercise in normal subjects and in COPD. *J Appl Physiol* 84:1573-1580.

40. Putman, C.T., N.L. Jones, L.C. Lands, T.M. Bragg, M.G. Hollidge-Horvat, and G.J.F. Heigenhauser. 1995. Skeletal muscle pyruvate dehydrogenase activity during maximal exercise in humans. *Am J Physiol* 269:E458-E468.

41. Killian, K.J., P. Leblanc, D.H. Martin, E. Summers, N.L. Jones, and E.J.M. Campbell. 1992. Exercise capacity and ventilatory, circulatory, and symptom limitation in patients with airflow limitation. *Am Rev Respir Dis* 146:935-940.

42. Mahler, D.A., and A. Harver. 1988. Prediction of peak oxygen consumption in obstructive airway disease. *Med Sci Sports Exerc* 20:574-578.

43. Serres, I., V. Gautier, A.L. Varray, and C.G. Préfaut. 1998. Impaired skeletal muscle endurance related to physical inactivity and altered lung function in COPD patients. *Chest* 113:900-905.

44. Shuey, C.B., A.K. Peirce, and R.L. Johnson. 1969. An evaluation of exercise tests in chronic obstructive lung disease. *J Appl Physiol* 27:256-261.

45. Jones, N.L., G.L. Jones, and R.H.T. Edwards. 1971. Exercise tolerance in chronic airway obstruction. *Am Rev Respir Dis* 103:477-491.

46. Casaburi, R., A. Patessio, F. Ioli, S. Zanaboni, C.F. Donner, and K. Wasserman. 1991. Reductions in exercise lactic acidosis and ventilation as a result of exercise training in patients with obstructive lung disease. *Am Rev Respir Dis* 143:9-18.

47. Maltais, F., S. Bernard, J. Jobin, R. Belleau, and P. Leblanc. 1997. Lactate kinetics during exercise in chronic obstructive pulmonary disease. *Can Respir J* 4:251-257.

48. Beaver, W.L., K. Wasserman, and B.J. Whipp. 1986. Bicarbonate buffering of lactic acid generated during exercise. *J Appl Physiol* 60:472-486.

49. Jones, N.L., and G.J.F. Heigenhauser. 1996. Getting rid of carbon dioxide during exercise. *Clin Sci* 90:323-335.

50. Mainwood, G.W., and J.M. Renaud.1985. The effect of acid-base balance on fatigue of skeletal muscle. *Can J Physiol Pharmacol* 63:403-416.

51. Hultman, E., S. Carale, and H. Sjoholm. 1985. Effect of induced metabolic acidosis on intracellular pH, buffer capacity and contraction force of human skeletal muscle. *Clin Sci* 69:505-510.

52. Westerblad, H., J.A. Lee, J. Lannergren, and D.G. Allen. 1991. Cellular mechanisms of fatigue in skeletal muscle. *Am J Physiol* 261:C195-C209.

53. Simpson, K., K. Killian, N. McCartney, D.G. Stubbing, and N.L. Jones. 1992. Randomised controlled trial of weightlifting exercise in patients with chronic airflow limitation. *Thorax* 47:70-75.

54. Decramer, M., R. Gosselink, T. Troosters, M. Verschueren, and G. Evers. 1997. Muscle weakness is related to utilization of health care resources in COPD patients. *Eur Respir J* 10:417-423.

55. Wilson, D.O., R.M. Rogers, E.C. Wright, and N.R. Anthonisen. 1989. Body weight in chronic obstructive pulmonary disease. The National Institutes of Health Intermittent Positive-Pressure Breathing Trial. *Am Rev Respir Dis* 139:1435-1438.

56. Rogers, M.A., and W.J. Evans. 1993. Changes in skeletal muscle with aging: effects of exercise training. In *Exercise and Sports Sciences Reviews,* ed. J.O. Holloszy. Philadelphia: Williams and Wilkins.

57. Casaburi, R. 1996. Deconditioning. In *Pulmonary Rehabilitation,* ed. A.P. Fishman. New York: Marcel Dekker.

58. Booth, F.W., and P.D. Gollnick. 1983. Effects of disuse on the structure and function of skeletal muscle. *Med Sci Sports Exerc* 15:415-420.

59. Coyle, E.F., W.H. Martin, S.A. Bloomfield, O.H. Lowry, and J.O. Holloszy. 1985. Effects of detraining on responses to submaximal exercise. *J Appl Physiol* 59:853-859.

60. Sargeant, A.J., C.T.M. Davies, R.H.T. Edwards, C. Maunder, and A.Young. 1977. Functional and structural changes after disuse of human muscle. *Clin Sci Mol Med* 52:337-342.

61. Berg, H.E., L. Larsson, and P.A. Tesch. 1997. Lower limb skeletal muscle function after 6 wk of bed rest. *J Appl Physiol* 82:182-188.

62. Larsson, L., and T. Ansved. 1985. Effects of long-term physical training and detraining on enzyme histochemical and functional skeletal muscle characteristics in man. *Musc Nerve* 8:714-722.

63. Maltais, F., P. Leblanc, and C. Simard, et al. 1996. Skeletal muscle adaptation to endurance training in patients with chronic obstructive pulmonary disease. *Am J Respir Crit Care Med* 154:442-447.

64. Baarends, E.M., A.M.W.J. Schols, D.L.E. Pannemans, K.R. Westerterp, and E.F.M. Wouters. 1997. Total free living energy expenditure in patients with severe chronic obstructive pulmonary disease. *Am J Respir Crit Care Med* 155:1549-1554.

65. Green, H.J., J.R. Sutton, A. Cymerman, P.M. Young, and C.S. Houston. 1989. Operation Everest II: adaptations in human skeletal muscle. *J Appl Physiol* 66:2454-2461.

66. Kayser, B., H. Hoppeler, H. Claassen, and P. Cerretelli. 1991. Muscle structure and performance capacity of Himalayan Sherpas. *J Appl Physiol* 70:1938-1942.

67. Fletcher, E.C., R.A Luckett, T. Miller, and J.G. Fletcher. 1989. Exercise hemodynamics and gas exchange in patients with chronic obstruction pulmonary disease, sleep desaturation, and a daytime PaO_2 above 60 mmHg. *Am Rev Respir Dis* 140:1237-1245.

68. Fletcher, E.C., C.F. Donner, and B. Midgren, et al. 1992. Survival in COPD patients with a daytime PaO_2 >60 mmHg with and without nocturnal oxyhemoglobin desaturation. *Chest* 101:649-655.

69. Sheahan, M.G., and P.J. Vignos. 1969. Experimental corticosteroid myopathy. *Arthr Rheum* 12:491-497.

70. Decramer, M., V. de Bock, and R. Dom. 1996. Functional and histologic picture of steroid-induced myopathy in chronic obstructive pulmonary disease. *Am J Respir Crit Care Med* 153:1958-1964.

71. Fiaccadori, E., E. Coffrini, and N. Ronda, et al. 1990. Hypophosphatemia in course of chronic obstructive pulmonary disease. Prevalence, mechanisms, and relationships with skeletal muscle phosphorus content. *Chest* 97:857-868.

72. Aubier, M., D. Murciano, and Y. Lecocguic, et al. 1985. Effect of hypophosphatemia on diaphragmatic contractility in patients with acute respiratory failure. *N Engl J Med* 313:420-424.

73. Moldawer, L.L., and F.R. Sattler. 1998. Human immunodeficiency virus-associated wasting and mechanism of cachexia associated with inflammation. *Semin Oncol* 25 (suppl. 1):73-81.

74. Balkwill, F., F. Burke, and D. Talbot, et al. 1987. Evidence for tumour necrosis factor/cachectin production in cancer. *Lancet* 2:1229-1232.

75. Levine, B., J. Kalman, L. Mayer, H.M. Fillit, and M. Packer. 1990. Elevated circulating levels of tumor necrosis factor in severe chronic heart failure. *N Engl J Med* 323:236-241.

76. Mitch, W.E., and A.L. Goldberg. 1996. Mechanism of muscle wasting. *N Engl J Med* 335:1897-1905.

77. Schols, A.M.W.J., W.A. Buurman, A.J. Staal-van den Brekel, M.A. Dentener, and E.F.M. Wouters. 1996. Evidence for a relation between metabolic derangements and increased levels of inflammatory mediators in a subgroup of patients with chronic obstructive pulmonary disease. *Thorax* 51:819-824.

78. Di Francia, M., D. Barbier, J.L. Mege, and J. Orehek. 1994. Tumor necrosis factor-alpha levels and weight loss in chronic obstructive pulmonary disease. *Am J Respir Crit Care Med* 150:1453-1455.

79. de Godoy, I., M. Donahoe, W.J. Calhoun, J. Mancino, and R.M. Rogers. 1996. Elevated TNF—a production by peripheral blood monocytes of weight-losing COPD patients. *Am J Respir Crit Care Med* 153:633-637.

80. Levine, S., L. Kaiser, J. Leferovich, and B. Tikunov. 1997. Cellular adaptation in the diaphragm in chronic osbtructive pulmonary disease. *N Engl J Med* 337:1799-1806.

81. Mercadier, J.J., K. Schwartz, and S. Schiaffino et al. 1998. Myosin heavy chain gene expression changes in the diaphragm of patients with chronic lung hyperinflation. *Am J Physiol* 274:L527-L534.

82. Heymsfield, S.B., C. McManus, J. Smith, V. Stevens, and D.W. Nixon. 1982. Anthropometric measurements of muscle mass: revised equations for calculating bone-free muscle area. *Am J Clin Nutr* 36:680-690.

83. Schols, A.M.W.J., E.F.M. Wouters, P.B. Soeters, and K.R. Westerterp. 1991. Body composition by bioelectrical-impedance analysis compared with deuterium dilution and skinfold anthropometry in patients with chronic obstructive pulmonary disease. *Am J Clin Nutr* 53:421-424.

84. Holloszy, J.O. 1967. Effects of exercise on mitochondrial oxygen uptake and respiratory enzyme activity in skeletal muscle. *J Biol Chem* 242:2278-2282.

85. Favier, R.J., S.H. Constable, M. Chen, and J.O. Holloszy. 1986. Endurance exercise training reduces lactate production. *J Appl Physiol* 61:885-889.

86. Casaburi, R. 1994. Physiologic responses to training. *Clin Chest Med* 15:215-227.

87. O'Donnell, D.E., M. McGuire, L. Samis, and K.A. Webb. 1995. The impact of exercise reconditioning on breathlessness in severe chronic airflow limitation. *Am J Respir Crit Care Med* 152:2005-2013.

88. Goldstein, R.S., E.H. Gort, D. Stubbing, M.A. Avendano, and G.H. Guyatt. 1944. Randomised controlled trial of respiratory rehabilitation. *Lancet* 344:1394-1397.

89. Ries, A.L., R.M. Kaplan, T.M. Limberg, and L.M. Prewitt. 1995. Effects of pulmonary rehabilitation on physiologic and psychosocial outcomes in patients with chronic obstructive pulmonary disease. *Ann Intern Med* 122:823-832.

90. Cockcroft, A.E., M.J. Saunders, and G. Berry. 1981. Randomised controlled trial of rehabilitation in chronic respiratory disability. *Thorax* 36:200-203.

91. Sinclair, J.M., and C.G. Ingram. 1980. Controlled trial of supervised exercise training in chronic bronchitis. *Br Med J* 1:519-521.

92. Belman, M.J., and B.A. Kendregan. 1981. Exercise training fails to increase skeletal muscle enzymes in patients with chronic obstructive lung disease. *Am Rev Respir Dis* 123:256-261.

93. Clark, C.J., L. Cochrane, and E. Mackay. 1996. Low intensity peripheral muscle conditioning improves exercise tolerance and breathlessness in COPD. *Eur Respir J* 9:2590-2596.

94. Serres, I., A. Varray, G. Vallet, J.P. Micallef, and C. Préfaut. 1997. Improved skeletal muscle performance after individualized exercise training in patients with chronic obstructive pulmonary disease. *J Cardiopulm Rehab* 17:232-238.

95. Belman, M.J. 1993. Exercise in patients with chronic obstructive pulmonary disease. *Thorax* 48:936-946.

96. Belman, M.J. 1986. Exercise in chronic obstructive pulmonary disease. *Clin Chest Med* 7:585-597.

97. Vyas, M.N., E.W. Banister, J.W. Morton, and S. Grzybowski. 1971. Response to exercise in patients with chronic airway obstruction. I. Effects of exercise training. *Am Rev Respir Dis* 103:390-400.

98. Mohsenifar, Z., D. Horak, H.V. Brown, and S.K. Koerner. 1983. Sensitive indices of improvement in a pulmonary rehabilitation program. *Chest* 83:189-192.

99. Bernard, S., F. Whittom, and P. Leblanc, et al. 1999. Aerobic and strength training in patients with COPD. *Am J Respir Crit Care Med* 159:896-901.

100. Wilson, D.O., R.M. Rogers, M.H. Sanders, B.E. Pennock, and J.J. Reilly. 1986. Nutritional intervention in malnourished patients with emphysema. *Am Rev Respir Dis* 134:672-677.

101. Goldstein, S.A., B.M. Thomashow, V. Kvetan, J. Askanazi, J.M. Kinney, and D.H. Elwyn. 1988. Nitrogen and energy relationships in malnourished patients with emphysema. *Am Rev Respir Dis* 138:636-644.

102. Efthimiou, J., J. Fleming, C. Gomes, and S.G. Spiro. 1988. The effect of supplementary oral nutrition in poorly nourished patients with chronic obstructive pulmonary disease. *Am Rev Respir Dis* 137:1075-1082.

103. Rogers, R.M., M. Donahoe, and J. Costantino. 1992. Physiologic effects of oral supplemental feeding in malnourished patients with chronic obstructive pulmonary disease. A randomized control study. *Am Rev Respir Dis* 146:1511-1517.

104. Lewis, M.I., M.J. Belman, and L. Dorr-Uyemura. 1987. Dietary supplementation and respiratory muscle performance in patients with COPD. *Am Rev Respir Dis* 135:1062-1068.

105. Knowles, J.B., M.S. Fairbarn, B.J. Wiggs, C. Chan-Yan, and R.L. Pardy. 1998. Dietary supplementation and respiratory muscle performance in patients with COPD. *Chest* 93:977-983.

106. Whittaker, J.S., C.F. Ryan, P.A. Buckley, and J.D. Road. 1990. The effects of refeeding on peripheral and respiratory muscle function in malnourished chronic obstructive pulmonary disease patients. *Am Rev Respir Dis* 142:283-288.

107. Donahoe, M., J. Mancino, H. Lebow, and R.M. Rogers. 1994. The effect of an aggressive nutritional support regimen on body composition in patients with severe COPD and weight loss. *Am J Respir Crit Care Med* 149:A313.

108. Schols, A.M.W.J., P.B. Soeters, R. Mostert, R.J. Pluymers, and E.F.M. Wouters. 1995. Physiologic effects of nutritional support and anabolic steroids in patients with chronic obstructive pulmonary disease. A placebo-controlled randomized trial. *Am J Respir Crit Care Med* 152:1268-1274.

109. Donahoe, M. 1997. Nutritional support in advanced lung disease. *Clin Chest Med* 18:547-561.

110. Bhasin, S., T.W. Storer, and N. Berman, et al. 1996. The effects of supraphysiologic doses of testosterone on muscle size and strength in normal men. *N Eng J Med* 335:1-7.

111. Casaburi, R., S. Goren, and S. Bhasin. 1996. Substantial prevalence of low anabolic hormone levels in COPD patients undergoing rehabilitation. *Am J Respir Crit Care Med* 153:A128(abstract).

112. Martins Ferreira, I., I.T. Verreschi, and L.E. Nery, et al. 1998. The influence of 6 months of oral anabolic steroids on body mass and respiratory muscles in undernourished COPD patients. *Chest* 114:19-28.

113. Burdet, L., B. de Muralt, Y. Schutz, C. Pichard, and J.W. Fitting. 1997. Administration of growth hormone to underweight patients with chronic obstructive pulmonary disease. A prospective, randomized, controlled study. *Am J Respir Crit Care Med* 156:1800-1806.

114. Casaburi, R., E. Carithers, J. Tosolini, J. Phillips, and S. Bhasin. 1997. Randomized placebo controlled trial of growth hormone in severe COPD patients undergoing endurance exercise training. *Am J Respir Crit Care Med* 155:A498.

115. Jakobsson, P., and L. Jorfeld. 1995. Long-term oxygen therapy may improve skeletal muscle metabolism in advanced chronic obstructive pulmonary disease with chronic hypoxaemia. *Resp Med* 89:471-476.

CHAPTER 10

Treatment of Skeletal Muscle Dysfunction With Anabolic Hormone Supplementation in Patients With Chronic Obstructive Pulmonary Disease

Richard Casaburi

Division of Respiratory and Critical Care Physiology and Medicine, Harbor-UCLA Medical Center, Torrance, California, USA

In the future, the 1990s will likely be viewed as a time when a clear rationale for pulmonary rehabilitation was defined. The decade began with a definite (though usually unspoken) conviction that pulmonary rehabilitation's goal was mainly to help patients cope with their debility. As the decade ends, the time has come to declare that a rehabilitation program should focus on improving the physiological ability of the patient to function. This is based on a series of investigations that have demonstrated that physiological improvements are both possible and beneficial.

Exercise Training and Peripheral Muscle Function

The key to reformulating the old concept of pulmonary rehabilitation was getting past an exclusive focus on lung pathology as mediating debility in patients with lung disease. Indeed, derangements in lung mechanics, lung gas exchange, and pulmonary vasculature are important sources of exercise intolerance and are not affected by pulmonary rehabilitation programs. However, the rehabilitative process can be viewed as an attempt to fix what is wrong with the patient outside of the lung. With this view, two effective rehabilitation targets can be defined. The first target is psychological improvement; teaching the patient that a diagnosis of lung disease need not mean a dramatic reduction in the quality of life yields practical benefits. The second target is muscle dysfunction; only recently has it been demonstrated that muscle function is abnormal in patients with chronic obstructive pulmonary disease (COPD). Further, these abnormalities are (at least in part) remediable and remediation results in improved function. It seems likely that dysfunction exists in respiratory and cardiac muscle, and that this dysfunction contributes to exercise intolerance in pulmonary patients. However, the most rapid progress has been made in defining dysfunction of (and therapy for) the muscles of ambulation.

A recent publication may prove important in reorienting rehabilitation programs. This is a joint statement of the American Thoracic Society and European Respiratory Society titled *Skeletal Muscle Dysfunction in Obstructive Lung Disease* (1). This document was composed by a group of experts in the fields of muscle biology, exercise physiology, and rehabilitation science. It provides a primer in muscle function, summarizes what is known regarding mechanisms of dysfunction of the muscles of ambulation in patients with COPD, and reviews progress in defining therapeutic strategies for this dysfunction. This document may well serve as a blueprint for the next burst of research investigating scientifically based rehabilitation strategies.

Four rehabilitative therapies are highlighted by this document as having the potential to modulate skeletal muscle dysfunction:

1. exercise training
2. nutritional supplementation
3. long-term oxygen therapy
4. anabolic hormone supplementation

Progress made to date in evaluating the potential of anabolic hormone supplementation will be reviewed. As a prelude to this discussion, it is necessary to note that all "anabolic" effects on the muscle are not the same. Using exercise training as the best-characterized paradigm of muscle anabolism, there are two distinct interventions that yield two distinct results. Endurance training induces a constellation of changes in the muscle (table 10.1) that improves oxygen delivery to the muscle mitochondria and improves the capacity of the mitochondria for aerobic respiration. In contrast, strength training changes in the muscle (table 10.2) yield hypertrophy of fibers needed for explosive tasks. Endurance training can be

Table 10.1 Muscle Adaptations to Endurance Training

Increased mitochondrial number in type I fibers
Increased concentration of aerobic enzymes in type I fibers
Type IIb fibers remodel into type IIa fibers
Modest hypertrophy
Increased capillarity
Decreased diffusion distances for oxygen
Increased peak muscle blood flow
Redistribution of blood flow from type II to type I fibers

Table 10.2 Muscle Adaptations to Strength Training

Muscle Adaptations to Strength Training
Increase in enzymes' facilitating ATP and creatine phosphate utilization
Substantial fiber hypertrophy, predominantly type II
Decreased mitochondrial concentration
Decreased capillary density
Increased force development
Optimization of fiber recruitment pattern

expected to improve exercise endurance and strength training can be expected to improve activities requiring strength. Given these distinct, and almost opposite, adaptations, it seems crucial to categorize any potential anabolic strategy. Does an anabolic drug induce changes in the muscle that more resemble strength or endurance adaptations? Failure to understand this distinction will predictably lead to misunderstanding of expected benefits. In fact, the anabolic hormones studied to date appear to induce hypertrophic changes; it may be illogical to expect improvements in exercise endurance. Rather, we should be assessing the changes in muscle strength and defining the benefits of rehabilitative interventions that improve strength (2).

Anabolic Hormone System

Two well-defined hormonal systems are anabolic for muscle. One is the growth hormone system. The pituitary, which is itself under hormonal control, secretes growth hormone in a pulsatile manner (3). The main consequence relevant to muscle is that growth hormone causes the liver and other organs (including the skeletal muscles) to secrete insulin-like growth factors. Insulin-like growth factor-1 (IGF-1) is the predominant mediator of growth hormone's actions on the skeletal muscles (4). Unlike growth hormone, its level in the circulating blood varies little on a minute-to-minute basis. The second hormonal system anabolic to muscle involves the anabolic steroids. Testosterone is the most important naturally occurring molecule, but other circulating anabolic steroids and many synthetic steroid molecules have been described. In men, the pituitary secretes follicle-stimulating hormone and luteinizing hormone that act on the testes to induce testosterone production. In women, circulating testosterone levels are roughly 10-fold lower than in men, yet it seems possible that testosterone plays an important role in muscle function in women, as well (5). Very few studies of the physiology of anabolic steroids in women have been conducted, and it is likely that other circulating substances (e.g., estradiol) may have a substantial influence on muscle function.

Anabolic Hormone Supplementation in Patients with COPD

When we consider therapeutic strategies for muscle dysfunction in patients with COPD, anabolic hormone supplementation seems an attractive target. Surveys of patients with COPD, both acutely ill and ambulatory, have shown that IGF-1 levels are often low (6) and, in men, testosterone levels are low (6,7). Of course, "normal values" must be related to a specified population. It is known that both IGF-1 and testosterone levels fall with age in healthy individuals (8,9). Preliminary results indicate that levels in COPD patients are low compared to those in healthy, age-matched individuals (6). The case may be made, however, that even the healthy elderly are relatively deficient of anabolic stimuli to the muscles. It seems reasonable to believe that restoring anabolic hormone levels to those seen in the healthy young may be a reasonable strategy. It is an attractive (though unproven) hypothesis that physiological hormonal replacement may be relatively free of adverse effects, as compared to administration of substantially supraphysiologic doses. Thus we may be able to avoid the toxicities experienced, for example, by athletes who self-administer huge doses of anabolic drugs.

Growth Hormone Supplementation

Review of the clinical experience with administration of anabolic hormones is instructive, though few reports to date have involved patients with lung disease. The use of growth hormone became common in the 1970s when growth hormone isolated from the pituitary glands of cattle was used to normalize stature of growth-hormone-deficient children. Unfortunately, in a few cases, prion-mediated diseases were transmitted by this practice. The availability of recombinant human growth hormone (starting in the late 1980s) obviated this problem. Since then a series of clinical trials have begun to define the effects of growth hormone supplementation. Clearly, when growth hormone is given to growth-hormone-deficient adults, their muscle mass increases and muscle strength improves (10,11). In healthy young subjects, administration of growth hormone causes muscle protein synthesis to increase (12). In healthy older subjects and in patient models of wasting syndromes (e.g., HIV wasting syndrome), growth hormone administration causes increases in muscle mass (13,14). However, studies of increase in functional capacity have yielded mixed results, with one study finding mild increases in measures of both strength and endurance (13), and other studies finding no such benefits (14). In patients with COPD, one uncontrolled study found that short-term growth hormone administration yielded an increase in maximum inspiratory pressure (15). A 3-week study of thrice-weekly growth hormone administration found evidence of increased muscle mass and decreased fat mass, but no change in endurance exercise capacity (16). There are growing doubts regarding growth hormone's potential as useful therapy for substantial numbers of patients with chronic disease (17). Growth hormone must be administered by injection several times per week and is quite expensive. The lack of consistent evidence that growth hormone increases exercise tolerance is troubling. However, future studies might focus on detecting improvements in strength-related outcomes, which might be a more rational expectation of a drug that predominantly induces muscle hypertrophy. Finally, it seems possible that the pulsatility of growth hormone secretion may be an important determinant of its anabolic effects (18). Approaches that amplify naturally occurring pulsatile growth hormone secretion might be more effective than current approaches that produce relatively constant blood levels.

Testosterone Supplementation

Testosterone was first synthesized in the 1930s. There is no question that administration of testosterone to men without adequate production by the testes increases muscle mass and strength (19,20). However, controversy over the widespread abuse of anabolic steroids by athletes and bodybuilders generated nearly a half century of debate. The underlying premise fueling this abuse was that supraphysiologic doses of testosterone produced muscle hypertrophy and improved performance. Anecdotal evidence, followed by reports from over a dozen clinical trials conducted mostly in the 1970s, failed to provide incontrovertible evidence for this premise (21). These clinical trials were seen as flawed in several respects. Safety concerns meant that only low doses were used. Concomitant strength training was often permitted, making it hard to isolate the hypertrophic responses to testosterone. Methods of determining body composition were often unsophisticated. Inadequate (or absent) control groups coupled with effort-dependent measures, made it difficult to assess performance gains. By the end of the 1980s, opinion was divided. Many endocrinologists argued that, on theoretical grounds, cellular testosterone receptors were saturated at physiological circulating testosterone levels and that further increases would be without effect (22). Most sports medicine experts felt that experimental evidence adequately demonstrated testosterone's anabolic effects (23). It was not until 1996 that the issue was settled by the publication of a randomized, placebo-controlled, double-blinded trial of supraphysiologic doses of testosterone in 40 healthy young men (24). Subjects were randomly assigned to receive a 10-week intervention consisting of placebo without exercise, testosterone (600 mg/week) without exercise, placebo with strength training (45-minute sessions thrice weekly), or testosterone with strength training. Compliance to the drug regimen and adherence to the training program were closely monitored. In the groups receiving testosterone, nadir levels (i.e., just before the next dose) were elevated roughly fivefold. Interestingly, the group receiving testosterone (without training) exhibited increases in lean body mass roughly comparable to those seen in the strength training (without testosterone) group. The group receiving both interventions exhibited impressive increases in lean body mass (averaging about

15%, as determined by underwater weighing) and in strength (averaging about 40%, as determined by one-repetition maximum testing of a squat weightlifting maneuver). The increases seen in this latter group were approximately additive with respect to those seen in those receiving the individual interventions. This study seems to have settled the issue; testosterone administration is now acknowledged to have anabolic effects in healthy men.

An accumulation of evidence indicates that older men whose circulating testosterone level is mildly low respond to short-term testosterone replacement with modest increases in muscle mass and strength (20,25-27). Recently, a 6-month placebo-controlled study of men with AIDS wasting syndrome and low testosterone levels was reported (28). Physiological testosterone replacement was found to increase lean body mass and quality of life; however, the change in 6-minute walk distance (an endurance task) was not different from the placebo group. Limited data is available thus far concerning the effects of anabolic steroid supplementation in patients with COPD. Schols et al. (29) administered a relatively low dose of nandrolone (an orally administered anabolic steroid) or placebo to 217 men and women with COPD. A small improvement in lean body mass (averaging roughly 1 kg) and an increase in respiratory muscle strength attributable to nandrolone was detected. In another study, 6 months of oral stanozolol produced a mean 1.8-kg increase in body weight in 10 underweight COPD patients, but significant increases in endurance exercise capacity (as assessed by 6-minute walk distance and maximum oxygen uptake) were not observed (30).

Several questions must be answered before anabolic steroids can be routinely prescribed for patients with COPD. Safety concerns must addressed (31), chief among them the concern that an undetected prostate malignancy might be stimulated to grow more quickly. Also, testosterone is known to stimulate red cell production (20,26,32), which may exacerbate the tendency toward polycythemia in hypoxemic patients with COPD. Researchers must determine whether testosterone is the preferable anabolic steroid, or whether testosterone analogs, some of which can be administered orally, have a better side effect profile (33). We also need to determine the dose-response relationship for these drugs (34) so that we can properly choose a dose that appropriately balances risk-benefit considerations.

Conclusion

It seems likely that neither growth hormone nor the anabolic steroids will prove to be the optimal agents for reversing the skeletal muscle dysfunction seen in patients with COPD. However, studies of these drugs will allow us to define the benefits of anabolic agents in this patient group. Meanwhile, it will be important to conduct basic science investigations to define the cellular mechanisms of muscle growth so that pharmacotherapy can be more appropriately focused. It seems likely that new molecules will be identified as anabolic agents (1). These developments should allow a new era of rehabilitative therapy, in which exercise and drug therapy interact to normalize muscle function in patients with COPD, allowing a higher level of function and a better quality of life.

References

1. American Thoracic Society/European Respiratory Society. 1999. Statement. Skeletal muscle dysfunction in chronic obstructive pulmonary disease. *Am J Resp Crit Care Med* 159:S1-S40.
2. Ory, M.G., K.B. Schechtman, J.P. Miller, E.C. Hadley, M.A. Fiatarone, and M.A. Province, et al. 1993. Frailty and injuries in later life: the FICSIT trials. *J Am Geriatr Soc* 41:283-296.
3. Casanueva, F.F. 1992. Physiology of growth hormone-secretion and action. *Endrocrinol Metab Clin N Am* 21:483-517.
4. LeRoith, D., M. Adama, H. Werner, and C.T. Roberts. 1991. Insulinlike growth factors and their receptors as growth regulators in normal physiology and pathologic states. *Trends Endocrinol Metab* 2:134-139.
5. Kenyon, A.T., K. Knowlton, I. Sandiford, F.C. Koch, and G. Lotwin. 1940. A comparative study of the metabolic effects of testosterone propionate in normal men and women and in eunuchoidism. *Endocrinol* 26:26-45.
6. Casaburi, R., S. Goren, and S. Bhasin. 1996. Substantial prevalence of low anabolic hormone levels in COPD patients undergoing rehabilitation. *Am J Resp Crit Care Med* 153:A128.
7. Semple, D.'A.P., G.H. Beastall, W.S. Watson, and R. Hume. 1980. Serum testosterone depression associated with hypoxia in respiratory failure. *Clin Sci* 58:105-106.
8. Davidson, J.M., J.J. Chen, and L. Crapo, et al. 1983. Hormonal changes and sexual function in aging men. *J Clin Endrocrinol Metab* 57:71-77.
9. Rudman, D., D.E. Mattson, and H.S. Nagraj. 1988. Plasma testosterone in nursing home men. *J Clin Epidemiol* 41:231-236.
10. Tanner, J.M., P.C.R Hughes, and R.H. Whitehourse. 1997. Comparative rapidity of response of height, limb muscle and limb fat to treatment with human growth hormone in patients with and without growth hormone deficiency. *Acta Endocrinol* 84:681-696.
11. Cuneo, R.C., F. Salomon, C.M. Wiles, R. Hesp, and P.H. Sonksen. 1991. Growth hormone treatment in growth hormone-deficient adults. I. Effects on muscle mass and strength. *J Appl Physiol* 70:688-694.
12. Fryburg, D.A., R.A. Gelfand, and E.J. Barrett. 1991. Growth hormone acutely stimulates forearm muscle protein synthesis in normal humans. *Am J Physiol* 260:E499-504.

13. Papadakis, M.A., D. Grady, D. Black, M.J. Tierney, G.A.W. Gooding, M. Schambelan, and C. Grunfeld. 1996. Growth hormone replacement in healthy older men improves body composition but not functional ability. *Ann Intern Med* 124:708-716.

14. Schambelan, M., K. Mulligan, C. Grunfeld, E.S. Daar, A. LaMarca, D.P. Kotler, J. Wang, S.A. Bozzette, J.B. Breitmeyer, and the Serostim Study Group. 1996. Recombinant human growth hormone in patients with HIV-associated wasting. *Ann Intern Med* 125:873-882.

15. Pape, G.S., M. Friedman, L.E. Underwood, and D.R. Clemmons. 1991. The effect of growth hormone on weight gain and pulmonary function in patients with chronic obstructive lung disease. *Chest* 99:1495-1500.

16. Burdet, L., B. deMuralt, Y. Schutz, C. Pichard, and J.W. Fitting. 1997. Administration of growth hormone to underweight patients with chronic obstructive pulmonary disease. *Am J Resp Crit Care Med* 156:1800-1806.

17. Mantzoros, C.S., and A.L. Moses. 1996. Whither recombinant human growth hormone? *Ann Intern Med* 125:932-934.

18. Gevers, E.F., J.M. Wit, and I.C.A.F. Robinson. 1996. Growth, growth hormone (GH)-binding protein and GH receptors are differentially regulated by peak and trough components of the GH secretory pattern in the rat. *Endrocrinol* 137:1013-1018.

19. Bhasin, S., T.W. Storer, N. Berman, K.E. Yarasheski, B. Clevenger, J. Phillips, W.P. Lee, T. Bunnell, and R. Casaburi. 1997. Testosterone replacement increases fat-free mass and muscle size in hypogonadal men. *J Clin Endocrinol Metab* 82:407-413.

20. Sih, R., J.E. Morley, F.E. Kaiser, H.M. Perry, P. Patrick, and C. Ross. 1997. Testosterone replacement in older hypogonadal men: a 12 month randomized controlled trial. *J Clin Endocrinol Metab* 82:1661-1667.

21. Casaburi, R., T. Storer, and S. Bhasin. 1996. Testosterone effects on body composition and muscle performance. In *Androgens: Biology, Pharmacology and Clinical Applications,* ed. S. Bhasin, H. Gabelnick, J. Spieler, R.D. Swerdloff, and C. Wang. New York: Wiley-Liss.

22. Wilson, J.D. 1988. Androgen abuse by athletes. *Endrocr Rev* 92:181-199.

23. American College of Sports Medicine. 1984. Position stand on the use of anabolic androgenic steroids in sports. *Sports Med Bull* 19:13-15.

24. Bhasin, S., T.W. Storer, N. Berman, C. Callegari, B. Clevenger, J. Phillips, T.J. Bunnell, L. Tricker, and R. Casaburi. 1996. The effects of supraphysiological doses of testosterone on muscle size and strength in normal men. *N Engl J Med* 335:1-7.

25. Urban, R.J., Y.H. Bodenburg, C. Gilkison, J. Foxworth, and A.R. Coggan, et al. 1995. Testosterone administration to elderly men increases skeletal muscle strength and protein synthesis. *Am J Physiol* 269:E820-826.

26. Tenover, J.S. 1992. Effects of testosterone supplementation in the aging male. *J Clin Endocrinol Metab* 75:1092-1098.

27. Morley, J.E., H.M. Perry, III, F.E. Kaiser, D. Kraenzle, J. Jensen, K. Houston, M. Mattammal, and M. Perry. 1993. Effects of testosterone replacement therapy in old hypogonadal males: a preliminary study. *J Am Geriatr Soc* 41:149-152.

28. Grinspoon, S., C. Corcoran, H. Askari, D. Schoenfeld, L. Wolf, and B. Burrows, et al. 1998. Effects of androgen administration in men with the AIDS wasting syndrome. *Ann Intern Med* 129:18-26.

29. Schols, A.M.W.J., P.B. Soeters, R. Mostert, R.J. Pluymers, and E.F.M. Wouters. 1995. Physiologic effects of nutritional support and anabolic steroids in patients with chronic obstructive pulmonary disease. A placebo-controlled randomized trial. *Am J Resp Crit Care Med* 152:1268-1274.

30. Ferriera, E.M., I.T. Verreschi, L.E. Nery, R.S. Goldstein, N. Zamel, D. Brooks, and J.R. Jardim. 1998. The influence of 6 months of oral anabolic steroids on body mass and respiratory muscles in undernourished COPD patients. *Chest* 114:19-28.

31. Bagatell, C.J., and W.J. Bremner. 1996. Androgens in men—uses and abuses. *N Engl J Med* 334:707-714.

32. Drinka, P.J., A.L. Jochen, and M. Cuisinier, et al. 1995. Polycythemia as a complication of testosterone replacement therapy in nursing home men with low testosterone levels. *J Am Geriatric Soc* 43:899-901.

33. Bhasin, S., and W.J. Bremner. 1997. Emerging issues in androgen replacement therapy. *J Clin Endocrinol Metab* 82:3-8.

34. Bhasin, S., R. Bross, T.W. Storer, and R. Casaburi. 1998. Androgens and muscles. In *Testosterone. Action—Deficiency—Substitution,* ed. E. Nieschlag and H.M Behre. Berlin: Springer.

PART V

Exercise in Cardiopulmonary Rehabilitation: Benefits and Special Considerations

CHAPTER 11

Putting the Risk of Exercise in Perspective: Implications for the Primary and Secondary Prevention of Heart Disease

Barry A. Franklin

Cardiac Rehabilitation and Exercise Laboratories, William Beaumont Hospital, Royal Oak, Michigan, USA; and Professor of Physiology, Wayne State University, School of Medicine, Detroit, Michigan, USA

Reports of acute myocardial infarction (MI) and cardiac arrest associated with physical exertion have appeared in the medical literature (1) as well as the lay press (2), suggesting that strenuous physical activity may precipitate cardiovascular events in some persons. The general acknowledgment of this association is exemplified by the uncomfortable and ever-present availability of a defibrillator in exercise stress testing laboratories and cardiac exercise training facilities.

The commonly held notion that vigorous physical activity can trigger cardiovascular complications has been substantiated by several recent reports (3-5). These alarming studies suggested that the additional risk of acute MI and cardiac arrest during exercise, compared with that at other times, may be more than 100-fold greater during or soon after exertion. Unfortunately, these findings have been misquoted or taken out of context, especially in the popular media: "Exercise can kill you; details at 11."

The purpose of this chapter is to put in perspective the concerns raised by these studies, with specific reference to the relative, absolute, and overall risk of acute MI and cardiac arrest in sedentary and habitually active persons; the influence of time of day (A.M. versus P.M.) on cardiovascular complications; high-risk activities (i.e., snow shoveling); identifying the person "at risk"; and practical recommendations to reduce the incidence of exercise-related cardiovascular events.

The Risk of Exercise

Persons who experience cardiovascular events during exercise generally have some form of heart disease. The incidence of cardiac arrest during exercise training in coronary patients is reported as 1 event per 59,142 hours. At this rate, a typical cardiac rehabilitation program that has 100 patients exercising 3 hours/week could expect a sudden cardiac death every 3.85 years (assuming 100% attendance). In contrast, one event occurs every 565,000 hours in the general population (6). Cardiac events (either acute MI or cardiac arrest) during physical exertion may represent manifestations of known or latent coronary artery disease (CAD), reflecting a sudden disparity between myocardial oxygen supply and demand, hemodynamic stresses that disrupt vulnerable atherosclerotic plaque, or both. Indeed, CAD is the most frequent autopsy finding in persons over 35 years of age who die suddenly during exercise (7). On the other hand, structural abnormalities of the heart, including ruptured aorta, anomalous origin of the left coronary artery, hypertrophic and/or right ventricular cardiomyopathy, mural left anterior descending coronary artery, mitral valve prolapse, and irregularities of the conduction system, are the major causes of sudden death during exercise in young people (8). Except in unusual circumstances, such as profound intra- and extracellular electrolyte derangements, or heat stroke secondary to exhaustive physical exercise (e.g., marathon or ultramarathon running), the healthy heart appears to be protected from the evolution of lethal arrhythmias. Thus, the combination of exercise and a diseased or susceptible heart, rather than exercise per se, seems to be the major acute cardiovascular risk of physical activity.

Cardiac Arrest

Pathophysiological evidence suggests that vigorous physical activity (increased myocardial oxygen consumption with simultaneous shortening of diastole and coronary perfusion time) may evoke a transient oxygen deficiency at the subendocardial level, which is exacerbated by venous pooling in recovery (figure 11.1). In addition, symptomatic or silent myocardial ischemia (9), sodium-potassium imbalance, increased catecholamine excretion, and circulating free fatty acids may all be arrhythmogenic. For patients with CAD, the relative risk of developing cardiac arrest during vigorous exercise is estimated to be 6 to 164 times greater than the risk at rest or during light activity (3).

Although it is difficult to identify individuals who may be predisposed to exertion-related sudden cardiac death, certain clinical characteristics have been noted. Persons with previous MI who have impaired left ventricular function (often manifested as exertional hypotension); significant exercise-induced ST-segment depression, angina pectoris, or both; threatening ventricular arrhythmias; or who have a very low or relatively high aerobic capacity appear to be at increased risk (10). However, because of the vagaries of the atherosclerotic process, accuracy in predicting which patients will experience a cardiac arrest during exercise remains unattainable.

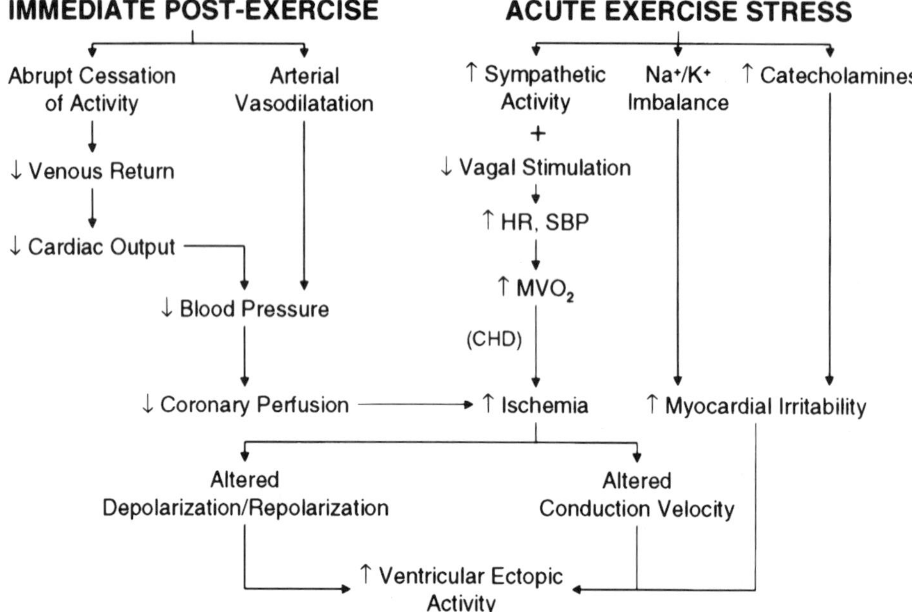

Figure 11.1 Physiological alterations accompanying acute exercise and recovery and their possible sequelae. HR = heart rate; SBP = systolic blood pressure; $M\dot{V}O_2$ = myocardial oxygen uptake; CHD = coronary heart disease.

Myocardial Infarction

Traditionally, it was believed that the degree of coronary artery stenosis determined the risk of acute coronary events. However, recent studies have shown that most acute MIs occur at sites in the coronary arteries that previously had only mild-to-moderate blockages (<70% obstruction) (11, 12). Such narrowings are not typically treated with revascularization procedures such as coronary artery bypass graft surgery or percutaneous transluminal coronary angioplasty. Consequently, the goals of contemporary prophylactic therapy have increasingly evolved to plaque stabilization and normalization of endothelial function via aggressive lipid lowering, especially low-density lipoprotein cholesterol (13).

Although the reasons that strenuous physical exertion sometimes can provoke plaque rupture and acute coronary thrombosis are unknown, several hypotheses have been suggested as triggering mechanisms (table 11.1) (14, 15). Apparently, a cascade of events can cause abrupt closure of a coronary artery, even at mild-to-moderate areas of plaque obstruction (figure 11.2), leading to acute MI (16).

Two recent studies, one in the United States and the other in Germany, reported that the "relative risk" of acute MI during or soon after strenuous physical exertion (≥6 metabolic equivalents [METs]) was two to six times greater than the risk during periods of lighter activity or no exertion (4,5). However, the relative risk

Table 11.1 Potential Triggering Mechanisms of Acute Myocardial Infarction by Strenuous Physical Exertion*

Exercise → coronary artery spasm in diseased segments → plaque rupture
Exercise → changes in cardiac dimensions → twisting of the epicardial coronaries → plaque rupture
Exercise → increased blood pressure (shear forces) → plaque disruption
Exercise → augmenting catecholamine-induced platelet aggregation

*Adapted from Thompson 1996 (14) and Kestin et al. 1993 (15).

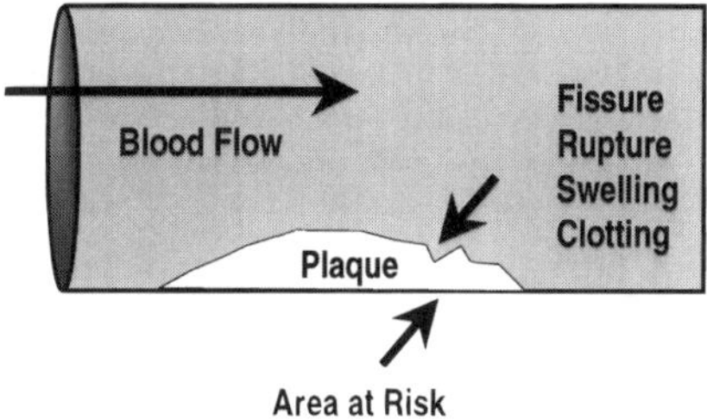

Figure 11.2 Atherosclerotic plaque can be either active and unstable or quiet and stable. If unstable, even mild-to-moderate sized plaques may fissure, rupture, and/or swell. This series of events at vulnerable regions can result in a sudden and complete obstruction of a coronary artery, causing an acute myocardial infarction. In some persons, it appears that vigorous exercise can trigger this sequence.

varied greatly depending on the patient's usual frequency of physical activity (table 11.2). Interestingly, both studies reported a protective effect of regular exercise in decreasing the risk of acute MI.

Relative Versus Absolute Risk

Although it appears that strenuous exercise increases the transient risk of acute MI (i.e., as compared with the risk during periods of lighter activity or no exertion), particularly among persons who are habitually inactive, it is important to clarify the difference between absolute risk and relative risk. Using data from the Framingham Heart Study, the absolute risk that a 50-year-old nonsmoking, non-diabetic man will have an acute MI during a given 1-hour period is approximately one in one million (17,18). Based on the U.S. findings of Mittleman et al. (4), if this man were habitually sedentary but engaged in strenuous physical activity during that hour, his relative risk would increase 107 times, but his absolute risk

Table 11.2 Relative Risk of Exertion-Related Myocardial Infarction According to the Usual Frequency of Strenuous Physical Exertion (≥6 METs)*

	Frequency of exertion	Relative risk
German study†	<4 times/week	6.9
	4 times/week	1.3
U.S. study‡	<1 times/week	107
	1-2 times/week	19.4
	3-4 times/week	8.6
	≥5 times/week	2.4

*1 metabolic equivalent (MET) = 3.5 ml O_2/kg/min; †Willich et al. 1993 (5); ‡Mittleman et al. 1993 (4).

during that hour would be only 1 in 9346. Accordingly, in a cohort of 60 previously sedentary men, average age 50 years, who initiated a vigorous exercise program 3 hours/week, one might expect one acute myocardial infarction per year (assuming 100% attendance).

Does the Benefit Outweigh the Risk?

The increased relative risk of exertion-related events seems to contradict the widely held belief that regular exercise reduces the risk of heart disease and its manifestations. The critical question, however, is whether the overall cardiovascular benefits of exercise outweigh the transient increased risk. To this end, Siscovick et al. (19) reported that the relative risk of cardiac arrest during exercise compared with that at other times was 56 times greater among sedentary men and only 5 times greater among men with high levels of habitual activity (figure 11.3). However, the total risk of cardiac arrest among habitually active men was only 40% of that for sedentary men. In other words, if a man exercises vigorously for 1 hour per day, he is more likely to experience a cardiac arrest during that period than during a comparable period of less vigorous activity, regardless of whether he is habitually active or sedentary. On the other hand, if he is a regular exerciser, as compared to a sedentary person, he is at a much lower overall risk for a cardiac arrest (i.e., over the remaining 23 hours of the day). These earlier findings agree with recent U.S. (4) and German (5) studies on the triggering of acute MI by strenuous physical exertion and support the hypothesis that exercise both protects against and provokes cardiovascular events (20). Unfortunately, similar data on women are lacking.

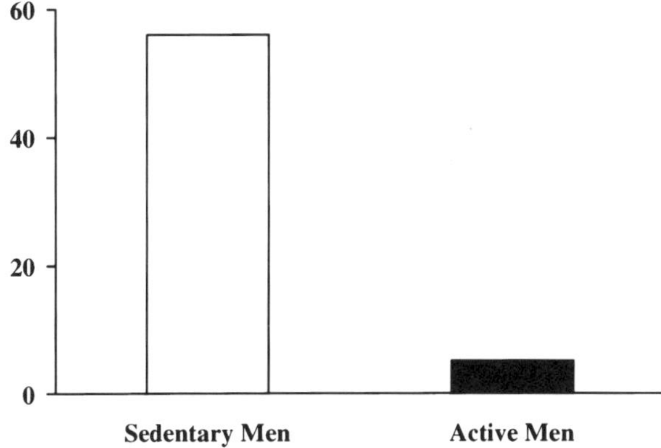

Figure 11.3 Relative risk of cardiac arrest during exercise among sedentary men versus men with high levels of habitual physical activity. Adapted from Siscovick et al. 1984 (19).

Morning Versus Afternoon Exercise?

During the early morning hours a variety of pathophysiological mechanisms for acute MI are more likely to be operative (21). These mechanisms include potential triggers of coronary artery plaque rupture and thrombosis such as circadian surges in heart rate, blood pressure, catecholamines, and cortisol; platelet aggregability; coronary vascular tone; plasma viscosity; and fibrinolytic activity associated with awakening and assuming an upright posture. It has been suggested that superimposed exercise training may accentuate these responses, and thus heighten the risk of cardiovascular events (22).

To date, two studies (23,24) have compared the rates of cardiovascular complications during exercise training in the morning versus afternoon/early evening. A retrospective review of cardiovascular events in our center over a 16-year period revealed that three of the five untoward events (three nonfatal MIs and two cardiac arrests) were during morning hours (23). However, during this period there were four to five morning and only two afternoon exercise classes, suggesting that time of day had little or no influence on the rate of complications. Similarly, an observational report (24) of outpatient exercise rehabilitation that compared morning-hours exercise with afternoon-hours exercise reported an overall cardiac complication rate (syncope, arrhythmia, MI, or sudden death) of 3.0 per 100,000 patient-hours for morning patients and 2.4 per 100,000 patient-hours for afternoon patients, an insignificant difference.

Snow Shoveling: A Trigger for Cardiovascular Events

During the winter months, an increased incidence of acute MI and sudden cardiac death has been reported in both the medical literature and lay press after heavy snowfalls: "At least 8 people died Wednesday in the Detroit area after snow-related exertion. In Wayne County alone, 17 heart attack deaths were attributed to exertion since the snow began Tuesday. Most of the victims were older men clearing their driveways and walks" (25). "On Saturday 8 December 1990, 35 cm of snow fell in Sheffield. The following day five patients were admitted to the coronary care unit with acute Q-wave myocardial infarction; this is much greater than the average admission rate of one to two infarctions a day in December" (26).

To clarify the physiological responses to manual snow shoveling in the cold (2°C), we studied 10 inactive men ($\overline{\chi} \pm$ SD age = 32.4 ± 2.1) with no history of cardiopulmonary or metabolic disease, hypertension, or other limiting orthopedic or musculoskeletal conditions, who were asked to clear a 10-cm-high tract of heavy, wet snow for 10 minutes using a lightweight plastic shovel (1.4 kg) on concrete pavement (27). The men were instructed to repetitively lift and throw snow at the rate they normally used to clear snow at home, which averaged 12 ± 2 loads per minute at approximately 7.3 kg per load (including the weight of the shovel).

The highest observed values for heart rate, systolic blood pressure, oxygen consumption, and perceived exertion during snow shoveling and treadmill testing are shown in table 11.3 (27). Oxygen consumption during snow shoveling (5.7 METs) was 39% lower than the energy expenditure of these subjects during maximal treadmill testing (9.3 METs). During the 10-minute bout of snow shoveling, the peak heart rate, blood pressure, and perceived exertion of our subjects increased to values that were comparable to or higher than the maximum values achieved by the same subjects during treadmill testing. The average subject lifted and threw nearly a ton of snow (12 lifts/minute × 7.3 kg/lift × 10 minutes = 876 kg or 1927 pounds), which is equivalent to the weight of a midsize automobile! It was concluded that heavy snow shoveling elicits myocardial demands that rival maximal treadmill testing in sedentary men. These responses may contribute to the plethora

Table 11.3 Cardiorespiratory Measurements During Maximal Treadmill Testing and Snow Shoveling (Mean ± SD)

Variable	Treadmill testing	Snow shoveling*
Heart rate (bpm)	179 ± 17	175 ± 15
Systolic blood pressure (mmHg)	181 ± 25	198 ± 17
Oxygen consumption (METs)†	9.3 ± 1.8‡	5.7 ± 0.8
Rating of perceived exertion (6-20 scale)	17.9 ± 1.5	16.7 ± 1.7

*Shoveling rates were self-paced (12 ± 2 loads/minute) during a 10-minute bout of work.
†METs = metabolic equivalents; 1 MET = 3.5 ml/kg/min.
‡$p < 0.01$ versus snow shoveling.

of cardiovascular events commonly reported in middle-aged and elderly persons after heavy snowfalls.

Our findings, in healthy untrained men, indicate that heavy snow shoveling may cause marked increases in heart rate and blood pressure. Accordingly, middle-aged and older persons who have CAD, or have symptoms suggestive of CAD, as well as those at risk for heart disease, especially smokers and those with a history of hypercholesterolemia, systemic hypertension, and diabetes mellitus, should be cautioned regarding the potentially threatening myocardial demands of this activity.

Identifying the Person at Risk

It is extremely difficult to identify persons who may be predisposed to exercise-related cardiovascular complications. Neither superior athletic ability nor regular physical training, nor the absence of coronary risk factors guarantees protection against being fatally stricken during exercise (28). One important clue, however, has emerged. Individuals who experience nonfatal and fatal cardiovascular complications during or soon after exercise often experience prodromal symptoms in the weeks or months before the event. Table 11.4 summarizes the prodromal symptoms reported by 45 subjects within 1 week of their exercise-related sudden cardiac death (29). Sixteen of the 45 reported multiple symptoms, yet only 20% of the entire group (n = 9) consulted a physician. Similarly, Noakes, Opie, and Rose (30) reported a high prevalence of premonitory symptoms in marathon runners who experienced exercise-related cardiovascular events: 81% developed

Table 11.4 Prodromal Symptoms Reported by 45 Subjects Within 1 Week of Their Sudden Death*

Symptom	No.
Chest pain/angina	15
Increasing fatigue	12
Indigestion/heartburn/gastrointestinal symptoms	10
Excessive breathlessness	6
Ear or neck pain	5
Vague malaise	5
Upper respiratory tract infection	4
Dizziness/palpitations	3
Severe headache	2

*Adapted from Northcote et al. 1986 (29).

warning symptoms, yet the majority of these runners continued to train without seeking medical advice. It has been suggested that highly trained individuals may deny prodromal symptoms, perhaps because they mistakenly believe that their superior aerobic fitness confers "immunity" to cardiac disease (31).

According to an earlier statement by the American Heart Association's Committee on Exercise (32), "The risk of strenuous exercise in the sedentary population may be minimized or perhaps even eliminated through proper preliminary testing and the individualized prescribing of exercise programs." Although exercise stress testing is often recommended to establish the safety of vigorous exercise participation, several studies have reported normal exercise ECG responses in persons who subsequently experienced cardiovascular complications during exercise (28,33). Moreover, a truly positive exercise test requires a hemodynamically significant coronary lesion, whereas most acute coronary events occur at the site of previously nonobstructive atherosclerotic plaques (34). These findings, coupled with the extremely low rate of cardiovascular complications in asymptomatic exercisers, the high costs of mass exercise testing and expensive follow-up studies (e.g., exercise testing with myocardial perfusion imaging), as well as the uncertainties associated with exercise-induced ST-segment depression in persons with a low pretest likelihood (<10%) of CAD, suggest that it is impractical to use exercise testing to prevent untoward events in all asymptomatic persons who exercise.

In summary, the need for routine exercise testing for asymptomatic people remains controversial. Perhaps one alternative to exercise testing as a regular screening procedure lies in categorizing patients according to age, gender, coronary risk factors, symptoms, and the presence or suspicion of disease, with specific reference to anticipated exercise intensity. Moderate exercise has been defined as corresponding to 40%-60% $\dot{V}O_2max$, whereas vigorous exercise represents an intensity >60% $\dot{V}O_2max$ (35). The American College of Sports Medicine recommends peak or symptom-limited exercise testing for men over 45 and women over 55, persons with two or more major coronary risk factors, and those who have—or have symptoms suggestive of—cardiac, pulmonary, or metabolic disease who plan to start a vigorous exercise program (35).

Recommendations to Reduce the Incidence of Cardiovascular Events

The following is a list of selected recommendations to reduce the incidence of cardiovascular complications during exercise.

- Emphasize appropriate warm-up and cool-down procedures.

A disproportionate number of cardiovascular events have been reported during the warm-up and cool-down phases of exercise (36). A gradual warm-up may decrease the occurrence of ischemic ST-segment depression, ventricular ectopy, or abnormal left ventricular responses that can occur with sudden strenuous exertion (37,38). A cool-down enhances venous return during exercise, reducing the possibility of postexercise hypotension and related sequelae (39). Moreover, it combats the potential deleterious effects of the postexercise rise in plasma catecholamines.

- Use continuous or instantaneous ECG monitoring for selected patients.

The degree of ECG surveillance during exercise should be linked inversely with the cardiac stability of the patient. As an alternative to costly continuous ECG monitoring, we have employed instantaneous electrocardiography (recording ECG rate, rhythm, and repolarization through defibrillator paddles) to screen for ST-segment displacement, threatening ventricular arrhythmias, and exercise intensity violators (40). Because of potential inaccuracies in assessing myocardial ischemia with this technique, if new-onset ST-segment depression is detected, it should be verified with 12-lead electrocardiography during a simulated exercise session.

- Encourage a mild-to-moderate exercise intensity.

The lower the intensity, the less likely it is that an exercise-related cardiovascular complication will occur (36). A reduced training intensity may be partially or totally compensated for by more frequent or longer training sessions.

- Promote patient education.

It is important that patients know their prescribed heart rate range for training, how to take their pulse accurately, and that they be counseled to discontinue exercise and seek medical advice if they experience abnormal heart rhythms, chest pain or pressure, or dizziness.

- Emphasize strict adherence to prescribed training pulse rates.

Cardiac arrest victims are more likely than other patients to exceed their prescribed training heart rates during exercise (10). Patients should be advised to exercise at intensities that are at least 10 to 15 beats/minute below the heart rate heralding the ischemic ECG (≥1.0-mm ST-segment depression) or anginal threshold during exercise testing (35). Staff should have periodic spot checks of suspected intensity violators and review training records to detect patients who consistently exceed the upper limit of their prescribed heart rate range.

- Modify recreational game rules and minimize competition.

The aerobic requirements and cardiac demands of game activities are influenced, to a large extent, by team members and opponent expertise. Moreover, the excitement of competition may increase sympathetic activity and catecholamine levels and lower the threshold to ventricular fibrillation (41). The exercise leader should minimize competition and modify game rules to decrease the energy cost and heart rate response to play.

- Adapt the exercise to the environment.

Cardiac patients can exercise safely in cold weather, if proper clothing is worn. For those who suffer from angina when inhaling cold air, discomfort can be reduced or alleviated by wearing a face mask to warm the inspired air (42). In contrast, hyperthermic conditions may constitute an even greater hazard for the exerciser with CAD. Simultaneous increases in body temperature and metabolism can result in disproportionate cardiac demands. Patients who are not acclimated to heat and who are exposed to temperatures higher than 24°C experience added heart rate increases of 1 beat/min/°C while exercising and 2 to 4 beats/min/°C with concomitant increased humidity (43). Consequently, in hot or humid weather, reduced exercise intensity (e.g., speed/grade or power output) will achieve the prescribed heart rate for training, so that the work of the heart remains unchanged.

These strategies, coupled with serial exercise testing, on-site medical supervision, the availability of a defibrillator and appropriate emergency drugs, and a regularly rehearsed plan of action in the event of a cardiac emergency, can help reduce the mortality rate of cardiac exercise therapy. Recent reports indicate that up to 90% of all people who experience cardiac arrests under such conditions are successfully resuscitated by nursing staff assisted by exercise physiologists-technologists and emergency medical service backup, without direct gymnasium supervision by a physician (i.e., in the exercise room) (23,44,45).

Conclusion

Although the literature suggests extremely low rates of cardiovascular complications during exercise, there appears to be an increased risk of acute MI and cardiac arrest in comparison with the risk at other times. This seems particularly true among persons with occult or known heart disease who are habitually sedentary. On the other hand, the overall risk of a cardiac event appears to be reduced in persons who are regular exercisers (46). At this time, considering the benefits and risks of exercise, the former outweighs the latter for most people, especially if one adopts a mild-to-moderate exercise intensity.

References

1. Cantwell, J.D., and G.F. Fletcher. 1969. Cardiovascular complications while jogging. *JAMA* 210:130-131.

2. "Doctors Urged Byron to Give Up Jogging," *The Baltimore Sun.* October 16, 1978: 1C-2C.

3. Cobb, L.A., and W.D. Weaver. 1986. Exercise: a risk for sudden death in patients with coronary heart disease. *J Am Coll Cardiol* 7:215-219.

4. Mittleman, M.A., M. Maclure, G.H. Tofler, J.B. Sherwood, R.J. Goldberg, and J.E. Muller. 1993. Triggering of acute myocardial infarction by heavy physical exertion. *NEJM* 329:1677-1683.

5. Willich, S.N., M. Lewis, H. Löwel, H.R. Arntz, F. Schubert, and R. Schröder. 1993. Physical exertion as a trigger of acute myocardial infarction. *NEJM* 329:1684-1690.

6. Fletcher, G.F., G. Balady, V.F. Froelicher, L.H. Hartley, W.L. Haskell, and M.L. Pollock. 1995. Exercise standards. A statement for healthcare professionals from the American Heart Association. *Circulation* 91:580-615.

7. Maron, B.J., S.E. Epstein, and W.C. Roberts. 1986. Causes of sudden death in competitive athletes. *J Am Coll Cardiol* 7:204-214.

8. Franklin, B.A., G.F. Fletcher, N.F. Gordon, T.D. Noakes, P.A. Ades, and G.J. Balady. 1997. Cardiovascular evaluation of the athlete. *Sports Med* 24(2):97-119.

9. Hoberg, E., G. Schuler, B. Kunze, A.L. Obermoser, K. Hauer, and H.P. Mautner. 1990. Silent myocardial ischemia as a potential link between lack of premonitoring symptoms and increased risk of cardiac arrest during physical stress. *Am J Cardiol* 65:583-589.

10. Hossack, K.F., and R. Hartwig. 1982. Cardiac arrest associated with supervised cardiac rehabilitation. *J Cardiac Rehab* 2:402-408.

11. Little, W.C., M. Constantinescu, R.J. Applegate, M.A. Kutcher, M.T. Burrows, F.R. Kahl, and W.P. Santamore. 1988. Can coronary angiography predict the site of a subsequent myocardial infarction in patients with mild to moderate coronary artery disease? *Circulation* 78:1157-1166.

12. Smith, S.C. 1996. Risk-reduction therapy: the challenge to change. *Circulation* 93:2205-2211.

13. Franklin, B.A. New insights into the value of cholesterol lowering. 1999. *ACSM's Health and Fitness J* 3:12-14.

14. Thompson, P.D. 1996. The cardiovascular complications of vigorous physical activity. *Arch Intern Med* 156:2297-2302.

15. Kestin, A.S., P.A. Ellis, M.R. Barnard, A. Errichetti, B.A. Rosner, and A.D. Michelson. 1993. Effect of strenuous exercise on platelet activation state and reactivity. *Circulation* 88:1502-1511.

16. Richardson, P.D., M.J. Davies, and G.V. Born. 1989. Influence of plaque configuration and stress distribution on fissuring of coronary atherosclerotic plaques. *Lancet* 2:941-944.

17. Anderson, K.M., P.W. Wilson, P.M. Odell, and W.B. Kannel. 1991. An updated coronary risk profile. A statement for health professionals. *Circulation* 83:356-362.

18. Anderson, K.M., P.M. Odell, P.W. Wilson, and W.B. Kannel. 1991. Cardiovascular disease risk profiles. *Am Heart J* 121:293-298.

19. Siscovick, D.S., N.S. Weiss, R.H. Fletcher, and T. Lasky. 1984. The incidence of primary cardiac arrest during vigorous exercise. *NEJM* 311:874-877.

20. Thompson, P.D., and J.H. Mitchell. 1984. Exercise and sudden cardiac death: protection or provocation? *NEJM* 311:914-915.

21. Muller, J.E. 1989. Morning increase of onset of myocardial infarction. Implications concerning triggering events. *Cardiology* 76:96-104.

22. Willich, S.N., M. Maclure, M. Mittleman, H.R. Arntz, and J.E. Muller. 1993. Sudden cardiac death: support for a role of triggering in causation. *Circulation* 87:1442-1450.

23. Franklin, B.A., K. Bonzheim, S. Gordon, and G.C. Timmis. 1998. Safety of medically supervised outpatient cardiac rehabilitation exercise therapy. *Chest* 114:902-906.

24. Murray, P.M., D.M. Herrington, C.W. Pettus, H.S. Miller, J.D. Cantwell, and W.C. Little. 1993. Should patients with heart disease exercise in the morning or afternoon? *Arch Intern Med* 153:833-836.

25. Shefer, J., J. Finkelstein, and M. Betzold. 1992. Icier weather on the way; 30 fatalities in Detroit area. *The Detroit Free Press,* January 16:A:1.

26. Heppell, R., S.K. Hawley, and K.S. Channer. 1991. Snow shoveler's infarction (letter). *BMJ* 302(6774):469-470.

27. Franklin, B.A., P. Hogan, K. Bonzheim, D. Bakalyar, E. Terrien, S. Gordon, and G.C. Timmis. 1995. Cardiac demands of heavy snow shoveling. *JAMA* 273:880-882.

28. Thompson, P.D., M.P. Stern, P. Williams, K. Duncan, W.L. Haskell, and P.D. Wood. 1979. Death during jogging or running. A study of 18 cases. *JAMA* 242:1265-1267.

29. Northcote, R.J., C. Flanningan, and D. Ballantyne. 1986. Sudden death and vigorous exercise—a study of 60 deaths associated with squash. *Br Heart J* 55:198-203.

30. Noakes, T.D., L.H. Opie, and A.G. Rose. 1984. Marathon running and immunity to coronary heart disease: fact versus fiction. In *Symposium on Cardiac Rehabilitation. Clinics in Sports Medicine,* ed. B.A. Franklin and M. Rubenfire, 527-543. Philadelphia: W.B. Saunders.

31. Friedwald, V.E., Jr., and D.W. Spence. 1990. Sudden cardiac death associated with exercise: the risk-benefit issue. *Am J Cardiol* 66:183-188.

32. American Heart Association's Committee on Exercise. 1972. *Exercise Testing and Training of Apparently Healthy Individuals: A Handbook for Physicians.* New York: American Heart Association.

33. Gibbons, L.W., K.H. Cooper, B.M. Meyer, and C. Ellison. 1980. The acute cardiac risk of strenuous exercise. *JAMA* 244:1799-1801.

34. Ambrose, J.A., M.A. Tannenbaum, and D. Alexopoulos, et al. 1988. Angiographic progression of coronary artery disease and the development of myocardial infarction. *J Am Coll Cardiol* 12:56-62.

35. American College of Sports Medicine. 2000. *ACSM's Guidelines for Exercise Testing and Prescription,* 6th ed. Baltimore: Lippincott, Williams and Wilkins.

36. Haskell, W.L. 1978. Cardiovascular complications during exercise training of cardiac patients. *Circulation* 57:920-924.

37. Barnard, R.J., G.W. Gardner, N.V. Diaco, R.N. MacAlpin, and A.A. Kattus. 1973. Cardiovascular responses to sudden strenuous exercise-heart rate, blood pressure, and ECG. *J Appl Physiol* 34:833-837.

38. Foster, C., D.S. Dymond, J. Carpenter, and D.H. Schmidt. 1982. Effect of warm-up on left ventricular response to sudden strenuous exercise. *J Appl Physiol* 53:380-383.

39. Dimsdale, J.E., L.H. Hartley, T. Guiney, J.N. Ruskin, and D. Greenblatt. 1984. Postexercise peril: plasma catecholamines and exercise. *JAMA* 251:630-632.

40. Franklin, B.A., P.S. Reed, S. Gordon, and G.C. Timmis. 1989. Instantaneous electrocardiography: a simple screening technique for cardiac exercise programs. *Chest* 96:174-177.

41. Lown, B., R.L. Verrier, and S.H. Rabinowitz. 1977. Neural and psychologic mechanisms and the problem of sudden cardiac death. *Am J Cardiol* 39:890-902.

42. Kavanagh, T. 1970. A cold weather "jogging mask" for angina patients. *Can Med Assoc J* 103:1290-1291.

43. Pandolf, K.B., E. Cafarelli, B.J. Noble, and K.F. Metz. 1975. Hyperthermia: effect on exercise prescription. *Arch Phys Med Rehabil* 56:524-526.

44. Vongvanich, P., M.J. Paul-Labrador, and C.N.B. Merz. 1996. Safety of medically supervised exercise in a cardiac rehabilitation center. *Am J Cardiol* 77:1383-1385.

45. Haskell, W.L. 1994. The efficacy and safety of exercise programs in cardiac rehabilitation. *Med Sci Sports Exerc* 26:815-823.

46. United States Department of Health and Human Services. 1996. *Physical Activity and Health: A Report of The Surgeon General.* Atlanta, GA: U.S. Department of Health and Human Services, Centers for Disease Control and Prevention, National Center for Chronic Disease Prevention and Health Promotion.

CHAPTER 12

Interaction Between Exercise Training and Remodeling in Patients With Left Ventricular Dysfunction and Chronic Heart Failure

Pantaleo Giannuzzi and Pier Luigi Temporelli
Division of Cardiology, Medical Center of Rehabilitation, Veruno, Italy

The potential value of rehabilitation with exercise in patients with coronary artery disease was recognized almost as early as the clinical description of the disease itself in the late 1700s. Ambulation early after myocardial infarction (MI) and the use of exercise-based cardiac rehabilitation are widely practiced because of their beneficial effects. Physical training is currently recommended for patients after acute MI, as well as for patients with other cardiac conditions such as compensated heart failure. However, although the effects of exercise training (ET) on exercise capacity and quality of life are well documented, the impact of ET on left ventricular (LV) function and remodeling are not well established, especially in patients with LV dysfunction. This chapter describes the results of the available studies and discusses the mechanisms underlying the effects of ET on LV remodeling in patients with poor LV function and chronic heart failure (CHF).

Physical Training in LV Dysfunction

Three decades ago, evidence that physical activity could promote beneficial cardiovascular and metabolic adaptations without significant untoward effects in patients with cardiac disease and normal LV systolic function gave rise to a new and very useful therapeutic tool. The beneficial effects of comprehensive cardiac rehabilitation and secondary prevention programs in patients with coronary artery disease are now well documented (1,2). Clinical benefits include improved exercise tolerance and quality of life, decreased mortality, and a possible decrease in health costs resulting from lower rehospitalization rates (1-4).

In the early 1980s, ET was found beneficial even for patients with impaired ventricular function in whom the increase in physical work capacity was not associated with deterioration of ventricular function (5,6). Animal studies (in the rat) confirmed that moderate exercise after myocardial infarction produces no significant detrimental effect on infarct size or on LV topography (7).

During the last decade, however, our understanding of the pathophysiological importance of LV volume after MI has been greatly enhanced by the recognition of the progressive nature of ventricular dilatation (8-11). Although the process of ventricular enlargement following MI begins with regional necrosis and infarct expansion, further distortion and global ventricular enlargement may continue during the chronic phase after the healing and scarring processes are complete. The combination of myocardial wall thinning, aneurysm formation, and an increase in the radius of the left ventricle has been termed "myocardial remodeling" and represents an important prognostic marker after infarction and a precursor of heart failure (11,12). Several factors may influence and modify the remodeling process, namely infarct size, ventricular wall stress, different loading conditions, continued ischemia, medications, and possibly others not well defined as yet. This is the case of physical training.

During the last few years questions have been raised about the possible deleterious effect of ET on LV remodeling after MI. Jugdutt, Michorowski, and Kappagoda (13) suggested that ET in patients with reduced LV function after an MI leads to further myocardial damage, including wall thinning, infarct expansion, and a reduction in ejection fraction (EF). Although the study was not randomized and other major limitations were present (i.e., standardization of timing of ET was lacking), it had considerable impact on clinical practice, raising the cautionary note that the potential to adversely alter ventricular size and function exists in selected patients with anterior MI. Several subsequent studies published in preliminary form failed to confirm these findings; in particular, the Exercise in Anterior Myocardial Infarction (EAMI) trial (14). This study was designed as a randomized, controlled trial to determine whether long-term ET influenced ventricular size and remodeling after anterior MI. The primary objective was to assess the effects of a long-term ET program (lasting 6 months) on global ventricular cavity dimension, function, and topography. The secondary aim was to define the role of myocardial ischemia in the possible deterioration of LV function. Patients with no contraindications to exercise were studied by echocardiography 4 to 8 weeks after anterior Q-wave MI and 6 months later. A computerized system was used to derive echocardiographic variables of ventricular size, function, and topography. After the initial study, patients were randomly allocated to a 6-month exercise training program ($n = 49$) or control ($n = 46$). After 6 months, a significant ($p < 0.01$) increase in work capacity was observed only in the training group, while global ventricular size, regional dilatation, and shape distortion did not change in either the control or training group. However, patients with <40% EF, compared to those with >40% EF, had more significant ($p < 0.001$) ventricular enlargement at entry and demonstrated further ($p < 0.01$) global and regional dilatation after 6 months, irrespective of whether they were in the control or training group. Ventricular size and topography did not change in patients with >40% EF. To summarize, the EAMI study demonstrated that patients with poor LV function 4 to 6 weeks after anterior MI are prone to further global and regional dilatation but, in contrast to previous findings, ET did not appear to influence this spontaneous deterioration. Nevertheless, because the group of patients with LV dysfunction in this trial was not large enough to draw a definite conclusion, further studies were recommended to verify whether there were any subsets of the MI population in whom ET may be harmful.

In fact, in a more recent study, Dubach et al. used magnetic resonance imaging to evaluate changes in myocardial wall thinning, thickness, global LV size, volumes, and EF in response to ET in 25 patients with reduced ventricular function (mean EF 32 ± 6%) after MI (15). A high-intensity, 2-month residential cardiac rehabilitation program started 1 month after infarction resulted in substantial increases in exercise capacity with no deleterious effects on LV volumes, function, or wall thickness regardless of infarct area. These data strongly supported the results of the EAMI study but, in view of the small number of patients enrolled, further studies were warranted to clearly elucidate the interaction between ET and remodeling in postinfarct patients with systolic dysfunction.

To fill this information gap, the Exercise in Left Ventricular Dysfunction (ELVD) study—a multicenter, randomized, controlled study carried out in 15 cardiac rehabilitation centers throughout Italy—was designed (16). Postinfarct patients with LV dysfunction (as defined by an echocardiographic EF <40%) underwent functional evaluation at 3 to 5 weeks after MI and then at the end of the study, 6 months later. After the initial evaluation, patients were randomly allocated to a 6-month ET program (n = 40) or control group (n = 40). All data were collected and analyzed at the coordinating center. As in the EAMI study, digital echocardiographic images were acquired and a computerized system was used for the automatic detection and quantification of regional wall motion, LV function, and remodeling. After 6 months, a significant increase in work capacity was observed only in the training group ($p < 0.01$), while LV volumes had increased in the control group ($p < 0.01$ for both end-diastolic and end-systolic volumes) but not in the training group (p = NS). Conversely, EF had improved in the training group ($p < 0.01$) but not in the control group. In other words, in postinfarct patients with systolic dysfunction, long-term ET attenuated the unfavorable remodeling response with a slight improvement in ventricular function over time. Thus, the ELVD study confirmed that a simple home-based exercise program is feasible and effective in improving exercise tolerance and quality of life in patients with LV dysfunction after an uncomplicated MI. Such patients may benefit from physical training without any additional clinical deterioration or deleterious effect on the remodeling process. On the basis of these data, cardiac rehabilitation ET in uncomplicated postinfarct patients with LV systolic dysfunction should clearly be encouraged as a useful adjunct to the existing medical therapy, not only to attain symptomatic and functional improvement but also to prevent the progression of LV dysfunction and its attendant morbidity and mortality.

Physical Training in Heart Failure

Given the favorable results in patients with large transmural MI, more recent research has cautiously broached the issue of exercise rehabilitation also in patients with CHF.

CHF is a serious and growing worldwide public health problem involving progressive clinical deterioration and dependency, poor quality of life, and unfavorable prognosis. Rest, salt restriction, diuretics, and cardiac glycosides were for a long time the mainstay of treatment. More recently, angiotensin-converting enzyme (ACE) inhibitors and β-blockers have been included in the drug armamentarium. Although a significant reduction in morbidity and mortality has been achieved with the newer pharmacological strategies, there remains a considerable burden of disability and unrelieved symptoms even in optimally treated patients, with corresponding poor quality of life and prognosis.

In recent years, increasing evidence indicates that restricting physical activity may be counterproductive in that it could lead to further disability. Although the effects of exercise training have been examined in a relatively low number of patients with CHF, the results are promising. A medically prescribed and supervised ET regimen has been found to reduce symptoms, improve exercise tolerance, and enhance quality of life with no significant cardiovascular complications or other serious adverse events (17-20). However, the safety of ET in patients with CHF has not been extensively examined because of the limited number of patients enrolled in randomized studies. Moreover, the impact of ET on LV function and remodeling has still to be established.

The Exercise in Left Ventricular Dysfunction and Chronic Heart Failure (ELVD-CHF) study was designed to address this issue. This multicenter, randomized, controlled trial (21) was actually aimed to determine whether long-term moderate ET could improve functional capacity in patients with stable CHF and LV systolic dysfunction (EF <40%). The effects on LV volumes and EF and on clinical status were also determined to assess safety. Ninety CHF patients with severely depressed systolic function (mean EF 25% ± 4%) were randomly assigned to a 6-month ET (50% of peak $\dot{V}O_2$) program ($n = 45$) or control ($n = 45$). At entry, clinical, functional, and echocardiographic characteristics were similar in the two groups. After 6 months, a significant improvement in work capacity ($p < 0.0001$), peak $\dot{V}O_2$ ($p < 0.006$), and walking distance ($p < 0.001$) was observed in the training group but not in the control group. At the same time, echocardiographic LV volumes had diminished and EF slightly improved in the training group, whereas in the control group LV volumes had slightly increased ($p < 0.01$ interaction) and EF showed no change ($p < 0.01$ interaction). In other words, the ELVD-CHF study clearly demonstrated that long-term moderate intensity ET was effective in improving both maximal and submaximal exercise tolerance and quality of life without any detrimental effect on LV size and function even in patients with CHF.

Mechanisms

How can we explain such a favorable effect on the remodeling process? Enhanced vasoconstrictor activity, decreased vagal tone, and impaired arterial baroreflex activity have all been described in patients with LV dysfunction with and without heart failure (22-24). The endogenous release of vasoconstrictor neurohormones may eventually play a deleterious role in the progression of ventricular dysfunction and development of congestive heart failure by increasing the loading conditions of the dysfunctioning heart, worsening the remodeling process (particularly in patients with low EF), and favoring the development of complex arrhythmias (25). Exercise training has been shown to reduce catecholamines and vascular peripheral resistance and enhance heart rate variability and baroreflex gain in patients with LV dysfunction and CHF (16,18,21).

Thus, possible mechanisms of the training-induced attenuation of the remodeling process and improvement in ventricular performance are a lessened increase in wall tension mediated by the antiadrenergic effect, favorable adaptations in the coronary circulation, or both. The beneficial changes in autonomic balance induced by ET may limit the deleterious effects of sympathetic hyperactivity on LV remodeling and function. The favorable control on LV wall stress after training, as documented by a decrease in submaximal rate-pressure product in trained patients (16,21), may attenuate the deterioration of LV size and function over time and ultimately reverse the unfavorable remodeling process. On the other hand, regular exercise has been shown to favorably affect whole blood flow rheology and enhance vascular function and structure (collaterals and microvasculature), and thereby may be of benefit to peripheral and myocardial perfusion (26,27). Physical training may also retard progression of coronary disease, and patients participating in regular physical exercise may achieve improvement in myocardial perfusion independent of regressive changes in coronary lesions (28). The improvement in myocardial blood flow of the infarcted area, even late after acute MI, may lead to a consistent recovery of both regional and global LV function (29). The decrease in ventricular wall stress, through peripheral adaptations, and possibly the improvement in myocardial perfusion may facilitate functional recovery of dysfunctioning but still viable myocardial regions.

It should be noted that the large majority of patients with LV dysfunction and CHF receive ACE inhibitors, and a considerable number are also treated with β-blockers. Thus, patients undergoing regular exercise on "maximal" medical therapy may well derive additional functional benefits from physical training. Similar observations have been reported recently in patients with CHF (20). Because there is a strong resemblance between the systemic and peripheral effects of ACE inhibitors and β-blockers and those of ET, the possibility should be considered that the long-term effects of a physical conditioning program may be mediated and even enhanced by these drugs, and vice versa. In this setting, newer β-blockers, such as carvedilol and bucindolol, are effective in improving cardiac function, and recent data with carvedilol suggest that there may also be a substantial survival benefit (30,31).

Carvedilol is a β-blocking agent with vasodilating properties: in CHF it improves left ventricle ejection fraction and reduces heart size and systemic vascular resistance. Patients improve in symptoms and ventricular function, although no significant changes in exercise tolerance have been demonstrated. The combination of long-term β-adrenergic blockade therapy and ET in stable CHF may potentially exert additional favorable effects on cardiac function and remodeling. To address this intriguing and so far unexplored issue, the Carvedilol and Training in Heart Failure Trial (CaT-HeFT) has recently started.

The CaT-HeFT is an ongoing Italian multicenter, randomized, parallel, controlled study. The aims of the study are to evaluate whether (a) the beneficial effect of ET on exercise tolerance can be maintained in the presence of a concomitant β-blocking agent (carvedilol) therapy; (b) the beneficial effect of a long-term (lasting 6 months) ET program on symptoms may be potentiated by carvedilol, which has been shown to have a favorable impact on NYHA functional class; and (c) ET has an additive effect to the third generation β-blocking agent, carvedilol, on LV function and remodeling. Patients with stable CHF resulting from either ischemic or idiopathic dilated cardiomyopathy with echocardiographic LVEF ≥35% and in NYHA functional class II-III are enrolled. All patients at enrollment are required to have been on chronic oral therapy with carvedilol for at least 6 months and treated at the maximum tolerated dose or at target daily dose 50-100 mg for at least 2 months. First results will be available early in 2000. The new challenge is on.

Conclusion

The available data provide evidence that in postinfarct patients with LV dysfunction, ET is beneficial in terms of improved exercise tolerance and quality of life with no detrimental effects on LV function and remodeling. In addition, recent data suggest that in clinically stable patients with LV dysfunction and CHF, regular exercise may result in attenuation of the unfavorable LV remodeling.

References

1. Wenger, N.K., E.S. Froelicher, and L.K. Smith, et al. 1995. Cardiac Rehabilitation. Clinical Practice Guideline No. 17. Rockville, MD: U.S. Department of Health and Human Services, Public Health Service, Agency for Health Care Policy and Research and the National Heart, Lung, and Blood Institute; AHCPR Publication No. 96-0672, October 1995.
2. Fletcher, G.F., G. Balady, and N.B. Steven, et al. 1996. Statement on exercise: benefits and recommendations for physical activity programs for all Ameri-

cans: a statement for health professionals by the Committee on Exercise and Cardiac Rehabilitation of the Council on Clinical Cardiology, American Heart Association. *Circulation* 94:857-862.

3. Specchia, G., S. De Servi, A. Sciré, et al. 1996. Interaction between exercise training and ejection fraction in predicting prognosis after a first myocardial infarction. *Circulation* 94:978-982.
4. Oldridge, N., W. Furlong, and D. Feeny, et al. 1993. Economic evaluation of cardiac rehabilitation soon after acute myocardial infarction. *Am J Cardiol* 72:154-161.
5. Lee, P.A., R. Ice, R. Blessey, and M.E. Sanmarco. 1979. Long-term effects of physical training on coronary patients with impaired ventricular function. *Circulation* 60:1519-1526.
6. Cobb, F.R., R.S. Williams, P. McEwan, R.H. Jones, R.E. Coleman, and A.G. Wallace. 1982. Effects of exercise training on ventricular function in patients with recent myocardial infarction. *Circulation* 66:100-108.
7. Hochman, J.S., and B. Healy. 1986. Effects of exercise on acute myocardial infarction in rats. *J Am Coll Cardiol* 7:126-132.
8. Erlebacher, J.A., J.L. Weiss, M.L. Weisfeldt, and B.H. Bulkley. 1984. Early dilatation of the infarcted segment in acute transmural myocardial infarction: role of infarct expansion in acute left ventricular enlargement. *J Am Coll Cardiol* 4:201-208.
9. Warren, S.E., H.D. Royal, J.E. Markis, W. Grossman, and R.G. Mckay. 1988. Time course of left ventricular dilation after myocardial infarction: influence of infarct-related artery and success of coronary thrombolysis. *J Am Coll Cardiol* 11:12-19.
10. Picard, M.H., G.T. Wilkins, P.A. Ray, and A.E. Weyman. 1990. Natural history of left ventricular size and function after acute myocardial infarction. *Circulation* 82:484-494.
11. Pfeffer, M.A., and E. Braunwald. 1990. Ventricular remodeling after myocardial infarction. Experimental observations and clinical implications. *Circulation* 81:1161-1172.
12. Gaudron, P., C. Eilles, I. Kugler, and G. Ertl. 1993. Progressive left ventricular dysfunction and remodeling after myocardial infarction: potential mechanisms and early predictors. *Circulation* 87:755-763.
13. Jugdutt, B.I., B.L. Michorowski, and C.T. Kappagoda. 1988. Exercise training after anterior Q wave myocardial infarction: importance of regional left ventricular function and topography. *J Am Coll Cardiol* 12:362-372.
14. Giannuzzi, P., L. Tavazzi, and P.L. Temporelli et al. 1993. Long-term physical training and left ventricular remodeling after anterior myocardial infarction: results of the Exercise in Anterior Myocardial Infarction (EAMI) trial: EAMI Study Group. *J Am Coll Cardiol* 22:1821-1829.

15. Dubach, P., J. Myers, and G. Dziekan, et al. 1997. Effect of exercise training on myocardial remodeling in patients with reduced left ventricular function after myocardial infarction. *Circulation* 95:2060-2067.

16. Giannuzzi, P., P.L. Temporelli, and U. Corrà et al. 1997. Attenuation of unfavorable remodeling by exercise training in postinfarction patients with left ventricular dysfunction. Results of the Exercise in Left Ventricular Dysfunction (ELVD) Trial. *Circulation* 96:1790-1797.

17. Coats, A.J.S., S. Adamopoulos, T.E. Meyer, J. Conway, and P. Sleight. 1990. Effects of physical training in chronic heart failure. *Lancet* 335:63-66.

18. Coats, A.J.S., S. Adamopoulos, and A. Radaelli, et al. 1992. Controlled trial of physical training in chronic heart failure: exercise performance, hemodynamics, ventilation, and autonomic function. *Circulation* 85:2119-2131.

19. Sullivan, M.J., M.B. Higginbotham, and F.R. Cobb.1989. Exercise training in patients with chronic heart failure delays ventilatory anaerobic threshold and improves submaximal exercise performance. *Circulation* 79:324-329.

20. Meyer, T.E., B. Casadei, and A.J.S. Coats, et al. 1991. Angiotensin-converting enzyme inhibition and physical training in heart failure. *J Intern Med* 230:407-413.

21. Giannuzzi, P., P.L. Temporelli, and U. Corrà et al., for the ELVD-CHF study group. 1997. Long-term exercise training in patients with chronic heart failure: results of the ELVD-CHF (Exercise in Left Ventricular Dysfunction and Chronic Heart Failure) Trial. *Circulation* 96: I-711.

22. Leimbach, W.H., G. Wallin, R.G. Victor, P.E. Aylward, E. Sundlof, and A. Mark. 1986. Direct evidence from intraneural recordings for increased central sympathetic outflow in patients with heart failure. *Circulation* 73:913-919.

23. Eckberg, D.L., M. Drabinsky, and E. Braunwald. 1971. Defective cardiac parasympathetic control in patients with heart disease. *N Engl J Med* 285:877-883.

24. Francis, G.S. 1985. Neurohumoral mechanisms involved in congestive heart failure. *Am J Cardiol* 55:15A-21A.

25. Pilati, C.F., F.G. Bosso, and M.B. Maron. 1992. Factors involved in left ventricular dysfunction after massive sympathetic activation. *Am J Physiol* 263:H784-H791.

26. Froelicher, V., D. Jensen, and F. Genter, et al. 1984. A randomized trial of exercise training in patients with coronary heart disease. *JAMA* 252:1291-1297.

27. Niebauer, J., and J.P. Cooke. 1996. Cardiovascular effects of exercise: role of endothelial shear stress. *J Am Coll Cardiol* 28:1652-1660.

28. Schuler, G., R. Hambrecht, and G. Schlierf, et al. 1992. Myocardial perfusion and regression of coronary artery disease in patients on a regimen of intensive physical exercise and low fat diet. *J Am Coll Cardiol* 19:34-42.

29. Galli, M., C. Marcassa, and R. Bolli, et al. 1994. Spontaneous delayed recovery of perfusion and contraction after the first five weeks following anterior infarction: evidence for the presence of hibernating myocardium in the infarcted area. *Circulation* 90:1386-1396.

30. Packer, M., M.R. Bristow, and J.N. Cohn, et al. 1996. The effect of carvedilol on morbidity and mortality in patients with chronic heart failure. *N Engl J Med* 334:1349-1355.

31. Krum, H., J.D. Sackner-Bernstein, and R.L. Goldsmith, et al. 1995. Double-blind, placebo-controlled study of the long-term efficacy of carvedilol in patients with severe chronic heart failure. *Circulation* 92:1499-1506.

CHAPTER 13

Effect of Cold, Wind, and Hot Temperature in Patients With Cardiovascular Diseases

Martin Juneau
Department of Medicine, Montreal Heart Institute, Montreal, Québec, Canada

In most countries, patients with cardiovascular disorders have limited access to cardiac rehabilitation centers and very often train in their own environment. At our cardiac rehabilitation center, we were concerned with the effects of cold weather during exercise training in patients with different cardiovascular conditions. We then performed three studies on the effect of cold in patients with cardiovascular diseases and a fourth study on the effect of extreme heat exposure (sauna) in patients with stable coronary disease and exercise-induced ischemia.

Cold Studies

Many patients with angina report that their symptoms are worst in cold weather. The mechanism accounting for this phenomenon is still controversial (1-3). Most studies published on the effect of cold in coronary patients have used the cold pressor test to simulate the effect of cold exposure (4,5) but this method does not adequately reproduce the natural environment to which patients are exposed during the winter months.

At the Montreal Heart Institute Rehabilitation Center, we conducted three studies on the effect of cold temperature in patients with coronary disease and heart failure using a specially designed cold room. First, we studied the effect of cold on the ischemic threshold with or without antianginal medication. In a second study, we studied the effect of cold and wind in another group of patients with stable coronary disease. Finally, we studied the effect of cold on exercise tolerance in patients with heart failure. In all three studies, a temperature of –8°C was chosen because it represents the average temperature during winter months in our area.

Effect of Cold on the Ischemic Threshold

This study (6) was undertaken to determine the effect of cold temperature on the ischemic threshold of patients with stable coronary disease and exercise-induced myocardial ischemia. Included in this study were 24 patients with documented coronary artery disease defined as: (a) coronary stenosis of 70% or more of the lumen diameter at arteriography, (b) previously documented myocardial infarction, or (c) reversible perfusion defect on nuclear exercise testing. All patients had both angina and 1-mm or more ST-segment depression compared with baseline during standard exercise testing using the Bruce protocol. Eight patients reported a history of increased angina during cold weather; they were considered "cold-sensitive."

The study design was double blind, randomized, and placebo controlled. Its purpose was to compare the effect of cold temperature (–8°C) with that of normal room temperature (20°C) on exercise test parameters either with no active medication, after 80 mg propranolol, or after 120 mg diltiazem. For each patient, three treadmill tests were performed at –8°C, one with placebo, one with propranolol, and one with diltiazem; three treadmill tests were also performed at 20°C, also with placebo, propranolol, and diltiazem. The sequence of the six treadmill tests was randomized. All tests were performed 90 minutes after oral drug or placebo administration.

Treadmill exercise using a Bruce protocol was performed at approximately the same hour each day, with the patient fasting or at least 2 hours after a light meal.

A cold chamber was used to perform treadmill tests at –8°C. The specially designed room (Foster Co., Canada) measured 12 × 10 × 8.5 feet and maintained a constant temperature during treadmill tests. A ventilation system recycled the air, and a large window allowed constant supervision by staff operating the electronic equipment, which was kept at room temperature outside the cold chamber. The patient, the nurse who recorded blood pressure, and the treadmill (Quinton Instrument, model 1854, Seattle, WA) were inside the cold chamber, and verbal communication with the patient and nurse inside the chamber was possible through an intercom system. All patients wore standardized clothing, a T-shirt and light pants, for the test at –8°C.

Results of the six treadmill tests in the 24 studied patients did not show any effect of cold on the ischemic threshold (table 13.1). Total duration also was not modified. Both medications prolonged time to ischemia at –8°C and at 20°C compared with placebo. The improvement produced by the two medications was similar at –8°C and at room temperature. However, in eight patients who were classified as cold-sensitive (table 13.2), time to ischemia appeared 30% sooner at –8°C compared with room temperature (169 seconds vs. 244 seconds, $p < 0.01$). Also, the double product at time to ischemia was significantly lower at –8°C (19×10^3 vs. 22×10^3, $p < 0.05$). In these cold-sensitive patients, both propranolol and diltiazem significantly improved time to ischemia and were effective to a similar degree at both temperatures. Time to angina was not influenced by cold in any patient.

Table 13.1 Effect of Cold Temperature on Ischemia and Angina: Response to Exercise in All Coronary Patients (n = 24)

	Placebo		Propranolol		Diltiazem	
	–8°C	+20°C	–8°C	+20°C	–8°C	+20°C
Time to onset						
ST ≥1 mm (sec)	222 ± 30	252 ± 22	320 ± 19*	341 ± 18*	304 ± 32*	339 ± 19*
Time to angina (sec)	306 ± 23	313 ± 25	343 ± 19	343 ± 19	375 ± 22*	374 ± 19*
Total exercise duration (sec)	396 ± 19	381 ± 18	380 ± 13	372 ± 16	426 ± 16*†	407 ± 14†§
At onset of 1-mm ST depression						
Heart rate	126 ± 3	129 ± 3	103 ± 2	106 ± 2	130 ± 4	135 ± 3
Systolic pressure	171 ± 5	175 ± 5	151 ± 5	163 ± 3	176 ± 6	182 ± 5
Rate-pressure product ($\times 10^{-3}$)	22.1 ± 1	22.6 ± 0.9	15.6 ± 0.5*†‡	17.3 ± 0.5*†	22.9 ± 1.3	24.6 ± 0.8§
Maximal ST depression (mm)	2.1 ± 0.2	2.1 ± 0.2	1.1 ± 0.2*†‖	0.8 ± 0.2*¶	1.7 ± 0.3§‖	1.2 ± 0.2*

Values are mean ± SEM. n = 24.

*$p < 0.01$ compared with placebo; †$p < 0.01$ compared with other drug; ‡$p < 0.01$ compared with 20°C; § $p < 0.05$ compared with placebo; ‖$p < 0.05$ compared with 20°C; ¶$p < 0.05$ compared with other drug.

Table 13.2 Effect of Cold Temperature on Ischemia and Angina: Response to Exercise in Cold-Sensitive Patients (n = 8)

	Placebo		Propranolol			
	–8°C	+20°C	–8°C	+20°C	–8°C	+20°C
Time to onset						
ST ≥1 mm (sec)	169 ± 41*	244 ± 38	312 ± 35†	349 ± 33†	262 ± 46‡	307 ± 36‡
Time to angina (sec)	292 ± 33	346 ± 39	351 ± 37	357 ± 31	388 ± 34‡	362 ± 41
Total exercise duration (sec)	420 ± 12	413 ± 24	400 ± 19	399 ± 23	453 ± 12§	422 ± 25
At onset of 1-mm ST depression						
Heart rate	117 ± 3	127 ± 6	104 ± 3	106 ± 4	125 ± 7	129 ± 5
Systolic pressure	164 ± 7	172 ± 6	148 ± 10	163 ± 6	165 ± 4	175 ± 7
Rate-pressure product ($\times 10^{-3}$)	19.3 ± 0.8‖	20 ± 1.6	15.3 ± 1.0†‖¶	17.3 ± 1.1†¶	207 ± 1.0‖	22.5 ± 1.1
Maximal ST depression (mm)	2.9 ± 0.4	2.7 ± 0.3	1.1 ± 0.3†§	1.1 ± 0.3†§	2.4 ± 0.6	1.9 ± 0.4‡

Values are mean ± SEM. n = 8.

*$p < .01$ compared with 20°C; †$p < .01$ compared with placebo; ‡$p < .05$ compared with placebo; § $p < .05$ compared with other drug; ‖$p < .05$ compared with 20°C; ¶$p < .01$ compared with other drug.

These results show that in a significant proportion (one-third) of coronary patients with stable angina, exposure to cold reduces the ischemic threshold by about 30%. Also, currently used antianginal medications (a β-blocker and a calcium antagonist) were equally effective in improving time to ischemia.

The Effect of Cold and Wind on Exercise-Induced Myocardial Ischemia in Stable Coronary Patients

This study was undertaken to measure the effects of cold and wind singly and in combination on myocardial ischemia (7). Fourteen patients with proven coronary disease, Canadian Cardiovascular Society class 1 or 2 angina, and exercise-induced angina and ST depression underwent four treadmill exercise tests in a randomized sequence using a Bruce protocol. Tests were performed off all antianginal medication at 20°C with and without a 15 mph headwind and at –8°C with and without wind. Temperature was controlled accurately in the specially designed cold room as previously described. The addition of wind at room temperature did not modify time to ischemia. In this study, exposure to cold alone did reduce time to ischemia but the largest reduction in time to ischemia was produced by the addition of wind at –8°C. As in the previous study, time to onset of angina was not influenced by cold or by wind. Contrary to the previous study, rate-pressure product at onset of ischemia was the same during all conditions.

Conclusions from the second study were as follows:

1. In coronary patients with stable angina, wind does not influence exercise capacity or ischemic threshold at normal temperature.
2. Exercise induces myocardial ischemia earlier (20%) in a cold environment, and this phenomenon is accentuated by wind (30%).
3. The earlier ischemia during cold exposure with and without wind occurs at the same rate-pressure product suggesting an increase in myocardial oxygen demand at comparable work rates.

Effect of Cold on Exercise Tolerance in Patients With Heart Failure

To investigate the effect of cold on exercise capacity in patients with compensated chronic heart failure, 11 patients with NYHA class 2 or 3 dyspnea and ejection fraction <35% (mean 25 ± 6) underwent four exercise tests (modified Naughton protocol), two at –8°C in a cold chamber and two at 20°C with the same equipment. Placebo or lisinopril 5 mg/day for 3 days was given in a double-blind fashion

12 hours before the test at each temperature. The test order was randomized and the end point of all tests was dyspnea. Exercise duration was 506 ± 156 seconds at 20°C and 419 ± 182 seconds at –8°C ($p < 0.01$). This difference of 87 seconds represents a 17% decrease in exercise tolerance in the cold environment. The estimated number of METs achieved according to a modified Naughton protocol was 4.3 ± 1.3 at 20°C and 3.6 ± 1.4 at –8°C ($p < 0.01$). The rate of increase in the rate-pressure products was significantly steeper at –8°C than at 20°C ($p < 0.001$). Exercise duration was increased significantly from 419 seconds to 475 seconds ($p < 0.01$) at –8°C when patients were treated with lisinopril. During testing at 20°C, lisinopril did not increase exercise tolerance (498 seconds vs. 506 seconds) (8).

From this study, we concluded that, in patients with compensated chronic heart failure, cold exposure reduces exercise tolerance by approximately 17%. Angiotensin-converting enzyme (ACE) inhibition improves this reduction of exercise tolerance at a dose that does not improve exercise tolerance at normal temperature.

Effect of Extremely Hot Temperature

Sauna bathing is a popular leisure activity in which individuals are exposed to supraphysiologic temperatures exceeding 85°C. In the United States, there are over 1 million saunas, whereas in Finland, with a population of approximately 5 million people, an estimated 1.4 million saunas are in regular use (9,10). Many cardiac rehabilitation centers, including our own, are equipped with saunas. Although sauna bathing is generally considered to be safe, there have been reports of syncope, myocardial infarction, and sudden death associated with its use. Studies on cardiac populations have included predominantly asymptomatic patients with a history of prior myocardial infarction or patients with dilated cardiomyopathy (11). This study was undertaken to assess the effects of sauna bathing on individuals with coronary artery disease and documented reversible ischemia. The first objective was to determine if sauna bathing is clinically well tolerated, and the secondary objective of the study was to assess whether heat exposure of sauna bathing can induce myocardial ischemia. Sixteen patients with known coronary artery disease and documented reversible exercise-induced myocardial ischemia were submitted to three conditions (rest, exercise, and sauna bathing) with continuous electrocardiographic monitoring and regular blood pressure measurements. For each condition, patients were injected with technetium 99 sestamibi followed by nuclear scintigraphic imaging, which enabled calculation of a perfusion defect score (PDS).

Results

Sauna bathing was clinically well tolerated. There was a 32% rise in heart rate in the sauna (resting mean heart rate = 60 vs. sauna mean heart rate = 79, $p < 0.001$) and a 13% drop in systolic blood pressure (resting mean systolic blood pressure = 142 vs. sauna mean systolic blood pressure = 123, $p < 0.001$). There were no arrhythmia or ECG changes in the sauna. Nuclear scintigraphy demonstrated exercise-induced ischemia (average rest PDS = –0.44 vs. average exercise PDS = –1.46, $p < 0.001$). Compared to rest, there was significant ischemia during sauna bathing (average rest PDS = –0.44 vs. average sauna PDS = –0.93, $p < 0.001$). The perfusion score in the sauna was worse than the resting PDS for 14 out of 15 patients. The degree of sauna-associated ischemia was highly correlated with exercise-induced ischemia (correlation coefficient $R^2 = 0.65$, $p < 0.001$).

We concluded that in patients with stable coronary disease, sauna use is clinically well tolerated but is associated with scintigraphically demonstrated myocardial ischemia. These observations need to be considered when advising patients with coronary artery disease about their safety while sauna bathing.

Conclusions

From these four studies, we conclude the following:

1. Cold weather (–8°C) can reduce time to ischemia in a significant proportion (one-third) of patients with stable coronary disease.
2. Wind has no effect on these patients at room temperature but causes a 30% reduction in time to ischemia when present at –8°C.
3. Cold weather can reduce exercise tolerance in patients with heart failure by about 20%, and this effect of cold is partially reversed by ACE inhibition.
4. Sauna use at 85°C provokes asymptomatic myocardial ischemia in patients with stable coronary disease.

These observations may be useful when advising patients who are involved in home-based or unsupervised cardiac rehabilitation programs.

References

1. Epstein, S.E., M. Stampfer, G.D. Beiser, R.E. Goldstein, and E. Braunwald. 1969. Effects of a reduction in environmental temperature on the circulatory response to exercise in man. *N Engl J Med* 280:7-11.
2. Lassvik, C.A., and N. Areskog. 1979. Angina in cold environment: reaction to exercise. *Br Heart J* 42:396-401.
3. Lassvik, C.A., and N.H. Areskog. 1983. Angina pectoris during inhalation of cold air: reactions to exercise. *Br Heart J* 43:661-667.

4. Nabel, E.G., P. Ganz, J.B. Gordon, R.W. Alexander, and A.P. Selwyn. 1988. Dilatation of normal and constriction of atherosclerotic coronary arteries caused by the cold pressor test. *Circulation* 77:43-52.

5. Raizner, A.E., R.A. Chahine, and T. Ishimori, et al. 1980. Provocation of coronary artery spasm by the cold pressor test. *Circulation* 62:925-932.

6. Juneau, M., M. Johnstone, E. Dempsey, and D.D. Waters. 1989. Exercise-induced myocardial ischemia in a cold environment: effect of antianginal medications. *Circulation* 79:1015-1020.

7. Juneau, M., L. Larrivée, M. de Guise, M. Smilovitch, J. Perrault, and D. Waters. 1993. Effects of wind and cold on exercise capacity and exercise-induced myocardial ischemia in stable angina patients. *J Am Coll Cardiol* 21(suppl A):96A.

8. Juneau, M., D. Waters, M. de Guise, M. Smilovitch, L. Belanger, M.J. Rey, and L. Larrivée. 1993. A cold environment reduces exercise capacity in patients with chronic heart failure: Reversal by ACE inhibitor. *J Am Coll Cardiol* 21(suppl A):378A.

9. Press, E. 1991. The health hazards of saunas and spas and how to minimize them. *Am J Public Health* 81:1034-1037.

10. Larrivée, O.J. 1992. The sauna and the heart. *J Intern Med* 231:319-320.

11. Giannetti, N., M. Juneau, A.Arsenault, M.A. Behr, J. Grégoire, M. Tessier, and L. Larrivée. 1999. Sauna-induced myocardial ischemia in patients with coronary artery disease. *Am J of Med* 107:228-233.

CHAPTER 14

Feasibility and Efficacy of a Home-Based Rehabilitation Program in Patients With Chronic Obstructive Pulmonary Disease

Pierre LeBlanc[1,2] and Richard Debigaré[1]

[1]Hôpital Laval, Institut Universitaire de Cardiologie et de Pneumologie de l' Université Laval, Québec, Canada

[2]Unité de Recherche, Centre de Pneumologie de l'Hôpital Laval Sainte-Foy, Québec, Canada

A national survey reported by *Statistics Canada* in 1995 estimated that 750,000 Canadians were suffering from chronic obstructive pulmonary disease (COPD) (1). This survey showed that COPD was the fifth leading cause of death in Canada and that the prevalence of the disease was 4.7%, 5.4%, and 8.3% for the age groups of 50-64 years, 65-74 years, and >75 years, respectively. It also showed that hospital admissions increased dramatically from 119.1 admissions per 100,000 persons in 1981-1982 to 239.6 admissions per 100,000 persons in 1993-1994. This increase represents more than 60,000 hospitalizations per year in Canada. When COPD is diagnosed, it is usually at an advanced and irreversible stage, and most medical interventions are aimed at improving symptoms, mostly dyspnea. Apart from oxygen therapy, treatment does not improve survival.

Increasing evidence indicates that pulmonary rehabilitation improves dyspnea, exercise capacity, and quality of life in patients with COPD (2-4). Rehabilitation favors a multidisciplinary approach, which includes exercise training, education, and psychosocial support of the patient, and, according to a recent meta-analysis (4), exercise is the most effective component of this multidisciplinary approach. Physiological studies have also shown that exercise training improves peripheral muscle function and reverses the possible deconditioning effects related to chronic inactivity (5). Based on this literature, there is little doubt that patients with COPD can benefit and should be submitted to exercise programs as part of the comprehensive treatment of their disease.

According to a recent survey, it is estimated that there are approximately 40 active rehabilitation programs across Canada (6) and of those, about 75% are directly supervised programs in hospitals. It has also been estimated that only 1% of all Canadian patients with COPD will participate in a rehabilitation program at least once in their lifetime. Several reasons, such as age, ignorance, and skepticism of the medical community about the positive effects of rehabilitation and lack of patient motivation, explain this low level of participation. Poor availability of these programs can also explain why only very few patients benefit from rehabilitation. In a large country such as Canada, individuals often live at great distances from specialized centers, and it is difficult for them to travel the necessary distances to attend rehabilitation programs.

To improve the accessibility of rehabilitation, some European centers have developed a community-based approach. In 1977, McGavin et al. reported the results of a randomized controlled study done in 24 patients with COPD (mean age: 59, mean FEV_1: 1.06 L) (7) in which a home-based training regimen was compared to no intervention. The 12 patients in the exercise group trained at home at the rate of five sessions per week, and, although the exact structure of the exercise program was not reported, subjects were asked to walk or to climb stairs. Patients were seen 2 weeks after starting the program and once a month thereafter. The authors reported improvement in symptoms and a significant improvement in the 12-minute walking distance (6%) and in the maximal power output on an ergocycle (23%).

In 1980, Sinclair and Ingram reported the results of a controlled, randomized study done in 33 patients with COPD (mean age: 65; mean FEV_1: 1.06 L) submitted to either home training during a 10 to 12-month period or to conservative treatment (8). The training group was asked to walk and to climb stairs, and the patients were visited at home weekly and had to fill out a diary. The authors reported a significant increase in the 12-minute walking distance (23%) and improvements in dyspnea. Although the results of these studies are interesting, they have not included exercise prescription, progression of training, or compliance to treatment. Moreover, patient symptomatology was not evaluated with validated tools. In 1988, Busch and McClements reported on the results of a controlled and randomized study done in 20 patients with COPD, in which they compared patients who underwent home training to a control group who did not train (9). Ten home-trained patients did not improve significantly their working capacity (improvement was only 3%) but the control group decreased its working capacity by 34%.

In 1996, two groups from the Netherlands reported the results of a home-based rehabilitation program. Strijbos et al. compared three groups of patients: one group training under supervision, one group training at home, and one control group (10). Both groups undergoing training were submitted to the same program consisting of upper limb exercise, respiratory exercise, ergocycle exercise, and relaxation. The authors reported similar improvements for exercise tolerance on ergocycle and the 4-minute walking distance in both exercise groups. Wijkstra et al. were unable to obtain significant improvements with a home-based program (11). During the 18-month duration of these two studies, home supervision was important, and patients had to regularly visit a local gymnasium to exercise under supervision as well as see their family doctor. In addition, they were visited at home once a month by a nurse practitioner.

From these studies, it seems that home-based training is feasible. However, the degree of supervision is often significant, the intensity of training is variable and not uniform, and no study has yet reported the compliance of patients participating in such programs. Because of these drawbacks, we became interested in designing a home-based exercise program that would not only be feasible, but also securely and efficiently improve capacity and quality of life in patients with COPD who could not attempt a supervised in-hospital program.

The results of this study have already been published (12). In this paper, we therefore present the design of this program with particular emphasis on patient evaluation, the training program itself, and the supervision carried out during the program.

Home-Based Exercise Training Program

Patient Selection

Twenty-three consecutive emphysema patients evaluated for possible lung volume reduction surgery (LVRS) were recruited (15 M/8 F, age = 61 ± 6, FEV_1 = 30 ± 6% of predicted). Patients were excluded if they had adverse medical conditions such as symptomatic heart disease, significant pulmonary hypertension, uncontrolled systemic hypertension, and exercise-induced O_2 desaturation ($SaO_2 < 90\%$) despite 4 L/min of oxygen that could make home exercise hazardous.

Patient Evaluation

Patients were evaluated during 1 or 2 consecutive days before and at completion of the exercise program. At final evaluation, the investigator was unaware of baseline results. At mid-program, patients were seen to ensure compliance and to detect any potential problems related to the training program. Anthropometric measurements and pulmonary function studies were performed. Patients underwent a progressive stepwise exercise test on a cycle ergometer to maximal capacity. Patients performed an endurance test at 80% of the peak work rate achieved during the initial maximal exercise test, and the duration of the test was recorded. They also performed a 6-minute walking test. Three tests were done for each patient, and only the results of the best one were used for final data analysis (13). Measurement of maximal voluntary strength was done during dynamic contractions against a hydraulic resistance (HF Star, Hydrafitness Total Power, Henley Health Care, Belton, TX). Patients were instructed to perform maximal effort at high velocity, and two sets of measurements were obtained for each muscle group with the higher values being used. Three muscle groups were evaluated: lower limbs (mostly quadriceps) during bilateral knee extension, shoulder girdle during a seated press (mostly pectoralis major), and a bilateral movement combining elbow flexion and shoulder adduction (mostly latissimus dorsi). Quality of life was finally assessed with the Chronic Respiratory Questionnaire, which includes four dimensions (dyspnea, fatigue, emotion, and mastery) (14).

Exercise Training Program

The home-based exercise training program (HBETP) included three parts: stretching, strength training, and aerobic training. Individual teaching with practice and feedback took approximately 2 hours.

Strength Training Strength training was performed using gravity, elastic bands with three levels of resistance according to the color (Theraband: red, green, and blue), and free weights (1, 1.5, and 2 kg). Six exercises were done for the arms and five for the legs. These included flexion and extension of elbows; flexion, extension, and adduction of shoulders; push-ups on the knees; flexion and abduction of the hip with straight leg; contraction of the gluteus maximus; and flexion and extension of the knee. Three exercises for the abdomen were also performed: sit-ups and sit-ups with left and right rotation. For each exercise, 10 movements were initially performed but this number was progressively increased, until 30 movements were done. For arm and leg exercises, the same procedure was repeated.

Aerobic Training The aerobic training was done on a portable, calibrated, and magnetically braked ergocycle (Cateye Ergociser, model EC-3200, Cat Eye Co., Osaka, Japan). The work rate (watt) was adjusted using the position of the workload shift lever and pedaling speed (rpm). The rpm and the number of watts were displayed on a digital screen. With this system, the work rate varies from 0 to 999 watts and can be adjusted with an accuracy of ± 5 watts. The calibration of all ergocycles was verified using the electrically braked ergocycle (Quinton Corrival 400; A-H Robins Company) as a reference and was performed before the ergocycle was lent to the patient. The initial training intensity corresponded to 50% of the initial maximal work rate achieved during maximal exercise test for up to 45 minutes. Training duration was initially set at 15 minutes and progressively increased by 5-10 minutes as tolerated (dyspnea Borg score = 4) until a period of 45 minutes was reached. After the training target was reached, the intensity was increased by steps of 5 watts. Further increases in training intensity were done when the actual training intensity could be maintained for 45 min.

Training Sessions and Supervision Patients trained 5 times/week for 10 to 12 weeks. Supervision was done through weekly phone calls during which the comprehension and progression of the training program as well as the presence of any related problems were verified. A diary, mailed weekly, was filled out by each participant in order to report the intensity, duration, and frequency of training.

Results

The amount of work (Joules) done during a training session was calculated by multiplying training intensity (watts) to duration (seconds). The relative amount of work accomplished during a given training week was calculated by dividing the total work performed during that week by the total work scheduled.

Summary of Results

Nineteen of the 23 patients were able to complete the exercise program. An average of 0.5 ± 0.6 exacerbations of disease per patient required treatment with systemic oral steroids and/or oral antibiotics. The mean duration of the HBETP was 11 ± 2 weeks (range 8-15 weeks). According to the patients' diaries, the training frequency was 4.9 ± 0.5 and 5.1 ± 0.5 sessions/week for the strength and aerobic components, respectively. The patients completed 97% ± 5% of the recommended sessions. The mean training intensity increased progressively and corresponded to 51% ± 4%, 58% ± 10%, 69% ± 17%, and 73% ± 27% of the baseline peak exercise work rate at weeks 1, 4, 8, and 11, respectively, while the training duration quickly stabilized at 200 minutes/week at week 4. The amount of work achieved during the whole HBETP amounted to 101% ± 46% of the total amount of work expected. Peak work rate, peak $\dot{V}O_2$, and arterial lactate level increased, respectively, by 18% ($p = 0.02$), 11% ($p = 0.05$), and 21% ($p = 0.04$) after training. Endurance time also increased significantly from 202 ± 162 to 710 ± 668 seconds after training ($p = 0.002$). Six-minute walking distance increased significantly from 354 ± 116 meters to 425 ± 110 meters ($p < 0.001$). After HBETP, significant increases in strength of 7% and 6% ($p < 0.05$) were observed for pectoralis major and latissimus dorsi, respectively, while an increase of 5% in quadriceps strength did not reach statistical significance. Each dimension of the questionnaire of quality of life showed significant increase after training.

Interpretation of Results

In a group of patients with severe emphysema being prepared for LVRS, this study shows that home training with minimal supervision is safe and that most patients comply well with the program. It was possible to improve maximal exercise capacity, endurance capacity, walking distance, muscle strength, and quality of life despite the absence of close supervision. Furthermore, the magnitude of improvement in exercise capacity and quality of life is comparable to what has been historically observed following supervised training programs in specialized centers (15).

Home-based training programs are easy to implement even in remote areas. The evaluation and teaching of the training techniques can be completed over 1 day, and the equipment, which includes a safe portable bicycle with stable resistance that can be used at home, is simple. The initial teaching session is crucial to ensure that the program will be performed adequately, and the weekly contacts are also important to maintain patient motivation. By limiting our intervention to an initial 2-hour period of teaching, one phone call a week, and one postal invoice to transmit the diary, costly interventions were reduced to a minimum. The necessary level of supervision was also much less than what has been reported in previous home training studies, in which patients had to make one or more hospital visits per week or had to be home visited by specialized personnel once a week, a supervision that may be difficult to carry out in vast countries (7,10,11). If we except a minimal number of COPD exacerbations, no major injuries or incidents were documented during the time of this study.

In order to avoid injury and to improve tolerance of submaximal exercise such as walking, we emphasize the need for a longer duration and lower intensity of training. Although high-intensity training as defined by Casaburi et al. in 1991 (80% of maximal workload) (3) was not attained during most of the training periods in this study, significant improvements in many aspects of exercise performance were obtained. Our results are in agreement with previous studies, which have shown that decrease in training intensity may be compensated for by an increase in its duration (16,17).

It can finally be argued that patients included in this study were highly motivated because they were part of an LVRS program. Our interpretation, however, is that these patients were severely obstructed and constituted a representative sample of patients with COPD for whom rehabilitation may be beneficial. A similar study should be done in a large group of heterogeneous patients with COPD who are not being proposed for LVRS.

We conclude that it is possible to train patients with advanced emphysema at home and without direct supervision. In motivated patients, compliance to the program was excellent. This exercise program improved performance of endurance tests and efficiently improved quality of life.

References

1. Lacasse, Y., D. Brooks, and R.S. Goldstein. 1999. Trends in epidemiology of chronic obstructive pulmonary disease in Canada, 1980-95. *Chest* 116: 306-313.

2. Ojanen, M., A. Lahdensuo, J. Laitinen, and J. Karvonen. 1993. Psychosocial changes in patients participating in a chronic obstructive pulmonary disease rehabilitation program. *Respiration* 60:96-102.

3. Casaburi, R., A. Patessio, F. Ioli, S. Zanaboni, C.F. Donner, and K. Wasserman. 1991. Reductions in exercise lactic acidosis and ventilation as a result of exercise training in patients with obstructive lung disease. *Am Rev Respir Dis* 143:9-18.

4. Lacasse, Y., R.S. Goldstein, E. Wong, G.H. Guyatt, D. King, and D.J. Cook. 1996. Meta-analysis of respiratory rehabilitation in chronic obstructive pulmonary disease. *Lancet* 348:1115-1119.

5. Casaburi, R. 1993. Exercise training in chronic obstructive lung disease. In *Principles and Practice of Pulmonary Rehabilitation,* ed. R. Casaburi and T.L. Petty. New York: W.B. Saunders.

6. Brooks, D., Y. Lacasse, and R.S. Goldstein. 1999. Pulmonary rehabilitation programs in Canada: national survey. *Can Resp J* 6:55-63.

7. McGavin, C.R., S.P. Gupta, E.L. Lloyd, and J.R. McHardy. 1977. Physical rehabilitation for chronic bronchitis: results of a controlled trial of exercises in the home. *Thorax* 32:307-311.

8. Sinclair, D.J.M., and C.G. Ingram. 1980. Controlled trial of supervised exercise training in chronic bronchitis. *Br Med J* 1:519-521.

9. Busch, A.J., and J.D. McClements. 1988. Effects of a supervised home exercise program on patients with severe obstructive pulmonary disease. *Phys Ther* 68:469-474.

10. Strijbos, J.H., D.S. Postma, P. van Altena, R. Gimeno, and G.H. Koëter. 1996. A comparison between an outpatient hospital-based pulmonary rehabilitation program and a home-care pulmonary rehabilitation program in patients with COPD. A follow-up of 18 months. *Chest* 109:366-372.

11. Wijkstra, P.J., T.W. Van der Mark, J. Kraan, R. van Altena, G.H. Koëter, and D.S. Postma. 1996. Long-term effects of home rehabilitation on physical performance in chronic obstructive pulmonary disease. *Am J Respir Crit Care Med* 153:1234-1241.

12. Debigaré, R., F. Maltais, F. Whittom, J. Deslauriers, and P. LeBlanc. 1999. Feasibility and efficacy of home exercise training before lung volume reduction. *J Cardiopulmonary Rehabil* 19:235-241.

13. Guyatt, G.H., S. Pugsley, M.J. Sullivan, P.J. Thompson, L.B. Berman, N.L. Jones, E.L. Fallen, and D.W. Taylor. 1984. Effect of encouragement on walking test performance. *Thorax* 39:818-822.

14. Guyatt, G.H., L.B. Berman, M. Townsend, S.O. Pugsley, and L.W. Chambers. 1987. A measure of quality of life for clinical trials in chronic lung disease. *Thorax* 42:773-778.

15. Maltais, F., P. LeBlanc, J. Jobin, C. Bérubé, J. Bruneau, L. Carrier, M.-J. Breton, G. Falardeau, and R. Belleau. 1997. Intensity of training and physiological adaptation in patients with chronic obstructive pulmonary disease. *Am J Respir Crit Care Med* 155:555-561.

16. Casaburi, R., T.W. Storer, C.S. Sullivan, and K. Wasserman. 1995. Evaluation of blood lactate elevation as an intensity criterion for exercise training. *Med Sci Sports Exerc* 27:852-862.

17. American College of Sports Medicine. 1990. The recommended quantity and quality of exercise for developing and maintaining cardiorespiratory and muscular fitness in healthy adults. *Med Sci Sports Exerc* 22:265-274.

CHAPTER 15

Quality of Life in Patients With Chronic Obstructive Pulmonary Disease on Long-Term Oxygen Therapy: Role of Exercise Training

Christian Préfaut, Véronique Gautier-Dechaud, Déborah Fuchs-Climent, and Magali Poulain

Département de Physiologie, Université Montpellier, Hôpital Arnaud de Villeneuve, Montpellier, France

Long-term oxygen therapy (LTOT) is an integral part of the treatment of patients with chronic obstructive pulmonary disease (COPD) and severe hypoxemia. In the early 1980s, two randomized trials, the British Medical Research Council Trial (1) and the Nocturnal Oxygen Therapy Trial (NOTT) (2), showed that LTOT for at least 15 hours per day has a substantial beneficial effect on survival of patients with COPD with severe hypoxemia (PaO_2 <60 mmHg).

The main goal in the management of any chronic disease, including COPD, is to improve the quality of life (QL) in patients. In order to assess the quality of life in the patient on LTOT, two main factors must be considered. On the one hand, life expectancy is improved, which should improve QL. On the other hand, the patient is "chained" to a stationary oxygen source at least 15 hours per day, which would seem to impair QL not only directly, but also by increasing the patient's sedentary lifestyle. Good questions can therefore be raised about the actual quality of life for these patients and about whether a comprehensive rehabilitation program that includes exercise training, which is well known to improve COPD (3), is feasible in patients on LTOT. If so, would such a program be able to optimize and even substantially improve the quality of life in patients on LTOT?

Quality of Life in Patients With COPD on Long-Term Oxygen Therapy

In an ancillary study of the NOTT (4), quality of life was not improved over a 6-month period as assessed using a general questionnaire, the Sickness Impact Profile (SIP). In contrast, another study showed that patients felt that their general well-being was improved by LTOT (5). It is well known, however, that these questionnaires have poor responsiveness to differences among treatment groups, though these differences are detected with disease-specific QL instruments (6).

Recently, Okubadejo et al. (7) assessed the effect of LTOT on quality of life using both a generic instrument, the SIP, and a specific instrument, the St. George's Respiratory Questionnaire (SGRQ). Twenty-three hypoxemic patients with COPD were studied before and after starting LTOT at 2 weeks and 3 and 6 months. A control group included 18 patients with COPD with less severe hypoxemia and almost the same FEV_1. Whatever the questionnaire, the authors did not observe a beneficial effect on QL over 6 months of LTOT provided by an oxygen concentrator.

None of these works studied quality of life in the patient on LTOT for more than 6 months, and it is unknown whether QL remains steady or is altered over a longer period. In order to determine this, we investigated 50 patients with severe COPD. Twenty-nine had been under LTOT for at least 1 year (1.7 ± 0.6; *M* ± SD) and the others served as control subjects (table 15.1). Each patient was asked to complete two questionnaires: a generic, the Nottingham Health Profile (NHP) (8), and a specific, the St. George's Respiratory Questionnaire (SGRQ) (9), both validated in the French language (10,11). There were no differences between the groups in terms of demography, clinical state, or lung function, except for blood gases. In the LTOT group, PaO_2 was significantly lower and $PaCO_2$ was slightly higher than in the control group. The Nottingham Health Profile showed only a trend ($p < 0.10$) toward impaired emotional reaction and social isolation in patients on LTOT as compared with control patients, but it showed a very significant decrease in physical mobility and a high impairment in energy in the patients on LTOT. The St. George's Respiratory Questionnaire showed that all item scores were significantly altered and that the total score was very significantly impaired in patients on LTOT in comparison with control patients. It is worth noting that, whether generic or specific, both questionnaires were able to discriminate between the two populations.

The data from these two questionnaires are consistent and indicate that after 1.5 years of long-term oxygen therapy, quality of life in patients with severe COPD is reduced. Indeed, almost all scores, and especially those concerning physical activity, were altered with a parallel increase in the emotional impact of the disease. This probably indicates an impairment in the activities of daily living (ADL) in patients on LTOT, as Okubadejo et al. (12) found that, in 23 patients on LTOT compared to 19 patients with COPD, the patients on LTOT were significantly less independent in activities of daily living than the control group. However, they also found that impairment of activities of daily living was significantly related to the percentage of the predicted FEV_1. Because the patients on LTOT had a lower FEV_1 than those not on LTOT, a possible explanation for this decrease in ADL was a more severe COPD in the patients on LTOT. In the present study, we did not measure ADL. However, the highly significant alteration in activity score on the St. George's Respiratory Questionnaire and the very significant impairment in physical mobility and energy on the Nottingham Health Profile were observed only in the LTOT group, whereas the FEV_1 was the same in both LTOT and control groups. This seems

Table 15.1 Characteristics and Quality of Life of COPD Patients Under Long-Term Oxygen Therapy for 1.7 Years Versus Non-LTOT Patients (*M* ± SD)

	With LTOT (n = 29)	Without LTOT (n = 21)
Age (yr)	61.9 (7.9)	65.8 (7.05)
Body mass (kg)	62.9 (11.6)	71.2 (16)
Height (cm)	164.8 (7)	168.1 (9.5)
FEV_1 (L)	.835 (.33)	.871 (.30)
FEV_1 (% pred.)	30.1 (10)	32.6 (8.7)
FVC	1.99 (.64)	2 (.83)
PaO_2 (mmHg)	51.1 (5.4)**	58.9 (6.8)
$PaCO_2$ (mmHg)	40.5 (5.8)*	37.7 (4.4)
St. Georgés Respiratory Questionnaire		
Symptom	65.4 (15.4)*	51.6 (21.1)
Impact	60.4 (18.4)**	43.5 (20.2)
Activity	83.7 (9.9)***	68.8 (17.8)
Total	68.3 (13)***	52.7 (16.7)
Nottingham Health Profile		
Physical mobility	55.5 (19.0)**	37.0 (20.5)
Emotional reaction	34.6 (26.1) [*]	21.8 (22)
Energy	80.5 (27.8)***	61.7 (34.8)
Social isolation	33.6 (34.4) [*]	17 (28.6)
Sleep	31 (31.4)	42.7 (35.2)
Pain	28.9 (24.5)	21.2 (24)

[*]$p < 0.10$; *$p < 0.05$; **$p < 0.01$; ***$p < 0.001$.

to rule out the exclusive role of obstruction suggested in the Okubadejo et al. study. The second explanation for their results was that LTOT in itself restricts daily activities. Based on the results of the present study, this latter hypothesis should be taken into consideration.

In summary, even though long-term oxygen therapy increases life expectancy in patients with COPD, it does not improve quality of life over a 6-month period. Furthermore, after 1.5 years of LTOT this quality of life decreases, probably as a result of a decrease in physical mobility and activities of daily living. We can reasonably assume that oxygen therapy confines patients to home more and reduces their overall exercise level. In turn, this decrease in physical activity increases the psychosocial impact of the disease.

Feasibility and Effects of Exercise Training in Patients on LTOT

The main goal of any rehabilitation program is to improve quality of life. As reported previously, this is not the result of LTOT rehabilitation in patients with COPD, probably because of the restriction in movement imposed by the stationary oxygen device and by the resulting poor psychosocial status. Exercise training programs are well known to improve exercise tolerance and quality of life in patients with moderate to severe COPD (3). There is therefore a strong rationale for hypothesizing that exercise training would improve exercise tolerance and quality of life, thereby allowing greater independence in the activities of daily living for patients with very severe COPD who are on LTOT. Unfortunately, we were unable to find any study on this topic in the literature. The aim of the present preliminary study was to investigate (a) the feasibility and (b) the effects of a rehabilitation program including exercise training on exercise tolerance and quality of life in patients with COPD who are on LTOT.

Methods

The methods that we employed in evaluating the feasibility and effects of exercise training are briefly discussed below.

Patients Thirty patients with COPD on long-term oxygen therapy were enrolled in this study. Ten were trained at the hospital as outpatients, 10 others were trained at home, and the last 10 served as controls. Baseline characteristics of these patients are reported in table 15.2.

Evaluation Exercise tolerance was evaluated by an incremental exercise test and by the 6-minute walking test performed under oxygen.

The incremental exercise test was performed on a calibrated cycle ergometer (Ergolyne 900, Germany) according to our individualized protocol (13,14). Briefly, the maximal predicted work rate was calculated according to the equation of Jones et al. (15) and then adapted to the patient by multiplying it by the ratio FEV_1/FEV_1 predicted. The 3-minute warm-up was conducted at 20% of this estimated maximal work rate. The work rate was then increased 8% of this estimated value every minute. This method allowed us to obtain maximal work rate in 7 to 10-minute increases of very small increments. The incremental exercise test allowed us to record symptom-limited maximal workload and dyspnea threshold. This latter was defined as the breakpoint in the dyspnea-vs.-work rate relationship. The dyspnea was evaluated on a visual analogic scale. The 6-minute walking test allowed us to report the maximal distance covered in 6 minutes. Finally, both tests were conducted

Table 15.2 Characteristics of LTOT Patients: Rehabilitation and Control Groups (*M* ± SD)

	Outpatients	At-home patients	Control patients
Age (yr)	64.1 (8.6)	61.3 (12)	62.4 (11.5)
Height (cm)	168.1 (9.7)	166.5 (6.8)	162.4 (9)
Body mass (kg)	66.5 (10.9)	69 (9.4)	61.3 (11.6)
FEV_1 (L)	0.82 (0.21)	0.96 (0.18)	0.91 (0.16)
FEV_1 /FVC (%)	41.8 (13.3)	38.9 (10.9)	39.3 (8.2)
PaO_2 (mmHg)	52.6 (5.2)	53.6 (5.3)	54.2 (4.5)
$PaCO_2$ (mmHg)	40.2 (5.3)	45.2 (5.4)*	40.5 (4.5)

*$p < 0.05$ vs. control.

under oxygen in order to maintain hemoglobin saturation in oxygen (SpO_2) greater than 90%.

Quality of life was studied using two questionnaires, the generic Nottingham Health Profile and the specific St. George's Respiratory Questionnaire. They were administered before and after the formal rehabilitation program.

Training Program Patients were instructed to perform one session of stationary bicycle exercise per day, 2 days per week, over an 8-week period. The target exercise intensity level was based on the heart rate recorded at the dyspnea threshold. The training schedule consisted of a 5-minute warm-up followed by 10 minutes of work and 5 minutes of active recovery repeated twice (30-minute session). During training, heart rate was continuously monitored by a heart rate meter (Sport tester PE3000, Finland). The patient was instructed to exercise within ± 5 beats per minute^{-1} of the target heart rate. An alarm ensured that the patient trained within the preselected range.

Rehabilitation Program

All patients received educational and psychosocial support and breathing exercise instruction.

At-Home Protocol A stationary bicycle, a heart rate meter, and documentation were given to the patient for the 2-month period. The first session at home was done under the supervision of a physician and nurse in the presence of the patient's physical therapist. The physician or nurse then followed the session at day 8 and then every 15 days. Between visits the patients were asked to record training information in a notebook.

Table 15.3 Exercise Tolerance in all Patient Groups Before and After Rehabilitation Program (M ± SD)

	Outpatients		At-home patients		Control patients	
	Before	After	Before	After	Before	After
6-minute walk test distance (m)	296.5 (93)	335.4* (86)	305 (73)	345.2* (86.6)	294.5 (79.6)	311 (99.8)
W max SL (% predicted)	18.7 (12.5)	26.4* (13.9)	25.5 (12)	38** (13.2)	26.6 (12.5)	27.2 (11.3)
Dyspnea threshold (% W max predicted)	11.3 (5.6)	18.6** (7.1)	13.1 (5.2)	24.7*** (7)	13.6 (7.7)	14.2 (6.5)

*p < 0.05; **p < 0.01; ***p < 0.001 vs. control.

Results

Exercise Tolerance

Exercise tolerance was significantly improved both in terms of 6-minute walking distance and symptom-limited maximal work load in both exercising groups but not in the control group. The dyspnea threshold was shifted to the right; that is to say, to higher work rates, in both exercising groups but, again, not in the control group (table 15.3).

Quality of Life

The outpatient data showed significant improvement ($p < 0.05$) only in the activity score of the SGRQ. With the same questionnaire, there was no change at all for the at-home patients, although there was a significant decrease ($p < 0.05$) in emotional reaction and a trend ($p < 0.10$) toward improvement in energy and sleep in the NHP. Finally, when both groups were pooled in order to increase the number of patients, we observed a significant decrease ($p < 0.05$) in impact score and a trend toward improvement in activity and total score ($p < 0.10$) in the SGRQ. In the NHP, we observed a significant decrease ($p < 0.05$) in emotional reaction and a trend ($p < 0.10$) to improvement in energy (table 15.4). There was no change at all in the control group.

Although this is not a questionnaire item, an interesting side point is that 7 out of 10 patients in the at-home group bought a training cycle at the end of the formal training program.

Table 15.4 Quality of Life Before and After a Rehabilitation Program in COPD Patients Under LTOT

	Rehabilitation groups		Control group	
	Before	After	Before	After
St. George's Respiratory Questionnaire				
Symptom	52.8 (18.9)	58.3 (23.9)	67.6 (27.9)	58.6 (22.5)
Impact	49.9 (19.9)	45.2 (17.4)*	56.8 (25)	56.6 (22.5)
Activity	75 (14.5)	72.3 (15.5)[*]	84.4 (10.2)	86 (9.8)
Total	57.9 (16)	55.1 (15)[*]	65.8 (18.6)	67 (19.8)
Nottingham Health Profile				
Physical mobility	41.9 (18.7)	39.2 (22.5)	54.2 (35)	47.7 (36.9)
Emotional reaction	25.4 (19.5)	18.5 (26.7)*	17.7 (25.5)	21.5 (24)
Energy	71.2 (34.3)	56.7 (41.4)[*]	63.3 (42.4)	73 (35)
Social isolation	11.7 (15)	12.4 (19.5)	6.15 (12.3)	11.2 (13)
Sleep	34.4 (35.6)	29.8 (31.6)	35.7 (31.4)	34.1 (28.2)
Pain	16.4 (12.7)	15.4 (18.5)	19.1 (13.8)	17.8 (13.7)

*p < 0.10; [*]p < 0.05.

Discussion

This study showed that exercise training in patients on LTOT (a) is feasible, (b) induces an increase in exercise tolerance, and (c) seems to improve, at least partially, quality of life.

All patients completed the entire program, which was well tolerated. Following training each patient experienced a subjective enhancement of well-being. The notebooks were well kept by the home patients, and no incidents or side effects were reported. Compliance with training was excellent. Therefore, an individualized training program at the level of the dyspnea threshold in patients on LTOT seems to be entirely feasible.

We observed an increase in distance of about 40 meters in the 6-minute walk test in both training groups, which was statistically significant. Recently, Redelmeier et al. (16) showed that the clinically significant difference was 54 meters. In fact, these authors observed that patients were able to detect a positive difference of about 40 meters but a negative difference of about 70 meters. This can be explained by the fact that individuals may view positive and negative differences asymmetrically because they are not equally sensitive to gains and losses. Therefore, this raises the question of whether a value that is the sample average of positive and negative evaluation is a good indicator of clinical improvement. We believe that the clinical reference should be the value reported for a given direction: 40 meters when we are looking for an improvement, 70 meters when we have to evaluate an impairment. Based on this reasoning, we observed a clinically and statistically significant change in the 6-minute walking distance after training in the patients on LTOT. These results were consistent with both the general clinical improvement described by the patients and the observed increase in the maximal symptom-limited workload after training. Furthermore, we observed a significant shift to the right in the dyspnea threshold, which indicated that dyspnea appeared for higher work levels and which would allow patients to increase the activities of daily living.

The improved exercise tolerance observed in these patients emphasizes the importance of the choice of intensity level in these patients. There are two global approaches to the prescription of exercise intensity in a training program. The first is a physiological approach at a very high intensity level (80% $\dot{V}O_2$ symptom limited), proposed by the Casaburi group (17). The rationale is that at high levels the improvement will be greater and will last longer. Our approach is more behavior based. We usually train our patients at the intensity of the ventilatory threshold because it allows an individualized prescription at an intensity level that avoids excessive dyspnea, thus maximizing compliance. It is difficult to precisely determine ventilatory threshold during an incremental exercise test under oxygen. However, it is relatively easy to determine the level at which there is an abrupt increase (breakpoint) in the dyspnea. This specific approach to training, which is always individualized, was well accepted by the patients and induced measurable improvement in exercise tolerance of these patients.

The present results seem to indicate that the exercise training program slightly improved some of the scores on the quality of life questionnaires, especially when we pooled the data of both training populations. It is interesting to note that, although the changes were small, they appeared in the components that were the most altered in the patients on LTOT for 1.5 years. These included the components related to activity and energy, as well as those related to disease impact and emotional reaction. In this study, both the generic and specific questionnaires were able to detect changes in the time course of quality of life. However, it is clear that we need a study with many more patients in order to demonstrate conclusively that such an exercise training program is able to significantly and clinically improve quality of life in patients on LTOT. With this in mind, we have devised a randomized multicentric study to investigate the true benefits of such a program in a larger number of patients with COPD (100) on LTOT.

References

1. MRC Working Party. 1981. Long-term domiciliary oxygen in chronic hypoxic cor pulmonale complicating chronic bronchitis and emphysema. *Lancet* i:681-686.

2. Nocturnal Oxygen Therapy Group. 1980. Continuous or nocturnal oxygen therapy in hypoxemic chronic obstructive lung disease: a clinical trial. *Ann Intern Med* 93:391-398.

3. Lacasse, Y., E. Wong, G.H. Guyatt, D. King, D.J. Cook, and R.S. Goldstein. 1996. Meta-analysis of respiratory rehabilitation in chronic obstructive pulmonary disease. *Lancet* 348:1115-1119.

4. Heaton, R.K., I. Grant, and A.J. McSweeney, et al. 1984. Psychologic effects of continuous and nocturnal oxygen therapy in hypoxemic chronic obstructive pulmonary disease. *Arch Intern Med* 143:1941-1947.

5. Dilworth, J.P., C.M.B. Higgs, P.A. Jones, and R.J. White. 1990. Acceptability of oxygen concentrators: the patient's view. *Br J Gen Pract* 40:415-417.

6. Lacasse, Y., E. Wong, G. Guyatt, and R.S. Goldstein. 1997. Health status measurement instruments in chronic obstructive pulmonary disease. *Can Respir J* 4:152-164.

7. Okubadejo, A.A., E.A. Paul, P.W. Jones, and J.A. Wedzica. 1996. Does long-term oxygen therapy affect quality of life in patients with chronic obstructive pulmonary disease and severe hypoxemia? *Eur Respir J* 9:2335-2339.

8. Hunt, S.M., S.P. McKenna, J. McEven, E.M. Backett, J. Williams, and E. Papp. 1980. A quantitative approach to perceived health status: a validation study. *J Epidemiol Comm Health* 34:281-286.

9. Jones, P.W., F.H. Quirk, and C.M. Baveystock. 1991. The St. George's Respiratory Questionnaire. *Respir Med 85* (suppl. B):25-31.

10. Bucquet, D., S. Condon, and K. Ritchie. 1990. The French version of the Nottingham Health Profile. A comparison of item weights with those of the source version. *Soc Med Sci* 7:829-835.

11. Bouchet, C.H., F. Guillemin, T.H. Hoang Thi, A. Cornette, and S. Briançon. 1996. Validation du questionnaire St. Georges pour mesurer la qualite de vie chez les insuffisants respiratoires chroniques. *Rev Mal Resp* 13:43-46.

12. Okubadejo, A.A., L. O'Shea, P.W. Jones, and J.A. Wedzicha. 1997. Home assessment of activities of daily living in patients with severe chronic obstructive pulmonary disease on long-term oxygen therapy. *Eur Respir J* 10:1572-1575.

13. Vallet, G., S. Ahmaidi, I. Serres, C. Fabre, D. Bourgouin, J. Desplan, A. Varray, and C. Préfaut. 1997. Comparison of two training programmes in chronic airway limitation patients: standardized versus individualized protocols. *Eur Respir J* 10:114-122.

14. Varray, A., and C. Prefaut. 1995. Exercise training in patients with respiratory disease: procedures and results. *Eur Respir Rev* 5:25, 51-58.

15. Jones, N.L., L. Markrides, and C. Hitchcock, et al. 1985. Normal standards for an incremental progressive cycle ergometer test. *Am Rev Resp Dis* 131:700-708.

16. Redelmeier, D.A., A.M. Bayoumi, R.S. Goldstein, and G.H. Guyatt. 1997. Interpreting small differences in functional status: the six minute walk test in chronic lung disease patients. *Am J Respir Crit Care Med* 155:1278-1282.
17. Casaburi, R., J. Porszasz, M.R. Burns, E.R Carithers, R.S.Y. Chang, and C.B. Cooper. 1997. Physiologic benefits of exercise training in rehabilitation of patients with severe chronic obstructive pulmonary disease. *Am J Respir Crit Care Med* 155:1541-1551.

PART VI

Psychosociological Aspects of Cardiopulmonary Rehabilitation

CHAPTER 16

Stress and Coronary Artery Disease: Should Stress Management Be Taken Into Consideration in the Rehabilitation of Patients With Coronary Artery Disease?

Dany-Michel Marcadet
Clinique Bizet, Paris, France

The aim of cardiac rehabilitation is to "limit the physiological and psychological effects of cardiac illness, reduce the risk of sudden death or reinfarction, control cardiac symptoms, stabilize or reverse the atherosclerosis process, and enhance the psychosocial and vocational status of selected patients"(1). Rehabilitation, based on exercise, improves functional capacity and reduces risk factors such as hypertension, diabetes, smoking, and high cholesterol levels.

Stress Factors and Coronary Artery Disease

Several factors influence the individual's perception of and response to stress.

Psychosocial Factors

Although the importance of psychosocial factors in coronary artery disease has long been underestimated, these factors should not be neglected. Indeed, increasing evidence indicates that psychiatric disorders may play an important role in patients with coronary artery disease, and numerous publications have shown that stress influences the cardiovascular system by way of neurohormonal regulators (2).

In his description of the "general adaptation syndrome," Hans Selye (3) defined stress as "the nonspecific response of the body to any demand upon it." This definition is, however, imprecise because all demands on the organism are not necessarily stressful.

It is difficult to satisfactory define stress because an adequate definition must include the stimulus, the organism's response to it, and the psychological state of the individual. Even if the definition of stress remains imprecise, it represents a recognizable state that patients can blame for their illness. For instance, patients will often say "Stress is the cause of my heart attack." Emotional stress is also associated with higher rates of subsequent cardiac events in patients with known coronary artery disease (4).

Stressors

The response to stress is variable and often depends on both the intensity of the stimulus and the individual's own characteristics. The stimulus can be violent and acute. For example, a natural catastrophe may result in a dramatic rise in rates of heart attacks or sudden deaths (5,6). In other cases, such as in certain stressful conditions, the stimulus is of lower intensity but more chronic. These situations may also result in an increase in coronary heart disease (7-9) through the stimulation of the hypothalamic-pituitary-adrenocortical and sympathetic systems (2).

Individual Characteristics

As shown in animal models (10), patients' responses to stress are at least in part a function of their genetic makeup, which can, on occasion, be modified by neonatal stress. An overactive gene may increase the production of the corticotropin-releasing factor (CRF) in the hypothalamus or may regulate several essential neurotransmitters such as serotonin, adrenaline, noradrenaline, and dopamine. Neurotransmitters are involved in various mental diseases, and CRF levels are abnormally high in people with severe depression and in those who commit suicide (11). These responses to stress appear to be more frequent in people with certain personality types.

Early on, most research efforts were centered on the study of the type A behavior pattern, characterized by time urgency and free-floating hostility (12,13). However, findings are inconsistent regarding the association of this type of behavior with coronary artery disease (14). More recently, research has shifted to emotional distress and its possible effects on coronary heart disease. For example, a meta-analytic review of research on hostility and physical health confirmed that anger and hostility were potential risk factors for the development of coronary heart disease (15). It also suggested that the development of coronary heart disease was also associated with other negative emotional conditions (4). Higher levels of worry in specific areas such as social conditions may increase the risk of coronary heart disease in older men (16). The occurrence of coronary heart disease has also been associated with anxiety (17), emotional exhaustion (18), and hopelessness (19).

A large number of studies have established a clear relationship between depression and coronary heart disease. Depression is very common in the general population and more than 65% of cardiac patients are depressed after a myocardial infarction (20). Usually, these symptoms decrease within several days of the infarct and are considered benign reactions to an acute, traumatic episode. In 15%-20% of cases, however, the symptoms are more significant. They persist after the first few days and are indicative of severe depression (21-23). Diagnosing postmyocardial infarction depression may be difficult because its symptoms are vague and often confused with cardiac symptoms.

Depression is also responsible for higher levels of sick leave, repeated hospital admissions, and, most importantly, recurring cardiac events with fatal or nonfatal myocardial infarctions (24). Depression can predict coronary artery disease (21) and is therefore more important than type A categorizing as a behavior predictor (4). In 1993 and 1995, Frasure-Smith et al. (25,26) studied 222 patients hospitalized for acute myocardial infarction and showed that depression was a predictive factor of death regardless of left ventricular ejection fraction or extent of coronary lesions. The risk factor of depression was higher than other known risk factors such as age, sex, smoking, aspirin consumption, use of β-blockers, use of thrombolytics, and left ventricular ejection fraction. Patients with ventricular arrhythmias had a higher risk, which suggested the presence of a possible arrhythmogenic mechanism.

More recently, Denollet and colleagues (27,28) showed that type D personality, defined as one with negative affect and tendency to inhibit the expression of emotions, was a relevant factor in predicting death in coronary patients. Two hundred sixty-eight patients were studied during a period of 8-10 years. Of all patients who experienced cardiac death during the interval (n = 38), the rate of death was higher for type D patients (27%) than for those without type D personalities (7%). In that study, the authors also found a positive correlation between death and changes in left ventricular ejection fraction, extent of coronary lesions, a small exercise capacity, and absence of use of thrombolytics during the acute phase of the myocardial infarction. Statistical analysis, however, showed that type D personality was a significant predictor of long-term mortality, independent of histochemical risk factors. In a more recent study of 87 patients with myocardial infarction and changes in left ventricular function (<50%), Denollet and Brutsaert (28) found that type D personality was a risk factor for repeated cardiac events such as myocardial infarction and sudden death. In their analysis, type D personality was an independent predicting factor, just as an ejection fraction smaller than 30% was. According to the authors, patients with type D personality are particularly sensitive to emotions, which may induce coronary spasm, increased platelet aggregation, and decrease in heart rate variability linked to modifications of the sympathetic tone. These mechanisms are also thought to be responsible for the biological response to stress. Evidence also suggests that a number of other direct or indirect mechanisms may explain the association between psychosocial stress and coronary heart disease.

Cardiovascular Changes Related to Stress

Cardiovascular changes related to acute or chronic stress are complex because they involve several mechanisms transmitted through the sympathetic nervous, hypothalamic-pituitary-adrenocortical, parasympathetic nervous, or renin-angiotensin-aldosterone systems, or through systems involving vasopressin and endogenous opioids. The effect of each mechanism alone is known, but when these mechanisms interact, the overall results may be different for each individual.

Catecholamines play an important role in some of the changes occurring in the cardiovascular system, but their role in heart disease is still not yet fully understood. They also play a specific role in other coronary atherosclerosis risk factors such as hypertension, hyperlipidemia, smoking, obesity, and insulin resistance, and are responsible for a number of events in patients with known coronary disease (2). Fatal and nonfatal cardiac events in patients with coronary heart disease can be induced by the development of atherosclerosis, ischemia, or arrhythmia.

Mechanisms That Relate Stress and Coronary Artery Disease

Several mechanisms that relate stress and coronary artery disease are briefly described below.

Stress-Induced Arterial Endothelial Injury and Serum Lipid Levels

The activation of the sympathetic system or of the adrenocortical system can accelerate the development of atherosclerosis by raising the peak blood flow velocity and heart rate, which may result in turbulence, increased endothelial cell turnover, and arterial wall damage (29). Several studies have also shown that stress is associated with disturbances in the lipid metabolism such as excessive mobilization of the free fatty acids and a rise in triglyceride and cholesterol levels (30-32).

Ischemia

Several authors have demonstrated the role of stress in the occurrence of severe myocardial ischemia (33,34) with left ventricular dysfunction (35) in patients with cardiac disease. It is possible that in those cases, ischemia remains silent (36) because of a parallel rise in β-endorphin levels (37). The presence of mental stress-induced ischemia is associated with significantly higher rates of subsequent fatal or nonfatal cardiac events independent of age, baseline left ventricular ejection fraction, or previous myocardial infarction. It is also associated with higher rates of predicted events over and above exercise-induced ischemia (38).

The mechanism of ischemia appears to be that of a paradoxical vasoconstriction of diseased coronary arteries probably related to decreased levels of endothelium-derived relaxing factor (EDRF). Serotonin released from aggregating platelets and thrombin formed by the coagulation cascade, have been shown to dilate normal coronary arteries through the release of endothelium-derived relaxing factor (EDRF). Atherosclerotic arteries, which are deficient in EDRF, are paradoxically constricted by serotonin and thrombin (39,40).

Mental stress-induced myocardial ischemia also occurs at lower heart rates than during exercise-induced stress. In this setting, there is a significant increase in systemic vascular resistance with relatively minor increases in heart rate and rate-pressure product when compared to ischemia induced by exercise. These hemodynamic responses to mental stress are thought to be mediated by the adrenal secretion of adrenaline (41).

In myocardial ischemia, there is also a rise in blood viscosity and levels of fibrinogen with secondary hemoconcentration favoring hypercoagulability and platelet activation (42-47). A reduction in fibrinolytic capacity in exhausted individuals has been noted by Kop et al. (43). All of these changes seem to be caused by higher levels of catecholamines, which would explain the higher frequency of myocardial infarction in the morning when the catecholamines are at their circadian peak (48). This phenomenon decreases when patients are treated with b-blockers (49).

Arrhythmia

In patients with coronary heart disease, stress has been found to induce ischemic and arrhythmic responses. When compared with standard exercise tests, stress caused more arrhythmic reactions than ischemic ones. Stress appears to induce these reactions through increased cardiac dynamics probably mediated through the direct action of catecholamines or other stress hormones on the myocardium and coronary arteries (50). Psychological stress in coronary patients increases ventricular ectopic activity and risk of ventricular fibrillation (51-53).

Interestingly, although the onset of increased vulnerability in response to stress occurs rapidly, the return to normal electrophysiological status after the removal of stress is more prolonged (54). Myocardial ischemia is the most significant factor in ventricular instability, and the myocardium is electrically destabilized by increased adrenergic tone (54). Modifications of ventricular repolarization may mediate the generation of stress-provoked arrhythmias in electrically unstable hearts (55). A significant body of clinical and experimental data supports the concept that ventricular fibrillation is the most common cause of sudden cardiac death among patients with previous coronary artery disease (56), and that stress provokes cardiac arrhythmia (57) and diminishes the threshold of ventricular fibrillation (58). Hypokalemia induced by adrenaline can increase the risk of arrhythmias, and signs of the activation of the sympathetic system often precede arrhythmia (51).

Conclusion

Stress management programs are currently popular but their overall effect on cardiovascular disease is still unclear. It is therefore important to consider individual psychosocial factors and their role in coronary heart disease.

Many unsolved problems remain, however, and represent a challenge for the future. For example, what medication should be given in the treatment of anxiety and depression? Are psychotherapies and behavioral therapies efficient? Does treatment reduce the risk of coronary artery disease and its complications?

Indeed, there is a great need for additional research because some studies have shown a correlation between stress and cardiac disease (59,60), whereas others have shown conflicting results (61). In order to increase treatment efficiency, cardiac rehabilitation needs the support of specialized teams that include physiotherapists, cardiologists, nurses, and perhaps neuroendocrinologists.

References

1. American Association of Cardiovascular and Pulmonary Rehabilitation. 1995. *Guidelines for Cardiac Rehabilatation Programs,* 2nd ed. Champaign, IL: Human Kinetics.
2. Goldstein, D.S. 1995. *Stress, Catecholamines, and Cardiovascular Disease.* New York: Oxford University Press.
3. Selye, H. 1946. The general adaptation syndrome and the diseases of adaptation. *J Clin Endocrinol* 6:117.
4. Booth-Kewley, S., and H.S. Friedman. 1987. Psychological predictors of heart disease: a quantitative review. *Psychol Bull* 101:343-362.
5. Leor, J., W.K. Poole, and R.A. Kloner. 1996. Sudden cardiac death triggered by an earthquake. *N Engl J Med* 334(7):460-461.
6. Suzuki, S., S. Sakamoto, and M. Koide, et al. 1977. Hanshin-Awaji earthquake as a trigger for acute myocardial infarction. *Am Heart J* 134(5):974-977.
7. Bosma, H., R. Peter, J. Siegrist, and M. Marmot. 1998. Two alternative job stress models and the risk of coronary heart disease. *Am J Public Health* 88(1):68-74.
8. Warheit, G.J. 1974. Occupation a key factor in stress at the manned space center. In *Stress and the Heart,* ed. R.S. Eliot. Mt. Kisko, NY: Futura Publishing Company.
9. Niedhammer, I., M. Goldberg, A. Leclerc, S. David, I. Bugel, and M.F. Landre. 1998. Psychosocial work environment and cardiovascular risk factors in occupational cohort in France. *J Epidemiol Comm Health* 52(2):93-100.

10. Walker, C.D. 1995. Chemical sympathectomy and maternal separation affect neonatal stress responses and adrenal sensitivity to ACTH. *Am J Physiol* 268(5 Pt 2): R1281-1288.
11. Stokes, P.E., and C.R. Sikes. 1988. The hypothalamic-pituitary-adrenocortical axis in major depression. *Neuro Clin* (6):1-19.
12. Friedman, M., and R.H. Rosenman. 1959. Association of specific overt behavior pattern with blood and cardiovascular findings. *JAMA* 169:1286.
13. Dembroski, T.M., J.M. MacDouglall, and P.T. Costa, et al. 1989. Components of hostility as predictors of sudden death and myocardial infarction in the Multiple Risk Factor Intervention Trial. *Psychosom Med* 51:514-522.
14. Dimsdale, J.E. 1998. A perspective on Type A behavior and coronary disease. *N Engl J Med* 318:110-112.
15. Miller, T.Q., T.W. Smith, C.W. Turner, M.L. Guijarro, and A.J. Hallet. 1996. A meta-analytic review of research on hostility and physical health. *Psychol Bull* 119:322-348.
16. Kubzansky, L.M., I. Kawachi, and A. Spiro, et al. 1997. Is worrying bad for your heart? A prospective study of worry and coronary heart disease in the normative aging study. *Circulation* 95(4):818-824.
17. Kawachi, I., D. Sparrow, P.S. Vokonas, and S.T. Weiss. 1994. Symptoms of anxiety and risk of coronary heart disease: the normative aging study. *Circulation* 90:2225-2229.
18. Appels, A., and P. Mulder. 1988. Excess fatigue as a precursor of myocardial infarction. *Eur Heart J* 9:758-764.
19. Anda, R.F., D.F. Williamson, D. Johns, C. Macera, E. Eaker, A.H. Glassman, and J. Marks. 1993. Depressed affect, hopelessness, and the risk of ischemic heart disease in a cohort of US adults. *Epidemiology* 4:285-294.
20. Cassem, H., and T.P. Hackett. 1971. Psychiatric consultation in a coronary care unit. *Ann Intern Med* 75:9-14.
21. Carney, R.M., K.E. Freedland, and A.S. Jaffe. 1990. Insomnia and depression prior to myocardial infarction. *Psychosom Med* 52:603-609.
22. Forrester, A.W., J.R. Lipsey, M.L. Teitelbaum, J.R. DePaulo, P.L. Andrzejewski, and R.G. Robinson. 1992. Depression following myocardial infarction. *Int J Psychiatr Med* 22:33-46.
23. Ladwig, K.H., W. Lehmacher, R. Roth, G. Breithhardt, T. Budde, and M. Borggrefe. 1992. Factors which provoke post-infarction depression: results from the post-infarction late potential study. *J Psychosom Res* 36:723-729.
24. Glassman, A.H., and P.A. Shapiro. 1998. Depression and the course of coronary artery disease. *Am J Psychiatr* 155:4-11.
25. Frasure-Smith, N., F. Lespérance, and M. Talajic. 1993. Depression following myocardial infarction. Impact on 6-month survival. *J Am Med Assoc* 270:1819-1825.

26. Frasure-Smith, N., F. Lespérance, and M. Talajic. 1995. Depression and 18-month prognosis after myocardial infarction. *Circulation* 91:999-1005.

27. Denollet, J., S.V. Sys, N. Stroobant, H. Rombouts, T.C. Gillebert, and D.L. Brutsaert. 1996. Personality as independent predictor of long-term mortality in patients with coronary heart disease. *Lancet* 347:417-421.

28. Denollet, J., and D.L. Brutsaert. 1998. Personality, disease severity, and the risk of long-term cardiac events in patients with a decreased ejection fraction after myocardial infarction. *Circulation* 167-173.

29. Pauletto, P., G. Scannapieco, and A.C. Pessina. 1991. Sympathetic drive and vascular damage in hypertension and atherosclerosis. *Hypertens* 17(suppl. III):III75-III81.

30. Cathey, M.S., H.B. Jones, and J. Naughton, et al. 1962. The relationship between life stress and concentration of serum lipids in patients with coronary artery disease. *Am J Med* 244:421-441.

31. Taggart, P., and M. Carruthers. 1971. Endogenous hyperlipidemia induced by emotional stress of racing driving. *Lancet* 1:363-366.

32. Thomas, C.B., and E.A. Murphy. 1967. The precursors of hypertension and coronary disease: statistical consideration of distributions in a population of medical students. II. Blood pressure. *Johns Hopkins Med J* 120(1):1-20.

33. Gottdiener, J.S., D.S. Krantz, and R.H. Howell, et al. 1994. Induction of silent myocardial ischemia with mental stress testing: relation to the triggers of ischemic functional severity. *J Am Coll Cardiol* 24:1645-1651.

34. Legault, S.E., M.R. Freeman, A. Langer, and P.W. Armstrong. 1995. Pathophysiology and time course of silent myocardial ischaemia during mental stress: clinical, anatomical, and physiological correlates. *Br Heart J* 73:242-249.

35. Jain, D., M. Burg, R. Soufer, and B.L. Zaret. 1995. Prognostic implications of mental stress-induced silent left ventricular dysfunction in patients with stable angina pectoris. *Am J Cardiol* 76:31-35.

36. Legault, S.E., A. Langer, P.W. Armstrong, and M.R. Freeman. 1995. Usefulness of ischemic response to mental stress in predicting silent ischaemia during ambulatory monitoring. *Am J Cardiol* 75:1007-1011.

37. Scheps, D.S., M.N. Ballenger, and G.E. De Gent, et al. 1995. Psychophysical responses to a speech stressor: correlation of plasma β-endorphin levels at rest and after psychological stress with thermally measured pain threshold in patients with coronary artery disease. *J Am Cardiol* 25:1499-1503.

38. Jiang, W., M. Babyak, and D.S. Krantz, et al. 1996. Mental stress-induced myocardial ischemia and cardiac events. *JAMA* 275(21):1651-1656.

39. Meredith, I.T., A.C. Yeung, and F.F. Weidinger, et al. 1993. Role of impaired endothelium-dependent vasodilation in ischemic manifestations of coronary artery disease. *Circulation* 93(suppl.):V56-V66.

40. Yeung, A.C., V.I. Vekshtein, and D.S. Krantz, et al. 1991. The effect of atherosclerosis on the vasomotor response of coronary arteries to mental stress. *New Engl J Med* 325:1551-1556.

41. Goldberg, A.D., L.C. Becker, and R. Bonsall, et al. 1996. Ischemic, hemodynamic, and neurohormonal responses to mental and exercise stress: experience from the Psychophysiological Investigations of Myocardial Ischemia Study (PIMI). *Circulation* 94:2402-2409.

42. Larson, P.T., P. Hjemdahl, and G. Olsson, et al. 1990. Platelet aggregability in humans: contrasting in vivo and in vivo findings during sympatho-adrenal activation and relationship to serum lipids. *Eur J Clin Invest* 20:398-405.

43. Kop, W.J., K. Hamulyak, C. Pernot, and A. Appels.1998. Relationship of blood coagulation and fibrinolysis to vital exhaustion. *Psychosom Med* 60(3):352-358.

44. Muldoon, M.F., T.B. Herbert, S.M. Patterson, M. Kameneva, R. Raible, and S.B. Manuck. 1995. Effects of acute psychological stress on serum lipid levels, hemoconcentration, and blood viscosity. *Arch Intern Med* 155(6):615-620.

45. Levine, S.P., B.L. Towell, A.M. Suarez, L.K. Knieriem, M.M. Harris, and J.N. George. 1985. Platelet activation and secretion associated with emotional stress. *Circulation* 7:1129-1134.

46. Grignani, G., F. Soffiantino, M. Zucchella, L. Pacchiarini, F. Tacconi, and E. Bonomi, et al. 1991. Platelet activation by emotional stress in patients with coronary artery disease. *Circulation* 83(suppl. II):II128-II136.

47. Malkoff, S.B., M.F. Muldoon, Z.R. Zeigler, and S.B. Manuck. 1993. Blood platelet responsivity to acute mental stress. *Psychosom Med* 55(6):477-482.

48. Tofler, G.H., D. Brezinski, and A.I. Schafer, et al. 1987. Concurrent morning increase in aggregability and the risk of myocardial infarction and sudden death. *N Engl J Med* 316:514-518.

49. Willich, R.B., T. Linderer, K. Wegcheider, A. Leizorovicz, I. Alamercery, and R. Schroder. 1989. Increased morning incidence of myocardial infarction in the ISAM study: absence with prior β-adrenergic blockade. *Circulation* 87:1442-1450.

50. Lyamina, N.P., E.S. Khalfen, and F.Z. Meerson. 1991. Effect of stress and exercise tests on cardiac performance and adrenergic regulation in patients with coronary heart disease. *Kardiologiya* 31:42-45.

51. Adgey, A.A.J., J.E. Delvin, and S.W. Webb, et al. 1991. Initiation of ventricular fibrillation outside hospital in patients with acute ischaemic heart disease. *Kardiologiya* 31:42-45.

52. Tavazzi, L., A.M. Zotti, and R. Rondanelli. 1986. The role of psychologic stress in the genesis of lethal arrhythmias in patients with coronary artery disease. *Eur Heart J* 7(suppl. A):99-106.

53. Follick, M.J., L. Gorkin, and R.J. Capone. 1988. Psychological distress as a predictor of ventricular arrhythmias in a post-myocardial infarction population. *Am Heart J* 116:32-36.

54. Lown, B., R.A. De Silva, and P. Reich, et al. 1980. Psychologic factors in sudden cardiac death. *Am J Psychiatr* 137:1325-1335.

55. Toivonen, L., K. Helenius, and M. Viitaselo. 1997. Electrocardiographic repolarisation during stress from awakening on alarm call. *Am J Cardiol* 30(3):774-779.

56. Lown, B., and R.L. Verrier. 1976. Neural activity and ventricular fibrillation. *N Engl J Med* 294:1165-1170.

57. Dolon, P.T., A. Meadow, and E. Amsterdam. 1979. Emotional stress as a factor in ventricular arrhythmias. *Psychosomatics* 20:233.

58. Lynch, J.J., D.A. Paskewitz, K.S. Guinbel, and S.A. Thomas. 1977. Psychological aspects of cardiac arrhythmia. *Am Heart J* 93:645.

59. Merz, C.N.B., D.S. Krantz, and A. Rozanski. 1993. Mental stress and myocardial ischemia: correlates and potential interventions. *Tex Heart Inst J* 20(3):152-157.

60. Friedman, M., C.E. Thorensen, and J.J. Gill, et al. 1986. Alteration of type A behavior and its effect on cardiac recurrences in post myocardial infarction patients: summary results of the recurrent coronary prevention project. *Am Heart J* 112:653-665.

61. Jones, D.A., and R.R. West. 1996. Psychological rehabilitation after myocardial infarction: multicentre randomised controlled trial. *BMJ* 313(7071):1517.

CHAPTER 17

Effects of Illness and Adversity on Quality of Life

Markku Ojanen
Department of Psychology, University of Tampere, Finland

Concern about the quality of life of people suffering from illnesses and adversity has rightfully increased in recent years. This phenomenon is important because personal satisfaction or subjective well-being are of paramount importance to human life. Everybody wants to live a good and happy life. Good health is valuable, while lack of objective and subjective quality of life bestows pessimism and helplessness.

Indeed, one must take seriously the general critique of narrow medical specialization and aim at comprehensive care of individual needs. Treatment and especially rehabilitation are best understood in this context and must be considered as a mixture of biological, psychological, social, and cultural interventions. The addition of cultural considerations means that an understanding of personal habits, preferences, and values is also essential for health care that meets high standards. We must not give in to fiscal pressures that make this goal difficult if not impossible to reach.

Each illness or human adversity has its own research tradition as does research involving quality of life (QL). Each major illness requires its own QL measurements; many of these measurements are reliable and have been validated (1). In chronic obstructive pulmonary disease (COPD), good examples include the St. George's Respiratory Questionnaire (SGRQ) (2); Chronic Respiratory Questionnaire (CRQ) (3); Quality of Life for Respiratory Illness Questionnaire (QOL-RIQ) (4); and the Seattle Obstructive Lung Disease Questionnaire (SOLQ) (5).

This chapter discusses subjective QL, which could also be described as subjective well-being or life satisfaction, subjective indicating that individuals evaluate their own lives through comprehensive testing (total life satisfaction) or through numerous questions covering various aspects of human life (6).

Often these measurements are extracted by factor analysis, with the results being theoretically or conceptually inadequate. The principles used in measurements of QL are different, but they still provide the therapist with an adequate picture of important aspects of QL, especially health-related QL. The main reason measures are inadequate is that they are based on narrow and haphazard samples of items. Selection of items should have a basis on a theory, a model, or a conceptual schema. This schema should be so comprehensive that it covers major aspects of QL.

One difficulty in measuring QL is that there is no clear definition of what the major components of QL are or should be. Another difficulty is that factors that can lower QL scores have not been precisely determined. It is usually assumed that any illness such as COPD, asthma, or mental illness will lower QL, and although this is likely to be true, this hypothesis is poorly documented. In general, large patient samples show that patients with illnesses have lower QL scores than those who are healthy, but the correlation between illness and QL is far from perfect (7,8). The effects of trauma on QL are often severe and long lasting (9,10), and multiple traumas seem to have multiplying effects on QL (10).

When does an illness, injury, or any other adversity lower the QL? This chapter presents a general analysis of many human adversities. In addition, variables that seem to influence the QL and may be important in the planning of rehabilitation are analyzed. For example, psychosocial rehabilitation or psychotherapy is likely to be most useful when there is a clear decrease in QL after the misfortune. Individuals with problems must feel that they are lacking something that can be corrected or bestowed on them.

The results of COPD-related research on QL are illuminating. Some studies do show statistically significant differences from control groups (11,12), whereas others do not (13-15). Rehabilitation programs have produced positive results on some variables, but not in others (16). The positive results have been achieved mainly on health-related QL, such as symptoms, exercise capacity, and mood. What can be changed and what cannot? A rough generalization based on comparisons of QL levels between afflicted versus control groups and on rehabilitation research supports the use of a list of factors (table 17.1). In such a list, the first factors are easier to change and show significant differences between groups, whereas the last factors are more difficult to change and/or have smaller differences between groups.

A good example is our own rehabilitation study (17) which included the QL components 1-5 and 8 from table 17.1. Significant, although transient, changes were only observed on components 1, 2, and 3.

What are the essential components of QL? Is it possible to define the core areas of QL? Five levels of QL can be differentiated. These include behavioral, emotional, social, and self/cognitive components, as well as values corresponding to phylogenetic and human developmental stages. Maslow's hierarchy of needs is similar to these levels (18). The behavioral, emotional, and social levels are often well represented on QL scales, whereas the cognitive and value levels are not. In the QL scales, behavioral levels refer to measures of activities; emotional levels to measure mood and emotion; and social levels to measure social support or social contacts. Quality-of-life scales should include information on purpose of life, personal safety, self-control, self-esteem, hope, optimism, and self-efficacy. Our hypothesis is that only in acute phases of illness are health-related variables as important as these.

Table 17.1 Components of QL

1. Mood (emotional state)
2. Specific symptoms
3. General health evaluations
4. Self-care behavior
5. Mobility, ambulation
6. Activities, hobbies
7. Social contacts
8. Psychological or mental problems (depression and anxiety)
9. Satisfaction and happiness
10. Values, life philosophies

Table 17.2 Factors Involved in Effect of Illness, Injury, or Adversity (Stress Load Factors)

1. Severity: danger to life or deleterious effects on life.
2. Restrictiveness: physical, mental, environmental restrictions; loss of movement; deafness, phobia, and imprisonment are examples.
3. Unexpectedness: a sudden change; an injury or the unexpected loss of a close person.
4. Shame: an illness or adversity carries a negative label or stigma (e.g., violent criminals or the mentally ill).
5. Regression: illness or adversity that has a poor prognosis.
6. Uncertainty: diagnosis is not known or the effects of adversity are unpredictable.
7. Injustice: the illness or adversity is not justified; it is not right that a person has it.
8. Visibility: the condition can be easily observed.
9. Alienation: Not many persons have the same fate. A person is compelled to bear the illness or adversity alone.
10. Fear: the amount of fear illness or adversity causes.
11. Cumulativeness: presence of other illnesses or adversities.

If an illness or adversity has an effect on at least some of the factors included in the list, it is likely to be serious. We believe the effects of an illness, injury, or adversity depend on the 11 factors such as those listed in table 17.2, called "stress load factors."

We believe there is a larger decrease in QL when more of these 11 factors are present or if a certain factor is present at a very high level. Severity and restrictiveness are good examples of this phenomenon. Though the hardship and illness experience is always subjective, severe problems in life drastically lower QL scale values. Examples are death of a child, rape, serious crimes against one's child, and cancer diagnosis. Restrictiveness leads either to helplessness or anger. Closed institutions and prisons severely restrict personal freedoms and thus create negative emotions and unhappiness.

Because all of these stress load factors have a strong subjective component, we can classify illnesses and adversities more objectively through a group of evaluators (here, psychologists) who perform the rating. One must, however, not expect too much from these so-called objective ratings because often the most important variable is the individual's unique personal reaction to adversity. This means that although differences between groups may be small or nonexistent, there may be wide individual differences in QL. Thus, individuals having COPD or mental illness differ greatly in their QL evaluations. Their reactions to rehabilitation or psychotherapy are also different and often difficult to predict (17).

It is possible that QL differences can be better predicted by personality variables than by external conditions. Personality traits such as optimism, hardiness, purpose in life, and values may be the most important variables (19). When these variables are used to explain QL scores, this is the likely explanation when, for example, optimism correlates with happiness or satisfaction.

The purposes of the present study were twofold. We were first concerned with the stress load inflicted by illness and adversity. What caused a certain adversity to be difficult? Is it the cumulative load of many factors, or is it one particular factor that lowers QL score? Using the objective stress load factors, we described various illnesses and adversities to test these hypotheses. In order to describe the actual QL differences, we also drew from the results of several adversity groups collected in our research programs. We expected the differences between the groups to reflect the stress load factors.

Rating of Stress Load Factors

Ten scales and 12 illnesses and adversities were presented to 17 clinical psychologists with master's or doctoral degrees. Cumulativeness was not used because it is not a quality of a particular illness or adversity but rather a combination of many adversities. The illnesses or adversities were COPD, asthma, paralysis of the lower limbs, schizophrenia, unemployment, obesity (+30-50 kg), anorexia, diabetes, imprisonment, fibromyalgia, AIDS, and lung cancer. The raters were given definitions taken from medical textbooks for COPD and fibromyalgia.

The purpose of the evaluations by psychologists was to get an objective view of the stress load factors through expert opinions. These opinions reflect the opinions existing in the culture about those factors. The evaluations of the people actually experiencing the adversities could also be used, but those results would reflect their QL ratings. The aim was to get a view of the load factors independent of subjective QL evaluations.

Table 17.3 Means of 10 Adversity Factors for 12 Illnesses and Adversities: Ratings by 17 Clinical Psychologists

	COPD	Asth	Paral	Schiz	Unemp	Obes	Anor	Diab	Pris	Fibr	AIDS	Canc
1. Sever.	7.2	6.2	8.2	7.7	5.9	6.6	7.6	5.8	7.1	5.9	9.3	9.1
2. Restr.	6.5	5.6	8.6	6.6	5.4	6.1	5.4	4.1	8.7	5.8	6.4	7.1
3. Unexp.	3.2	4.5	7.8	3.8	5.4	1.4	3.9	5.1	3.1	3.4	5.6	4.7
4. Shame	2.7	1.5	2.5	6.3	4.6	5.8	4.3	0.9	8.8	2.1	8.0	2.6
5. Regr.	6.2	3.7	2.6	4.2	4.4	4.5	5.5	3.6	3.4	4.4	7.9	6.6
6. Uncer.	2.6	2.8	1.1	5.8	4.1	2.9	3.9	2.6	2.4	7.1	5.1	3.6
7. Injus.	2.6	5.9	7.2	6.4	7.2	2.2	4.4	5.1	1.9	6.4	6.8	5.5
8. Visib.	3.4	4.1	8.7	5.3	3.6	9.1	7.1	1.4	5.2	3.2	3.8	2.9
9. Alien.	2.9	3.2	5.4	6.6	5.0	4.2	6.5	1.6	4.7	4.0	6.3	4.0
10. Fear	2.4	1.9	3.0	6.3	1.6	1.9	3.4	1.5	6.4	2.1	8.0	5.4
TOTAL	4.9	3.9	5.5	5.8	4.7	4.5	5.2	3.2	5.2	4.4	6.7	5.1

Scale: 0 = not typical at all; 10 = describes very closely the adversity.

Results

The results are presented in table 17.3.

Two important conclusions emerge from the results. When total stress load is analyzed, the most difficult adversities are AIDS, schizophrenia, and paralysis, and according to the hypothesis, QL should be low in these groups. Some adversities also had high values on certain characteristics. For instance, COPD is high in severity, restrictiveness, and regression, while obesity is high on visibility and fibromyalgia is high in uncertainty. The psychologists had great sympathy toward the adversities because they saw them as quite stressful. One would therefore expect that QL evaluations of those having adversities would be lower when compared to the control groups, which included people selected because they did not belong to any adversity group. However, it must be remembered that any control group selected from a general population always includes a few persons that have serious adversities. To some degree this could diminish the differences between the adversity groups and control groups.

The analysis of standard deviations shows that evaluation was fairly difficult. Of the adversities, paralysis and AIDS had particularly large standard deviations, and of the stress load factors, injustice and fear also had large standard deviations. Injustice gave rise to the most comments by the psychologists. In this context, injustice is a philosophical question and thus difficult to evaluate. Is there any adversity that is justified? It is difficult to establish an average picture of illnesses and adversities that is very heterogeneous. The raters can adopt many roles when they fill out the questionnaire. They can be experts, sympathizers, or representatives of a community. From the point of view of the people having these adversities, it might mean that these particular factors (injustice and fear) are subject to variable interpretations.

Results of Empirical QL Data

During the last 15 years, we have collected data on QL and well-being and have used descriptive visual analogue scales (DVAS; see example in appendix 17.1 on page 207). The DVAS have a range of 0-100, 100 denoting a very high level of a given attribute and 0 a very low level or lack of it. In the similar visual analogue scales (VAS) the 0-100 range is used but only the end points are described. The Global Assessment of Functioning Scale (GAF) in the DSM-IV classification is similar to the DVAS. Both scale types (VAS and DVAS) are reliable, correlate well with traditional scales, and are easy to use. There are about 20 available QL scales of which only a few are currently used in most studies.

During the last 10 years, numerous QL studies have been carried out in the Department of Psychology at the University of Tampere. The groups pertinent to this article are listed in table 17.4. The number of respondents are mentioned in parentheses after each group. The DVAS used most often were well-being, mood, anxiety, and self-confidence. Usually 8 to 16 scales were completed. The respondents completed the scales independently. Most of the respondents, except for the control group and the unemployed people, were undergoing treatment or rehabilitation when they participated in the QL studies. After respondents had drawn their lines (see the directions in appendix 17.1 on page 207), scoring was done using the nearest full number between 0-100, which corresponded to the line drawn.

Of the total population studied, groups 4, 9, and 11 are representative because they include those patients or inmates being taken care of for a given period of time. The control group (group 13) is a random sample drawn from a large Finnish company. Groups 2 and 9 can be divided according to the severity of their condition. Group 4 consists mainly of long-term schizophrenic patients and 11 of acute psychotic patients. Group 9 includes two groups of prisoners—those in a maximum security prison and those in minimum security where they only stay at nights and during weekends. The paresis group includes 18 individuals with paraparesis or paraplegia and 11 with quadriparesis or quadriplegia. Obese persons were at least 30 kilograms overweight compared to ideal weight. The unemployed all had university degrees. Some groups included mainly (groups 1 and 3) or only (group 9) men while groups 7 and 10 were mostly women (see table 17.4).

The standard deviations of the four scales are about 15 in control groups and between 18-22 in adversity groups. Variation of QL is thus generally somewhat

Table 17.4 Means of Well-Being, Mood, Anxiety, and Self-Confidence by DVAS (With Range of 0-100) in 12 Adversity Groups and in a Control Group*

	Well-being	Mood	Anxiety	Self-confidence
1. COPD (40)	47	71**	—	—
2. Asthma				
(mild, 43)	71	69	33	—
(severe, 15)	54	68	44	—
3. Paralysis (29)	—	—	40	64
4. Schizophrenia (78)	64	60	48	56
5. Unemployment (58)	—	63	—	60
6. Obesity (23)	—	77	34	72
7. Anorexia (17)	—	47	58	62
8. Diabetes (139)	—	—	36	64
9. Imprisonment				
(open, 31)	79	67	33	70
(high security, 48)	72	61	45	72
10. Fibromyalgia (63)	—	64	41	63
11. Acute psychosis (402)	57	61**	—	—
12. Short-term therapy (60)	62	55	53	57
13. Control group (450)	82	75	31	74

*See references for this table on page 209.

**A scale based on adjectives (transformed to range 0-100).

larger in adversity groups. Regardless of the illness or adversity, there are always those who rate their lives very positively and those who give very negative ratings. A reason for these extreme variations might be the ability to adapt to adversities. An optimistic, hopeful attitude protects people from low moods and depression, and a pessimistic attitude makes life worse. Also, time heals. The most acute adversities are probably more difficult subjectively.

We like to give a lot of significance to the mean level of the QL, which is almost always over the midpoint of 50. In all scales, the midpoint is stated neutrally, such as "in-between," "both-and," or "either-or." In the scales we have been using, ordinary people having no major adversity choose a value between 70-75, and people belonging to an adversity group choose a value between 55-70. Usually, there is about a 10-15 point difference between control and adversity groups on 0-100 point scales. The distributions are thus positively skewed in almost all adversity groups included in the study. This points to a very good adaptability of human beings.

Our results can be summarized as follows:

1. Although adversities in life do generally lower QL, the dire expectations of laymen, patients, and experts are not fulfilled.
2. Some adversities such as mild asthma, obesity, and even imprisonment, if not overly restricting, seem to have only an insignificant effect on QL.
3. The drop seems to be larger in mental than in physical illnesses. This is predictable because negative moods must reflect in ratings of QL.
4. If the illness is severe, its effects will be seen in health-related well-being, but not necessarily on other scales. Ratings of severity by experts probably depend on the patients' own complaints. If a patient complains a lot, the condition is rated more severely. To a large extent, experts base their ratings on what the patient says the adversity feels like. The appearance, symptoms, and physical conditions also have an effect on these ratings.

Discussion

The great ability of humans to adapt has long been recognized, and Crocker and Major (21) have shown that even members of stigmatized groups have self-esteem that is about as high as that of the general population. Taylor and Brown (23) speak of positive illusion. Human beings are generally optimistic and believe they can control life. Only when these beliefs are challenged, as in depression or when too much is required, does this human adaptability break down. In unpublished data on 1200 women from our program, the number of negative life events during the previous year predicted life satisfaction almost linearly. The number of negative life events, or cumulativeness, is thus an important factor in QL.

We also predicted that the sum of adversity factors would explain QL scores. This is supported by the result that those who had severe asthma had somewhat lower values of QL than those having milder symptoms. Also, high security prisoners surely have more adversity factors than those in open prisons. Their mood and well-being are lower and their anxiety is higher than those who are in open prisons. Other studies point in a similar direction (23), although correlations between QL and physiological variables are generally low (24). Restrictiveness seems to have a marked effect on QL in the prisoner sample. Interestingly, self-confidence is at a normal level in both prisoner groups. COPD patients are also restricted in their movements because of their illness, but the meaning of this kind of restriction is subjectively different.

It must be recognized that most of the QL variance is individual, and, although some of this variance is explained by personality traits and personal values, the rest must result from unique factors often difficult to predict. It is almost self-evident that physical or mental pain correlates with QL. Each stress load factor is experienced differently by each person undergoing a particular adversity.

In what ways can QL research be of use?

1. It shows the power of human adaptability. It is common to underestimate this ability and to emphasize all kinds of problems. Many restrictions and difficulties can be overcome and transformed into strengths. Luckily, the dire expectations of both laymen and experts are not fulfilled. It can often implicitly be read from the research reports that researchers expected that the effects of a particular adversity would be more serious than they actually were.
2. Some groups require strong psychosocial support. Low level of QL is a clear sign of problems and the causes for it can be manifold. The illness or adversity may be severe, or help or treatment has not met the needs of the persons, or the whole life situation is difficult (loneliness, helplessness).
3. A special group requiring help consists of those who simultaneously have two or more serious adversities or negative life events. Cumulation of adversities can break the normal adaptation process. Rehabilitation efforts should be directed to this group.
4. QL results can document areas that are not in accordance with human rights. Even if the afflicted persons tolerate their condition well, their rights must be respected and upheld. QL studies can reveal the problems that must be acted on.
5. The QL approach makes the evaluation of treatment and rehabilitation more comprehensive and relevant from the individual's point of view. In addition to their symptoms, the afflicted persons are very much concerned about their life qualities. Often much more can be done with these other factors than with the illness itself.

In addition to these uses of QL research, we must also determine what the ultimate aim of rehabilitation is. The components of QL are not equal in value. Should one aim at general life satisfaction or happiness, or it is enough to achieve positive changes in mobility, symptoms, or skills? We must discuss our priorities openly.

Conclusion

Quality-of-life research has increased significantly during the last decade, and classically, this research follows one of two patterns: studies of general well-being and those related to particular illnesses and adversities. Each illness has its own research mode and measurements. The analysis of QL components has been very practical but lacks theory. There is a general expectation that adversities lower QL but it is not known what the most stressful factors in adversities are. These problems show up as conflicting results.

Appendix 17.1 Example of Descriptive Visual Analogue Scales: Mood

MOOD

What is your general disposition? This refers to the basic nature of your experiences and feelings. Is your general emotional state happy and good-humored or are you inclined to be gloomy and ill-humored? Draw a short line across the vertical line at the point that best describes you. The scale is a continuum; the line may be drawn between two descriptions.

Extremely good mood	100	I am almost always happy and in a good mood. I am practically never in a bad mood.
Very good mood	90	I am most often in a good mood. It is very rare that I am down. Any bad mood soon passes.
Good mood	80	My mood is generally light and positive. Although I know what gloom and bad mood are, they are so rare that they mean next to nothing in my life.
Fairly good mood	70	Mostly I am in a positive mood. Although I have a slight tendency to gloom, this is not very disruptive. I manage with it quite well.
Reasonably good mood	60	Despite some bad moods, there are more good moments. The gloom is not strong enough to affect my life significantly. My disposition is more good than bad.
Neutral	50	I sometimes feel in a bad mood, but then there are times when I am in a good mood. My disposition is not so good, although not so bad.
Fairly bad mood	40	Although inclined to melancholy, I can somehow manage with it. Bad mood and melancholy do not greatly affect my work.
Reasonably bad mood	30	I take reasonably good care of my work and my affairs, but I cannot escape my gloomy thoughts. There are good moments from time to time, but I have a tendency to gloom and to have a bad mood.
Bad mood	20	The gloomy mood will not let up. Momentarily it feels as if I have overcome it, but then it comes over me again. I can manage my work and my everyday affairs when I force myself into action. My mood is constantly bad.
Very bad mood	10	I am very strongly inclined to gloom. I am not completely down, but not far from it. Everything seems gloomy and hopeless. It's hard work to manage everyday affairs.
Extremely bad mood	0	My disposition is very gloomy and heavy. I feel so dreadful and hopeless that I feel as if I were falling down a bottomless pit. Nothing moves or interests me. I cannot work or take care of my affairs.

References

1. Jones. 1998. Testing health status (quality of life) questionnaires for asthma and COPD. *Eur Respir J* 11:5-6.
2. Jones, P.W., F.H. Quirk, C.M. Baveystock, and P. Littlejohns. 1992. A self-complete measure of health status for chronic airflow limitation. *Am Rev Respir Dis* 145:1321-1327.
3. Guyatt, G.H., L.B. Berman, M. Townsend, S.O. Pugsley, and L.W. Chambers. 1987. A measure of quality of life for clinical trials in chronic lung disease. *Thorax* 42:773-778.
4. Maillé, A.R., C.J. Koning, A.H. Zwinderman, L.N. Willems, J.H. Dijkman, and A.A.Kaptein. 1997. The development of the "Quality-of-Life for Respiratory Illness Questionnaire (QOL-RIQ)": a disease-specific quality-of-life questionnaire for patients with mild to moderate chronic non-specific lung disease. *Respir Med* 91:297-309.
5. Tu, S.P., M.B. McDonell, J.A. Spertus, B.G. Steele, and S.D. Fihn. 1997. A new self-administered questionnaire to monitor health-related quality of life in patients with COPD. *Chest* 112:614-612.
6. Bowling A. 1991. *Measuring Health. A Review of Quality of Life Measurement Scales.* Philadelphia: Open University Press.
7. Kainulainen, S. 1998. *Life Events and Satisfaction with Life in Different Social Classes.* Finland: Kuopio University Publications.
8. Isoaho, R. 1995. Astma ja krooninen obstruktiivinen keuhkosairaus iäkkäässä väestössä - vallitsevuus ja yhteydet toimintakykyyn. (Asthma and chronic obstructive pulmonary disease in the elderly—prevalence and associations with functional abilities). Oulu: *Acta universitatis ouluensis* D347.
9. Lehman, D.R., C.B. Wortman, and A.F. Williams. 1987. Long-term effects of losing a spouse or child in a motor vehicle crash. *J Pers Soc Psychol* 52:218-231.
10. Follette, V.M., M.A. Polusny, A.E. Bechtle, and A.E. Naugle. 1966. Cumulative trauma: the impact of child sexual abuse, adult sexual assault, and spouse abuse. *J Traum Stress* 9:25-35.
11. Schlenk, E.A., J.A. Erlen, and J. Dunbar-Jacob, et al. 1998. Health-related quality of life in chronic disorders: a comparison across studies using the MOSSF-36. *Qual Life Res* 7:57-65.
12. Monsó, E., J.M. Fiz, and J. Izquierdo, et al. 1998. Quality of life in severe chronic obstructive pulmonary disease: correlation with lung and muscle function. *Respir Med* 92:221-227.
13. Herbert, R., and F. Gregor. 1997. Quality of life and coping strategies of clients with COPD. *Rehabil Nurs* 22:182-187.

14. Kaptein, A.A., P.L. Brand, F.W. Dekker, H.A Kerstjens, D.S. Postma, and H.J. Sluiter. 1993. Quality-of-life in a long-term multicentre trial in chronic nonspecific lung disease: assessment at baseline. The Dutch CNSLD Study Group. *Eur Respir J* 6:1478-1484.
15. Engström, C.-P., L.-O. Persson, S. Larsson, A. Rydén, and M. Sullivan. 1996. Functional status and well being in chronic obstructive pulmonary disease with regard to clinical parameters and smoking: a descriptive and comparative study. *Thorax* 51:825-830.
16. Lacasse, Y., E. Wong, G.H. Guyatt, D. King, D.J. Cook, and R.S. Goldstein. 1996. Meta-analysis of respiratory rehabilitation in chronic obstructive pulmonary disease. *Lancet* 348:1115-1119.
17. Ojanen, M., A. Lahdensuo, J. Laitinen, and J. Karvonen. 1993. Psychosocial changes in patients participating in a chronic obstructive pulmonary disease rehabilitation program. *Respiration* 60:96-102.
18. Maslow, A.H. 1968. *Toward a Psychology of Being.* Princeton, NJ: Van Nostrand.
19. Lewinsohn, P.M., J.E. Redner, and J.R. Seeley. 1991. The relationship between life satisfaction and psychosocial variables: new perspectives. In *Subjective Well-Being. An Interdisciplinary Perspective,* ed. F. Strack, M. Argyle, and N. Schwarz. Oxford: Pergamon.
20. American Psychiatric Association. 1994. Diagnostic and statistical manual of mental disorders. 4th ed. Washington, D.C.: APA.
21. Crocker, J., and B. Major. 1989. Social stigma and self-esteem: the self-protective properties of stigma. *Psychol Rev* 96:608-630.
22. Jones, P.W. 1993. Quality of life: specific problems associated with hypoxaemia. *Monaldi Arch Chest Dis* 48:565-573.
23. Taylor, S.E., and J.D. Brown. 1998. Illusion and well-being: a social psychological perspective on mental health. *Psychol Bull* 103:193-210.
24. Mishima, M., Y. Oku, and S. Muro, et al. 1996. Relationship between dyspnea in daily life and psychophysiologic state in patients with chronic obstructive pulmonary disease during long-term domiciliary oxygen therapy. *Intern Med* 35:453-458.

References for Table 17.4

1. Ojanen, M., A. Lahdensuo, J. Laitinen, and J. Karvonen. 1993. Psychosocial changes in patients participating in a chronic obstructive pulmonary disease rehabilitation program. *Respiration* 60: 96-102.
2. Koistinen, P. 1996. *Astma ja elämänlaatu* (Asthma and quality of life). Master's thesis, Department of Psychology, University of Tampere, Finland.

3. Kaarenoja, T. 1992. *Selkäydinvammaisten minäkäsitys, elämänhallinta ja selviytymisstrategiat* (Self concept, mastery, and coping of paralysed persons). Master's thesis, Department of Psychology, University of Tampere, Finland.

4. Ojanen, M., P. Helin, L. Leppänen, P. Koistinen, and M. Vuorinen. 1998. *Seinäjoen seudun mielenterveyskeskuksen tutkimustoiminta 1992-1996* (Research on Seinäjoki Mental Health Center). Seinäjoki: Etelä-Pohjanmaa District Publication.

5. Vikeväinen-Tervonen, L. 1998. *Akateemisten työttömien työnhakijoiden psyykkinen valmennus* (The mental training of academic unemployed). Doctoral dissertation, Department of Psychology, University of Tampere, Finland.

6. Kettunen, P. 1996. *Susceptibility of Anorexia Nervosa Versus Autonomy and Identity.* Master's thesis, Department of Psychology, University of Tampere, Finland.

7. Marttila, J. 1996. Insuliinihoitoisten diabeetikkojen sopeutumisvalmennuksen vaikuttavuus. (Effects of patient education program for diabetic patients treated with insulin). Licentiate's thesis, Department of Psychology, University of Tampere, Finland.

8. Nyman, M. Quality of life in open prison and in maximum security prison. Department of Psychology, University of Tampere, Finland. Unpublished.

9. Rantalaiho, I. *Rehabilitation Program for Persons Suffering from Fibromyalgia.* Department of Psychology, University of Tampere, Finland. Unpublished.

10. Ojanen, M. 1950. *Psykiatrisen akuuttihoidon kehittämisprojekti Hesperian sairaalassa vuosina 1983 ja 1984.* (Hesperia Acute Treatment Project 1983-1984). Helsinki, Finland: Helsingin kaupungin terveysviraston raportteja, sarja A/45, 1990.

11. Ojanen, M. *Effects of Short-Term Psychotherapy.* Tampere Short-Term Psychotherapy Project Group. Department of Psychology, University of Tampere, Finland. Unpublished.

12. Ojanen, M. 1994. *Liikunta ja psyykkinen hyvinvointi* (Exercise and psychological well-being). Helsinki: Liikuntatieteellisen seuran moniste no. 19.

CHAPTER 18

Economic Evaluation of Cardiopulmonary Rehabilitation

Neil Oldridge
Schools of Allied Health Sciences and Medicine, Regenstrief Institute for Health Care, Indiana University, Indianapolis, Indiana, USA

Identifying the most efficient use of limited and finite health care resources is a major challenge for health care systems. The trade-offs involved in choosing between alternative interventions are used in economic evaluations to examine the effectiveness of interventions designed to improve health. However, the evidence for the effectiveness of many current and emerging medical practices is often of poor quality, and in many cases entirely lacking (1). In addition, little is known about the cost effectiveness of many of our current interventions (2), making decisions about the choice of alternative health care services difficult.

Although rehabilitation is increasingly considered a standard practice for patients with heart disease and for patients with respiratory disease, this is not without some controversy. The key components of cardiopulmonary rehabilitation include exercise training, risk factor management counseling, appropriate behavioral intervention, and education (3,4). Controversy in cardiac rehabilitation (CR) focuses less on the effectiveness of the individual components of the services (3) and more on how services are delivered, as well as their cost effectiveness (5-8). Although respiratory rehabilitation (RR) with exercise training is generally considered effective (4,9-12), some controversy exists, particularly regarding the cost effectiveness of exercise training (13). With the dynamic nature of the changes in the current health care environment, the effectiveness and the cost effectiveness of both CR and RR need further documentation.

Effectiveness of Cardiopulmonary Rehabilitation

This chapter primarily reviews the cost-effectiveness data for CR and RR. Drummond et al. (14) have suggested that economic evaluations are most helpful when preceded by the demonstration of at least the effectiveness of a given health care service.

Cardiac Rehabilitation

Evidence for the benefits of CR has been documented rigorously in the Clinical Practice Guidelines on Cardiac Rehabilitation (3). Although largely based on evidence from patients with myocardial infarction, the most substantial benefits of CR include improvements in exercise tolerance, symptoms, blood lipid levels, psychological well-being, and reductions in stress, smoking, and mortality.

Given patient needs and expectations and the realities of the current health care environment, the traditional approach to the delivery of exercise-based CR services needs significant reform and restructure. It is argued that CR services need to be integrated more with primary care, focus more on the spectrum of cardiovascular disease risk reduction, and be evidence based, each of which should result in more effective and cost-effective care (5-8). This evolution will need considerable commitment on the part of the cardiac rehabilitation professional community. The challenge will be to see if these changes are seen as necessary—and useful!

Respiratory Rehabilitation

The joint American College of Chest Physicians/American Association of Cardiovascular and Pulmonary Rehabilitation guidelines (4) and a number of recent systematic overviews of RR (10,15-17) conclude that patients with COPD who are referred to RR programs demonstrate significant clinical benefit over and above that derived from conventional care. The most substantial benefits of RR include reduced dyspnea symptoms, improved health-related quality of life, and increased exercise tolerance.

The conclusion on the supporting side of a debate over the benefits of RR was that "evidence based on multidisciplinary studies from different continents has proved that RR that includes exercise training is highly effective in improving patients' outcomes" (9). The conclusion for the other side of the debate, based primarily on the paucity of the data, was summarized by the following quote (ascribed to John Maynard Keynes): "The real difficulty in changing [medical practice] lies not in developing new ideas but in escaping from old ones" (13).

Economic Evaluation

The basis of an economic evaluation is a balance sheet of advantages (benefits) and disadvantages (costs) associated with alternative health care services. Economic evaluation is defined as "the comparative analysis of alternative courses of action in terms of both costs and consequences" (14). With increasing awareness of the need to stay within a given budget, economic evaluation is one additional systematic evaluation strategy to assist decision makers to make rational choices about effective and efficient health care. Two key questions in the economic evaluation of health care services are:

- Is health care service A more cost effective than alternative B, typically usual care?
- How does the substitution of service A for B affect the costs to the health care system?

The calculation of a cost-effectiveness (C/E) ratio requires that data be collected on at least two alternatives: alternative A as the service under investigation and alternative B, typically "routine care" (18). The numerator term in the C/E ratio is the "net incremental" cost, expressed as the difference between the costs of service A and the comparison service B. The denominator term in the C/E ratio is the "net incremental" improvement, capturing the differences in the change in health outcomes with services A and B. Because the C/E analysis is comparative, cost effectiveness can be estimated as follows:

$$\text{Incremental cost effectiveness}_A = \frac{\text{Cost}_A - \text{Cost}_B}{\text{Effect}_A - \text{Effect}_B}$$

The efficiency of the service is estimated in a full economic evaluation where both costs and consequences are considered in the same study with a comparison of at least two alternative services (14). Conversely, a partial economic evaluation is one in which there is a description of the service with no comparison, or, if alternatives are compared, costs and consequences are not considered simultaneously; therefore, an efficiency estimate cannot be made.

Costs, the numerator term in the C/E ratio, reflect utilized resources. Direct costs are associated with the delivery of the health care (medical—activities of the hospital and health professionals and patients' own costs, and nonmedical—food, transportation, lodging, and family care). Indirect costs reflect the impact of the resources lost as a result of either mortality (premature death) or morbidity (time lost from production and/or consumption activities). It is difficult to estimate the intangible costs associated with pain and suffering, grief, and other nonmonetary outcomes of illness and health care.

The health effect or outcome of the intervention is the denominator term in the C/E ratio and determines the type of economic evaluation (2).

- Cost-minimization analysis: the less expensive intervention, provided the effectiveness of the alternative interventions is similar, will be preferred because it is considered the more efficient.
- Cost-benefit analysis: both costs and health effects are given a monetary value, permitting comparison across different health care services. The service with the most favorable cost-benefit ratio is the most efficient. Although it is perhaps the most comprehensive of the economic evaluations, cost-benefit analysis is

used infrequently because it is difficult to put a monetary value on complex health care outcomes such as life-years gained.
- Cost-effectiveness analysis: the outcome of an intervention is estimated in natural units (usually expressed in a single dimension, most commonly life-years gained or years of life saved) and the associated monetary costs. Incremental costs are determined per unit effect, and the lower the C/E ratio, the greater the cost effectiveness and efficiency. In cost-utility analysis, a form of cost effectiveness, the outcome of an intervention is estimated as a preference or utility score that reflects the individual's ranking of desirability for a specific health state or treatment outcome (2,19). The score is typically anchored at 0.00 (death) and 1.00 (full health) and is used to estimate the value of the time spent in a given health state as a "quality-adjusted life-year" (QALY) (20). The net incremental cost per QALY can be compared across diseases, conditions, and treatments, and the lower the cost-utility (C/U) ratio, the more efficient the service.

Cost-utility analysis, conducted from the societal perspective, has been accepted for making health care policy decisions in Canada (21) and Australia (22) and is now being recommended in the United States (23).

Economic Evaluation of Cardiopulmonary Rehabilitation

Patients with coronary heart disease and patients with respiratory disease are extensive users of the health care system (3,4). Although the costs of rehabilitation are only a small component of the total resource utilization, a better understanding of the efficiency of cardiopulmonary rehabilitation requires information about health care benefits and resource utilization during and subsequent to the intervention. This includes information on factors such as physician visits, emergency room visits, hospital inpatient days, allied health visits, and drug prescription utilization. A summary of full (both costs and consequences considered in the same study with a comparison of at least two alternative services) and partial (description of the service with no comparison of services or if alternative services are compared, costs and consequences are not considered simultaneously) economic evaluations of CR (24-31) and RR (32-38) discussed in this review is provided in table 18.1.

Cardiac Rehabilitation

Within certain limitations, the available economic evaluations of CR (24-31) suggest that it is cost effective. These limitations include (a) the sparse database on which to estimate the cost effectiveness of CR (3,39), (b) the fact that data from studies of CR with less rigorous designs demonstrate reductions in health care utilization, whereas data from the more rigorous randomized controlled trials (RCTs) of CR report increased costs with CR, and (c) the fact that most of the available information on the cost effectiveness of CR is derived from studies of patients with myocardial infarction.

Partial Economic Evaluation Partial economic evaluations are available in five studies with CR services, providing evidence of lower health care utilization rates and costs (25-28) or lower health care utilization rates (29). Cost data are available on a random sample of 25 CR programs in England and Wales but outcome data were not provided (40).

Full Economic Evaluations There are three reports of a full economic evaluation in CR. Data were collected in two RCTs, one with "post hoc" estimates of the costs in two experimental groups (24), another with an "a priori" cost-effectiveness hypothesis (30). In the third report, cost effectiveness was estimated with the use of computer modeling (31).

In the RCT of home and group exercise training after myocardial infarction (24), exercise tolerance was improved in the home training group by 36% (n = 33) compared to 35% for group training (n = 30). With no difference in outcome and an estimated cost of the group program over 12 weeks of $720 compared to $328 for at-home training, the at-home program is the more efficient intervention. Because medically directed at-home rehabilitation is less expensive than group intervention, it has the potential to increase the availability and to decrease the cost of rehabilitation for low-risk survivors of myocardial infarction (24).

An economic evaluation was included as a planned outcome in an RCT comparing usual care (n = 102) and an 8-week exercise and behavioral counseling intervention (n = 99) in patients with myocardial infarction and mild to moderate anxiety and/or depression (30). With an additional 0.052 QALYs per patient over 1 year attributable to the rehabilitation intervention and net direct incremental costs of $480 per rehabilitation patient, the best estimate C/U ratio for CR was $9200 per QALY gained per patient (i.e., $480 / 0.052 QALYs). With 0.022 life-years gained (LYG) per rehabilitated patient, estimated from meta-analyses of CR (41,42), the best estimate C/E ratio was $21,800 per life-year gained. The differences in QALYs were combined with the reduction in mortality providing a mean of 0.071 QALYs gained per patient attributable to CR, resulting in a best estimate comprehensive C/U ratio of $6800 per QALY gained. These data provide evidence that brief CR initiated soon after myocardial infarction for patients with mild to moderate anxiety and depression, or both, is an efficient use of health care resources and can be economically justified (30).

A computer-model cost-effectiveness analysis of CR after myocardial infarction was carried out using previously published data (31). With an estimated incremental life expectancy of 0.202 years during a 15-year period and 1985 net costs of $430 (direct costs = $1280; savings = $850), the C/E ratio is projected to be $4950/

Table 18.1 Partial and Full Economic Evaluations of Cardiac and Respiratory Rehabilitation; Cost Savings (Lower Utilization Rates), Net Costs, and Health Consequences With Rehabilitation

	Intervention	Cost savings	Net costs	Cost-effectiveness/utility ratio
Cardiac				
Partial evaluation				
Levin et al. (25)	Clinic-based for 2 years; then home & outpatient	SEK73,510 over 5 years		
Ades (26)	Clinic-based; outpatient	US $739 over 3 years		
Edwards et al. (27)	Clinic-based; outpatient	US $2597 over 1 year		
Allison et al. (28)	Clinic-based; outpatient	US $7358 over 6 months		
Bondestam et al. (29)**	Primary care clinic; outpatient	Lower utilization		
Full evaluation				
DeBusk et al. (24)	At-home vs. clinic-based; outpatient	US $392 over 12 weeks		Similar exercise tolerance increase
Oldridge et al (30)	Clinic-based; outpatient		US $480 over 1 year	0.052 QALYs gained with CR, C/U ratio = $9200/QALY gained; 0.022 LYG, C/E ratio = $21,800/LYG
Ades et al. (31)	Computer modeling		US $940 over 1 year	0.190 YOLS[¶] gained with CR, C/U ratio, $4950/YOLS[¶] gained

Respiratory				
Partial evaluation				
Sneider et al. (32)	Clinic-based; outpatient	US $2147 over 1 year		
Jensen (33)	Clinic-based; outpatient	Shorter LOS¶¶		
Ries et al. (34)	Clinic-based; outpatient	Similar utilization		
Lewis and Bell (35)	Rural medical center; outpatient	Similar utilization		
Reina-Rosenbaum et al. (36)	Home-based; outpatient		US $650 over 10 weeks	
Full evaluation				
Toevs et al. (37)	Home-based; outpatient		US $101,876 over 18 months	4.2 well-years gained with RR, C/U ratio, $24,256/well-year gained
Goldstein et al. (38)	Inpatient for 8 weeks; outpatient for 16 weeks		Can $11,597 over 6 months	C/E ratio = Can $16,567-$35,142 per unit difference in HRQL

*Comparison of distressed and nondistressed patients; **patients 65 years old and greater; ***computer modeling; ¶year of life saved; ¶¶length of stay.

life-year gained for 1995. Although CR is less cost effective than smoking cessation or statins for certain subgroups of patients, the authors point out that CR is as cost effective, or more cost effective, than thrombolytic therapy, coronary bypass surgery, and cholesterol-lowering drugs for certain subgroups of patients. The authors suggest that CR should stand alongside these therapies as standard of care in the postmyocardial infarction setting (31).

Respiratory Rehabilitation

Although the effects of RR on reducing health care utilization in patients with chronic obstructive pulmonary disease (COPD) were first reported as many as 30 years ago (43), there also are a number of limitations of the available evidence: (a) Electronic searches for RR economic evaluations between 1966 and 1999 identified only four studies (32,36-38) in which the costs associated with the intervention were estimated; (b) Of the 12 studies included in the recent RR guidelines that substantiated a reduction in the number, days, or length of hospitalization (4), eight were observational studies or reports, limiting their interpretability.

Partial Economic Evaluation There are five studies with a partial economic evaluation of RR services (see table 18.1). One provides evidence of lower health care utilization rates and costs (32); one provides evidence of lower (33) and two of similar (34,35) health care utilization rates; and the fifth reported costs of $650 for 10 weeks of RR with significant improvements in exercise tolerance, forced vital capacity (although not clinically meaningful), and the sensation of dyspnea (36).

Full Economic Evaluation There are two reports of a full economic evaluation in RR, one published in 1984 (37), the other 13 years later in 1997 (38).

Patients with COPD were randomized either to exercise plus behavioral interventions (n=47) or as controls (n=28) (37). Greater improvements in health status were observed in the intervention patients than in the control patients, and this translated into a total of 4.2 well-years attributable to the intervention with a C/U ratio of $24,256 per well-year gained. The authors concluded that the intervention is moderately cost effective as an adjunct for patients with COPD (37).

In the second RCT, patients with COPD were randomized to a 2-month, 5 days per week inpatient RR phase followed by 4 months of daily outpatient RR (n = 45) or to conventional community care (n = 44) (38). An economic evaluation was carried out and the incremental costs of the RR intervention amounted to Canadian $11,597 for a single patient, with 90% of this attributable to the inpatient phase (38). The improvement observed in health-related quality of life (HRQL) using the Chronic Respiratory Questionnaire (CRQ), which includes four domains and a 7-point Likert scale (45), was 0.70 for mastery, 0.61 for dyspnea, 0.44 for emotional function, and 0.33 for fatigue. Using these data, the C/E ratio per patient was estimated to be as little as \$16,567 (i.e., \$11,597/0.70) for improvement in the mastery domain and as high as \$35,142 for fatigue (38), suggesting that providing RR services is relatively efficient when compared to usual community care.

Discussion

Although the available evidence suggests that cardiopulmonary rehabilitation is probably at least relatively cost effective, the limited number of economic evaluations makes it difficult to make comparisons between cardiopulmonary rehabilitation and other interventions competing for the same limited resources. League tables provide a perspective from which to compare the results of cost-effectiveness analyses (46,47). One such classification scheme is summarized in table 18.2 with comparisons between CR, RR, and various cardiology interventions using data published in 1996 by Goldman et al. (48). However attractive they appear to be, the inherent variability of the methodological quality of the data included in league tables can mislead decision makers when attempting to assess the relative value for money of competing health care services (46,47). For example, CR economic evaluation data included in tables such as table 18.2 must be interpreted carefully as they were generated at different times, in different countries with different health care systems (e.g., the United States, Sweden, and Canada), using different study designs and analytic strategies (24-31). However, given these methodological provisos and the natural tendency to consider the relative cost effectiveness of competing health care services, the cost effectiveness per QALY or well-year gained with CR and RR services ranges from highly cost effective (<US \$20,000) to relatively cost effective (>\$20,000 to <\$40,000).

The collection of information on costs in RCTs of CR has been advocated (49). However, the role of RCTs in addressing cost effectiveness is unclear. High internal validity is a hallmark of RCTs as they are carried out under strictly controlled conditions, but this also limits generalizability to routine clinical practice (50,51). Although the health care savings reported in nonrandomized studies of cardiopulmonary rehabilitation might reflect routine clinical practice, costs were reported to have been incurred primarily in RCTs with full economic evaluations (table 18.1). This raises questions about the validity and interpretability of both sets of data. For example, the controlled but nonrandomized trials and observational studies generally demonstrate reduced health care utilization rates and lower costs with CR. However, in at least one RCT, there were no significant differences in annual utilization of physician or allied health visits, emergency room visits, hospital inpatient days, or drug-prescription utilization (30). As some proportion of the costs identified in an RCT is protocol driven, careful consideration must be given to both

Table 18.2 Cost-Effectiveness League Table for Cardiopulmonary Rehabilitation and Other Interventions for Heart Disease (Cost Effectiveness per Life-Year Gained Unless Otherwise Noted)

Cost per LYG or QALY	Description	Examples of cardiopulmonary interventions
<$20,000	Highly cost effective	Lovastatin: (2^{ary}, >250 mg/dl, 45-50 yr male), saves $ and lives
		Smoking cessation (MI), $250-$1300
		→ CR (post-MI), $6800-$9200/QALY
		CABG (severe angina, left main), $9200
		PTCA (severe angina), $8700-$10,200/QALY
		→ RR (COPD), $16,567 per unit HRQL (mastery)
		CABG (mild angina, 3 v), $18,200/QALY
$20,000 to $40,000	Relatively cost effective	β-blocker (MI), $20,200
		→ CR (post-MI), $21,800
		ECG exercise test (CAD), $30,200
		→ RR (COPD), $35,142 per unit HRQL (fatigue)
		Angiography (90% prob. CAD), $37,700/QALY
>$40,000 to $60,000	Borderline	Lovastatin: (2^{ary}, <250 mg/dl, 55-64 yr female), $41,800
		Nifedipene (hypertension), $48,900
>$60,000 to $100,000	Expensive	Angiography (60% prob. CAD), $71,300/QALY
		CCU (20% prob. MI), $88,700
>$100,000	Unattractive	Captopril (hypertension), $111,600
		CCU (5% prob. MI), $373,800

2^{ary} = secondary prevention; prob. = probability.

the feasibility and suitability of incorporating an economic evaluation within an RCT (51).

When planning for wider implementation of cardiopulmonary rehabilitation, an estimate of the number of patients that must be treated in order for one patient to benefit, in addition to information on costs and benefits, is likely to be helpful. As a measure of HRQL, the CRQ is scored on a 7-point Likert scale with a difference of 0.5-0.99 considered to be the equivalent of a minimal clinical important difference and 1.0 or more considered to be at least moderate (52). Using the CRQ to measure HRQL, Goldstein and colleagues (38) demonstrated that between

2.8 patients (mastery domain scores) and 6.9 patients (fatigue domain scores) would need to be treated with RR in order to have one patient gain at least a moderate benefit in HRQL.

In a trial of CR (53), we used the CRQ cut points for minimal important differences in the Quality of Life after Myocardial Infarction instrument (QLMI), which had been developed using the same approach and also is scored on a 7-point Likert scale (54,55). We calculated that 5.3 patients (global QLMI scores), 4.4 patients (emotional domain QLMI scores), and 7.7 patients (limitations domain QLMI scores) would need to be treated in order for one patient to demonstrate a moderate or greater improvement in HRQL by the end of the intervention. Knowing the number of patients who need to be treated in order to achieve a clinically important difference is an estimate of the effort required to gain benefit and would provide useful additional information to those making policy decisions about cardiopulmonary rehabilitation. This is likely to be important when the benefits of cardiopulmonary rehabilitation appear to be similar in different environments (e.g., inpatient, outpatient, physician's office, and home) (24,28).

The dynamics of change in the health care environment bring considerable pressure to deliver health care more efficiently (i.e., at lower cost without reducing effectiveness). As a strategy for evaluating the efficiency of health care services, cost-effectiveness data demonstrating the efficiency of alternative delivery systems for cardiopulmonary rehabilitation services should make those services more attractive and more widely available to all who need them.

Conclusions

A major challenge for all health care systems is to identify the most efficient use of limited and finite resources available for health care. Economic evaluation provides a balance sheet of the benefits, harms, and costs of alternative health care services and is used to decide how to get the greatest improvement in health from limited resources and how to choose between two or more different treatments for the same health problem. Evidence for the effectiveness of many current and emerging medical practices is often of poor quality and, in many cases, entirely lacking. Further, even less evidence is available regarding the cost effectiveness of many of our current interventions.

Economic evaluations of CR are encouraging and suggest that it is probably an efficient use of health care resources that can be economically justified. However, this tentative conclusion is based on only five observational studies, two randomized controlled trials, and one study modeling previously published data. The studies were carried out in the United States, Sweden, and Canada. With no universal approach to CR in the same country, let alone between different countries, the generalizability of the data on the cost effectiveness of comprehensive CR is uncertain. Although health care utilization may be reduced with RR, economic evaluations of RR are even more limited than those for CR with apparently only one formal economic analysis of RR.

This information, or lack of information, clearly demonstrates both the paucity of and the need for additional economic evaluations of cardiopulmonary rehabilitation services. Specifically, we do not have answers to either of the following two critical questions in either cardiac or RR:

1. If exercise is a key component of comprehensive rehabilitation, what is the incremental value of exercise when added to other cost-effective secondary prevention interventions?
2. Does either cardiac or pulmonary rehabilitation actually reduce costs and save scarce health care resources?

References

1. Eddy, D.M., and J. Billings. 1988. The quality of medical evidence: implications for quality of care. *Health Aff* (Spring):19-32.
2. Russell, L.B., M.R. Gold, J.E. Siegel, N. Daniels, and M.C. Weinstein, for the Panel on Cost-Effectiveness in Health and Medicine. 1996. The role of cost-effectiveness analysis in health and medicine. *JAMA* 276:1162-1177.
3. Wenger, N.K., E.S. Froelicher, L.K. Smith, P.A. Ades, K. Berra, and J.A. Blumenthal, et al. 1995. *Cardiac Rehabilitation.* Clinical Practice Guideline #17. Rockville, MD: U.S. Dept. of Health and Human Services, Public Health Service, Agency for Health Care Policy and Research and the National Heart, Blood, and Lung Institute. AHCPR # 96-0672.
4. American College of Chest Physicians/American Association of Cardiovascular and Pulmonary Rehabilitation. 1997. Pulmonary rehabilitation: joint ACCP/AACVPR evidence-based guidelines. ACCP/AACVPR pulmonary rehabilitation guidelines panel. *Chest* 112:1363-1396.
5. Mayou, R. 1996. Rehabilitation after heart attack. *BMJ* 313:1498-1499.
6. Dafoe, W., and P. Huston. 1997. Current trends in cardiac rehabilitation. *Can Med Assoc J* 156:527-532.
7. Franklin, B.A., L. Hall, and G.C. Timmis. 1997. Contemporary cardiac rehabilitation services. *Am J Cardiol* 79:1075-1077.
8. Gordon, N.F., and W.L. Haskell. 1997. Comprehensive cardiovascular disease risk reduction in a cardiac rehabilitation setting. *Am J Cardiol* 80:69H-73H.
9. Celli, B.R. 1997. Is pulmonary rehabilitation an effective treatment for chronic obstructive pulmonary disease? Yes. *Am J Respir Crit Care Med* 155:781-783.

10. Lacasse, Y., G.H. Guyatt, and R.S. Goldstein. 1997. The components of a respiratory rehabilitation program: a systematic overview. *Chest* 111:1077-1088.

11. Tiep, B.L. 1997. Disease management of COPD with pulmonary rehabilitation. *Chest* 112:1630-1656.

12. Resnikoff, P.M., and A.L. Ries. 1998. Maximizing functional capacity. Pulmonary rehabilitation and adjunctive measures. *Respir Care Clin N Am* 4:475-492.

13. Albert, R.K. 1997. Is pulmonary rehabilitation an effective treatment for chronic obstructive pulmonary disease? No. *Am J Respir Crit Care Med* 155:784-785.

14. Drummond, M.F., B.J. O'Brien, G.L. Stoddart, and G.W. Torrance. 1997. *Methods for the Economic Evaluation of Health Care Programmes.* Oxford: Oxford University Press.

15. Celli, B.R. Pulmonary rehabilitation in patients with COPD. *Am J Respir Crit Care Med* 152:861-864.

16. Lacasse, Y., E. Wong, G.H. Guyatt, D. King, D.J. Cook, and R.S. Goldstein. 1996. Meta-analysis of respiratory rehabilitation in chronic obstructive pulmonary disease. *Lancet* 348:1115-1119.

17. Cambach, W., R.C. Wagenaar, T.W. Koelman, A.R. van Keimpema, and H.C. Kemper. 1999. The long-term effects of pulmonary rehabilitation in patients with asthma and chronic obstructive pulmonary disease: a research synthesis. *Arch Phys Med Rehabil* 80:103-111.

18. Weinstein, M.C., J.E. Siegel, M.R. Gold, M.S. Kamlet, and L.B. Russell, for the Panel on Cost-Effectiveness in Health and Medicine. 1996. Recommendations of the panel on cost-effectiveness in health and medicine. *JAMA* 276:1253-1258.

19. Feeny, D., G.W. Torrance, and R. LaBelle. 1996. Integrating economic evaluations and quality of life assessments. In *Quality of Life Assessments in Clinical Trials,* ed. B. Spilker. New York: Lippincott-Raven Publishers.

20. Torrance, G.W., and D. Feeny. 1989. Utilities and quality-adjusted life years. *Int J Technol Assess Health Care* 5:559-575.

21. Canadian Coordinating Office for Health Technology Assessment. 1994. *Guidelines for the Economic Evaluation of Pharmaceuticals: Canada,* 1st ed. Ottawa: CCHOTA.

22. Commonwealth of Australia. 1993. Background document on the use of economic evaluation as a basis for the inclusion of pharmaceutical products on the Pharmaceutical Benefits Scheme. Canberra: Australian Government Publishing Service.

23. Gold, M.R., J.E. Siegel, L. Russell, and M. Weinstein, eds. 1996. *Cost-Effectiveness in Health and Medicine.* New York: Oxford University Press.

24. DeBusk, R.F., W.L. Haskell, N.H. Miller, K. Berra, C.B. Taylor, and W. Berger, et al. 1985. Medically-directed at-home rehabilitation soon after uncomplicated acute myocardial infarction: a new model for patient care. *Am J Cardiol* 55:251-257.

25. Levin, L.-A., J. Perk, and B. Hedback. 1991. Cardiac rehabilitation—cost analysis. *J Intern Med* 230:427-434.

26. Ades, P.A. 1993. Decreased medical costs after cardiac rehabilitation. A case for universal reimbursement. *J Cardiopulm Rehabil* 13:75-77.

27. Edwards, W.W., E. Glickman-Weiss, B.D. Franks, Y. Iyriboz, S.L. Dodd, and T.P. Quaid. 1993. Percutaneous transluminal coronary angioplasty rehabilitation. A cost-effectiveness analysis. *J Cardiopulm Rehabil* 13:172-181.

28. Allison, T.G., D.E. Williams, T.D. Miller, C.A. Patten, K.R. Bailey, and R.W. Squires, et al. 1995. Medical and economic costs of psychologic distress in patients with coronary artery disease. *Mayo Clin Proc* 70:734-742.

29. Bondestam, E., A. Breikks, and M. Hartford. 1995. Effects of early rehabilitation on consumption of medical care during the first year after acute myocardial infarction in patients >65 years of age. *Am J Cardiol* 75:767-771.

30. Oldridge, N., W. Furlong, D. Feeny, G. Torrance, G. Guyatt, J. Crowe, et al. 1993. Economic evaluation of cardiac rehabilitation soon after acute myocardial infarction. *Am J Cardiol* 72:154-161.

31. Ades, P.A., F.J. Pashkow, and J.R. Nestor. 1997. Cost-effectiveness of cardiac rehabilitation after myocardial infarction. *J Cardiopulm Rehabil* 17:222-231.

32. Sneider, R., J.A. O'Malley, and M. Kahn. 1988. Trends in pulmonary rehabilitation at Eisenhower Medical Center: An 11-year experience (1976-1987). *J Cardiopulm Rehabil* 8:453-461.

33. Jensen, P.S. 1983. Risk, protective factors, and supportive interventions in chronic airway obstruction. *Arch Gen Psychiatr* 40:1203-1207.

34. Ries, A.L., R.M. Kaplan, T.M. Limberg, and L.M. Prewitt. 1995. Effects of pulmonary rehabilitation on physiologic and psychosocial outcomes in patients with chronic obstructive pulmonary disease. *Ann Intern Med* 122:823-832.

35. Lewis, D., and S.K. Bell. 1995. Pulmonary rehabilitation, psychosocial adjustment, and use of healthcare services. *Rehabil Nurs* 20:102-107.

36. Reina-Rosenbaum, R., J.R. Bach, and J. Penek. 1997. The cost/benefits of outpatient-based pulmonary rehabilitation. *Arch Phys Med Rehabil* 78:240-244.

37. Toevs, C., R. Kaplan, and C. Atkins. 1984. The costs and effects of behavioral programs in chronic obstructive pulmonary disease. *Med Care* 22:1088-1100.

38. Goldstein, R.S., E.H. Gort, G.H. Guyatt, and D. Feeny. 1997. Economic analysis of respiratory rehabilitation. *Chest* 112:370-379.

39. Oldridge, N.B. 1998. Comprehensive cardiac rehabilitation: is it cost-effective? *Eur Heart J* 19:O42-49.

40. Gray, A.M., G.S. Bowman, and D.R. Thompson. 1997. The cost of cardiac rehabilitation services in England and Wales. *J R Coll Phys Lond* 31:57-61.

41. Oldridge, N.B., G.H. Guyatt, M. Fischer, and A.R. Rimm. 1988. Cardiac rehabilitation after myocardial infarction: combining data from randomized clinical trials. *JAMA* 260:945-980.

42. O'Connor, G.T., J.E. Buring, S. Yusuf, S.Z. Goldhaber, E.M. Olmstead, and R.S. Paffenbarger, et al. 1989. An overview of randomized trials of rehabilitation with exercise after myocardial infarction. *Circulation* 80:234-244.

43. Petty, T.L., L.M. Nett, M.M. Finigan, G.A. Brink, and P.R. Corsello. 1969. A comprehensive care program for chronic airway obstruction. Methods and preliminary evaluation of symptomatic and functional improvement. *Ann Intern Med* 70:1109-1120.

44. Goldstein, R.S., E.H. Gort, D. Stubbing, M.A. Avendano, and G.H. Guyatt. 1994. Randomised controlled trial of respiratory rehabilitation. *Lancet* 344:1394-1397.

45. Guyatt, G.H., L.B. Berman, M. Townsend, S.O. Pugsley, and L.W. Chambers. 1987. A measure of quality of life for clinical trials in chronic lung disease. *Thorax* 42:773-778.

46. Drummond, M.F., G.W. Torrance, and J. Mason. 1993. Cost-effectiveness league tables: more harm than good? *Soc Sci Med* 37:33-40.

47. Mason, J., M. Drummond, and G. Torrance. 1993. Some guidelines on the use of cost effectiveness league tables. *BMJ* 306:570-572.

48. Goldman, L., A.M. Garber, S.A. Grover, and M.A. Hlatky. 1996. Cost effectiveness of assessment and management of risk factors. *J Am Coll Cardiol* 27:1020-1030.

49. Taylor, R., and B. Kirby. 1997. The evidence base for the cost effectiveness of cardiac rehabilitation (editorial). *Heart* 78:5-6.

50. O'Brien, B. 1996. Economic evaluation of pharmaceuticals. Frankenstein's monster or vampire of trials? *Med Care* 34:DS99-108.

51. Coyle, D., L. Davies, and M.F. Drummond. 1998. Trials and tribulations. Emerging issues in designing economic evaluations alongside clinical trials. *Int J Technol Assess Health Care* 14:135-144.

52. Juniper, E.J., G.H. Guyatt, A. Willan, and L.E. Griffith. 1994. Determining a minimally important change in a disease-specific quality of life questionnaire. *J Clin Epidemiol* 4:81-87.

53. Oldridge, N., G. Guyatt, N. Jones, J. Crowe, J. Singer, and D. Feeny, et al. 1991. Effects on quality of life with comprehensive rehabilitation after acute myocardial infarction. *Am J Cardiol* 67:1084-1089.

54. Hillers, T.K., G.H. Guyatt, N.B. Oldridge, J. Crowe, A. Willan, and L. Griffith, et al. 1994. Quality of life after myocardial infarction. *J Clin Epidemiol* 47:1287-1296.

55. Oldridge, N.B., M. Gottlieb, G.H. Guyatt, N.L. Jones, D. Feeny, and D. Streiner. 1998. Predictors of health-related quality of life with cardiac rehabilitation after acute myocardial infarction. *J Cardiopulm Rehabil* 18:95-103.

PART VII

Quality of Life and Cardiopulmonary Rehabilitation

CHAPTER 19

Health-Status Measurement Instruments in Patients With Chronic Obstructive Pulmonary Disease

Yves Lacasse[1], Eric Wong[2], Gordon Guyatt[3], and Roger S. Goldstein[4]

[1]Centre de Pneumologie, de l'Hôpital Laval Sainte-Foy, Québec, Canada

[2]Department of Medicine, University of Alberta, Edmonton, Alberta, Canada

[3]Department of Medicine and Department of Clinical Epidemiology and Biostatistics, McMaster University, Hamilton, Ontario, Canada

[4]Department of Medicine, University of Toronto, Toronto, Ontario, Canada

Even though the focus of treatment of patients with chronic lung diseases often includes physiological measurements of expiratory flow or exercise capacity, the growing evidence that symptoms and overall health-related quality of life (HRQL) are poorly related to these physiological outcomes (1-3) has prompted investigators to include measurements of health status as end points into their clinical trials. Over the last 15 years, investigators have developed a number of instruments to measure health status in patients with chronic obstructive pulmonary disease (COPD). The availability of a large variety of questionnaires has sometimes led to confusion regarding the most appropriate instrument to use and how to interpret the results. The objective of this review was to describe and classify health status measurement instruments currently available for patients with COPD.

Methods

We have used our judgment in selecting the most popular and widely used instruments and in collecting the most salient data on their measurement properties.

This chapter is a shorter, updated version of an article published previously (Lacasse, Y., Wong, E., Guyatt, G.H., and Goldstein, R.S. 1997. Health-status measure instruments in chronic obstructive pulmonary disease. *Can Respir J* 4:152-164 [7]). Permission was granted by Dr. Norman Jones.

This report will assist individuals interested in recent articles and reviews of the measurement of HRQL in COPD (4-6). We also refer the reader to an Internet site designed by the American Thoracic Society for researchers, clinicians, industrial groups, and other interested parties who wish to learn about patient-oriented quality-of-life measures (**http://www.thoracic.org/qol/qoldata.htlm**).

To retrieve papers reporting on the measurement properties of the questionnaires included in our review, we conducted computer searches of the English-language medical literature in the Science Citation database using the reference of the original article describing the questionnaire. When information on the measurement properties of a particular questionnaire was limited, we contacted the authors of the original report on the instrument for more detailed information (7). The basic terminology related to health status measures has been defined elsewhere (8). In commenting on the responsiveness of the instruments, we gave priority to clinical trials that were randomized and controlled. Such trials usually provide stronger evidence of responsiveness than nonrandomized trials. Throughout this text, when interpreting the coefficients of correlation, we have qualified the strength of the correlations as follows: coefficients ranging from 0 to 0.20 denote a negligible correlation; 0.21 to 0.35, a weak correlation; 0.36 to 0.50, a moderate correlation; and larger than 0.50, a strong correlation.

Why Should We Measure Health-Related Quality of Life in COPD?

End-stage COPD is preceded by years of progressive disability and handicap associated with decreased exercise capacity (9,10) as well as a variety of symptoms not necessarily confined to the respiratory system. For instance, when specifically asked to describe their symptoms, patients have most frequently mentioned breathlessness, fatigue, sleep disturbance, irritability and sense of hopelessness (11,12). Typically, affected patients rapidly enter into the vicious cycle of dyspnea, inactivity, and physical deconditioning (13), with consequent potentially devastating emotional responses, including depression (14).

Many investigators have found that measures of exercise capacity (either maximal or functional) correlate only weakly or moderately with measures of quality of life (table 19.1). Consequently, exercise capacity cannot be used as a surrogate for quality of life. Quality of life should rather be measured directly.

A recent review of the health status instruments used in controlled clinical trials of respiratory rehabilitation (15) reflected the evolution of measurement in pulmonary medicine over the last 20 years. In early trials (16,17), HRQL was assessed by means of either

1. more or less structured interviews,
2. questionnaires related to fixed personality traits, or

Table 19.1 Correlations Between Fully Validated HRQL Measurement Instruments and Functional Exercise Capacity

Reference	Study population	HRQL measure instrument	vs.	Functional exercise capacity measure	Pearson's coefficients of correlation
Mahler et al. 1984 (1)	38 patients (32 COPD; 5 asthma, 1 interstitial fibrosis)	Baseline Dyspnea Index	vs.	12-minute walk test	$r = 0.60$ $p < 0.05$
Guyatt et al. 1987 (12)	43 patients (25 COPD; 18 chronic heart failure)	Chronic Respiratory Questionnaire (dyspnea)	vs.	6-minute walk test	$r = 0.46$ $p < 0.05$
Jones et al. 1992 (3)	141 patients (COPD and asthma, proportion not specified)	St. George's Respiratory Questionnaire (symptoms)	vs.	6-minute walk test	$r = -0.26$ $p < 0.01$

3. health status measurement instruments borrowed from the psychosocial sciences that had most often been developed to measure psychological status among psychiatric patients.

The most important limitation of these early strategies related to their validity (the capacity of an instrument to measure what it claims to measure) (18).

Recognizing that chronic lung disease is an important determinant of quality of life, some investigators developed their own questionnaires or adapted existing instruments (19). More recently, the availability of disease-specific questionnaires has highlighted the limitations of these strategies. For instance, trials of theophylline in patients with stable COPD, in which health status was measured with nonvalidated diary questionnaires, failed to show significant improvement in subjective effects of the drug (19). Subsequently several trials in which disease-specific questionnaires were used concluded that theophylline was associated with significant changes in quality of life (20-22).

Important Domains in Quality of Life in COPD

Defining "quality of life" remains a difficult task. Dimensions assessed by a representative group of quality-of-life instruments ranged from burden of symptoms to social functioning (23). The term "health-related quality of life" is often used when widely valued aspects of life not directly related to health, such as income and freedom, are not considered (18). The concept of HRQL usually refers to the patient's perception of performance in at least one of four important domains:

1. somatic sensation
2. physical function
3. emotional state
4. social interaction (24).

These domains allow us to classify the areas explored by health status measuring instruments currently used in COPD (1,25-50) (table 19.2).

Table 19.2 An Overview of Selected Health Status Measurement Instruments in COPD

	Quality of life domains				
Questionnaire	Overall quality of life	Somatic sensation	Physical function	Emotional function	Social interaction
Disease-specific questionnaires					
• Medical Research Council Dyspnea Scale (Fletcher et al. 1959 [25])		✓			
• American Thoracic Society Dyspnea Scale (American Thoracic Society 1978 [26])		✓			
• Oxygen Cost Diagram (McGavin et al. 1978 [27])		✓			
• Additive Activities Profile Test (ADAPT) quality-of-life scale (Daughton et al. 1992 [28])			✓		
• Baseline/Transition Dyspnea Index (Mahler et al. 1984 [1])		✓			
• Modified Dyspnea Index (Stoller et al. 1986 [29])		✓			
• Chronic Respiratory Questionnaire (Guyatt et al. 1987 [30])		✓		✓	
• Pulmonary Functional Status Scale (Weaver and Narsavage 1989 [31]; Weaver et al. 1998 [32])		✓	✓	✓	
• Chronic Disease Assessment Tool (Moody 1990 [33])		✓	✓	✓	

(continued)

Table 19.2 ***(continued)***

	Quality of life domains				
Questionnaire	Overall quality of life	Somatic sensation	Physical function	Emotional function	Social interaction
• COPD self-efficacy scale (Wigal et al. 1991 [34])				✓	
• Medico-Psychological Questionnaire for Lung Patients (Cox et al. 1991 [35])				✓	
• St. George's Respiratory Questionnaire (Jones et al. 1992 [3]; Jones et al. 1991 [36])		✓	✓		✓
• Pulmonary Functional Status and Dyspnea Questionnaire (Lareau et al. 1994 [37])		✓	✓		
• Pulmonary Functional Status and Dyspnea Questionnaire-Modified (Lareau et al. 1998 [38])		✓	✓		
• UCSD Shortness of Breath Questionnaire (Eakin et al. 1995 [39], 1998 [40])		✓			
• Seattle Obstructive Lung Disease Questionnaire (Tu et al. 1997 [41])		✓		✓	
Generic questionnaires					
Health profiles					
• Psychological Adjustment to Illness Scale (Morrow et al. 1978 [42]; Derogatis 1977 [43])				✓	✓
• Nottingham Health Profile (Hunt et al. 1980 [44])		✓	✓	✓	✓
• Sickness Impact Profile (Bergner et al. 1981 [45])			✓	✓	✓
• Medical Outcome Survey—Short Form (SF-36) (Ware and Sherbourne 1992 [46]; McHorney et al. 1993 [47])		✓	✓	✓	✓
Utility measures					
• Quality of Well-Being (Kaplan et al. 1976 [48])		✓	✓		✓
• Standard Gamble (Torrance 1976 [49])	✓				
• Time Trade-Off (Torrance 1976 [49])	✓				
• Rating Scale (Torrance 1976 [49])	✓				
• Health Utilities Index (Boyle et al. 1995 [50])	✓				

Disease-Specific Questionnaires in COPD

Disease-specific questionnaires focus on the areas of function that are relevant to a particular condition and, consequently, are likely to detect small changes. We selected 16 disease-specific questionnaires used in COPD populations (1,25-41) (see table 19.2) and reviewed their specifications and measurement properties. These questionnaires focus on one or more of the four major domains of HRQL and are presented accordingly.

Somatic Sensations

Dyspnea is the most frequent symptom presented by patients with COPD and is associated with a wide range of activities (11,12). Accordingly, most questionnaires measuring somatic sensations have focused on the measurement of dyspnea. Other somatic sensations reported by patients with COPD include fatigue and sleep disturbances (11,12).

Defining and Measuring Dyspnea

For clinical purposes, dyspnea may be defined as "an increased sense of respiratory effort" (51). In the questionnaires in which dyspnea was measured, the correlations between HRQL scores and indices of physiological functions were most often weak to moderate. We interpret this observation as reflecting that patients with COPD of similar severity have different perceptions of the effects of their disease.

Instruments applied to measure dyspnea are heterogeneous measures examining different components of dyspnea, ranging from the stimuli preceding the development of dyspnea to the consequences of dyspnea (5). For instance, the earliest health status measures used in COPD (those of the British Medical Research Council [25] and the American Thoracic Society [26]) were developed for discriminative purposes within the frame of epidemiological surveys. They focus on predetermined activities that provoke dyspnea. They offer little potential for the detection of small changes over time and are only useful in discriminating among patients according to the activities associated with dyspnea. On the other hand, the Transition Dyspnea Index (1) and the dyspnea domain of the Chronic Respiratory Questionnaire (30) focus on a set of activities selected as important by the individuals being tested. They offer the potential for responsiveness but are inappropriate as discriminative instruments because the dyspnea rating is derived from different sets of activities. A major limitation of most dyspnea scales (with the exception of the Chronic Respiratory Questionnaire) is their interpretability.

Measuring Other Symptoms

The Chronic Respiratory Questionnaire (30) contains a domain for measuring fatigue, a symptom that has been reported as important by patients with COPD (11,12). Cough, sputum production, and wheeze are measured by the St. George's Respiratory Questionnaire (3,36). Since the latter has been developed for patients with COPD and asthma, the inclusion of cough and wheeze is appropriate.

Physical Function

Functional status, as determined by the patient's ability to perform activities of daily living (6), often reflects the level of autonomy of affected patients and is of crucial importance in the delivery of health services. In a recent review, Lareau et al. (6) summarized the psychometric properties of the questionnaires measuring functional status in COPD. The disease-specific questionnaires that measure physical function in COPD include the ADAPT quality-of-life scale (28), the Pulmonary Impact Profile Scale (31), the St. George's Respiratory Questionnaire (3,36), the Pulmonary Functional Status and Dyspnea Questionnaire (PFSDQ) (37), and its modified version (PFSDQ-M) (38). Both the St. George's Respiratory Questionnaire and the Pulmonary Functional Status and Dyspnea Questionnaire have proved able to detect change over time.

Emotional Function

Irritability and hopelessness are frequent complaints in patients with COPD (11,12). The prevalence of depression in patients with moderate to severe COPD approximates 42% (14,52), with rates as high as 76% having been reported (53). The prevalence of anxiety disorders in COPD is less clear, with reported anxiety rates ranging from 2% (53) to 34% (54,55). Therefore, most clinicians consider the measurement of anxiety and depression in clinical trials of COPD to be relevant (56). The imprecision of depression and anxiety prevalence rates may stem from the heterogeneity of the populations.

Depression has been measured in COPD with the Center for Epidemiologic Studies' Depression Scale (CES-D) (57), the Beck Depression Inventory (58), and the Zung Self-Rating Depression scale (59). The level of anxiety has been assessed by Spielberger's State-Trait Anxiety Inventory (60) and the Zung Self-Rating Anxiety scale (59). These questionnaires are problem specific (i.e. "depression-specific" and "anxiety-specific") and have not been specifically developed for use in patients with COPD. As many have been developed and validated in the general population, their validity in patients with COPD is limited. Their usefulness as evaluative instruments is also unknown. A more complete review of these instruments was reported by Lader (61) and Mulrow et al. (62).

Self-Efficacy Negative attitudes and beliefs held by patients with COPD concerning themselves, their illness, and its treatment correlate with reduced functional capacity (63). This finding is congruent with Bandura's self-efficacy theory. Self-efficacy refers to the personal conviction people have regarding whether or not they feel that they can successfully execute particular behaviors in order to produce certain outcomes (34,64). According to this theory, people who entertain doubts about their capabilities give up their efforts; those who have a strong sense of efficacy persist (64). In COPD, self-efficacy may be a determinant of unnecessary activity restriction (34). Kaplan, Atkins, and Reinsch (65) demonstrated that in patients with COPD, efficacy expectations correlated significantly with health status and exercise tolerance.

The COPD Self-Efficacy Scale was developed by Wigal, Creer, and Kotses (34). In the original paper, the authors presented evidence of test-retest reliability, internal consistency, and the description of item aggregation of the scale. Validity of this questionnaire was then assumed on the basis of the apparent validity of the self-efficacy theory. Correlations with other health status instruments and physiological measures have recently provided support to the construct validity of the COPD Self-Efficacy Scale (66). Further explorations of the psychometric measurement properties of the instrument are necessary.

Other Disease-Specific Instruments Other disease-specific questionnaires include items or even full domains measuring emotional dimensions related to COPD (table 19.2). Data regarding the validity and responsiveness of the emotional function and mastery domains of the Chronic Respiratory Questionnaire (30) exist. Items specifically relating to anxiety and depression were not included in the St. George's Respiratory Questionnaire (3), the authors arguing that a number of established measures exist for this area of health.

Social Function

Social function refers to an individual's capacity to perform activities associated with his or her usual role, including employment, school work, or homemaking (7). Occupational function in patients with COPD is often irrelevant. Most patients with symptomatic COPD are elderly patients aged >65 years who have retired. The St. George's Respiratory Questionnaire (3,36) includes work-related items.

Disease-Specific Questionnaires in COPD: Summary

The currently used COPD-specific health status instruments usually focus on patients' perceptions of performance in four major domains of HRQL: somatic sensation, physical and occupational function, psychological state, and social function (table 19.2). A major limitation of many of the questionnaires is their unproved ability to detect change over time. Furthermore, when differences in scores have been demonstrated in the setting of clinical trials, the clinical relevance of these differences has been uncertain. Information regarding the interpretability of the Chronic Respiratory Questionnaire (30) and the St. George's Respiratory Questionnaire (3,36) currently exists. Although comparisons of these two questionnaires in a discriminative purpose, meaning used to distinguish between groups of patients, have suggested that both instruments are valid (67,68), a direct comparison of their responsiveness in the setting of a randomized trial remains unavailable.

Generic Measures for COPD

Generic measures of quality of life have been used extensively both in population research and in clinical research. They can be broadly divided into two groups: health profiles and utility measures. In this chapter, we review the measurement properties of four health profiles (42,47) and five utility measures (48-50) that are frequently used in research studies.

Health Profiles

Health profiles are useful because they provide information on many aspects of a patient's life. The Psychological Adjustment to Illness Scale (42) and the Self-Reported Psychological Adjustment to Illness Scale (43) focus only on the psychological aspects of health. The Nottingham Health Profile, the Sickness Impact Profile (SIP), and the Medical Outcome Survey—Short Form (SF-36) are multidimensional profiles that cover many health concepts (44-47).

All the instruments have proved helpful in distinguishing among different populations and among patients within the same population. The SIP, the SF-36, and the Nottingham Health Profile have been validated in patients with COPD. However, because the Nottingham Health Profile was designed to discriminate among patients with moderate to severe illness (69), it may not be able to discriminate among patients with mild disease. In an evaluative setting, the same three instruments have been validated against other measures. Only the SF-36 has not been validated in pulmonary patients. The other two instruments both showed weak correlations with physiological measures such as the FEV_1.

The Sickness Impact Profile has shown strong evidence of reliability (45). In the remaining questionnaires, there were a few domains in which measures of reliability correlated poorly (42,43,70,71). Trials in COPD patients in which the SIP or Nottingham Health Profile was used sometimes identified significant changes in physiological parameters such as the FEV_1 without accompanying changes in quality of life assessments (72-74). The SF-36 (75,76) and PAIS-SR

(77) are responsive in nonpulmonary patient populations. For the SF-36, some dimensions are responsive to self-perceived changes in HRQL. Whether PAIS-SR is responsive to changes in the quality of life of patients with COPD remains to be seen. The Sickness Impact Profile, the SF-36, and the Nottingham Health Profile have distinctive profiles for COPD patients as compared with the normal population, with the SIP (78) and the SF-36 (79) having different profiles at different levels of impairment. However, the minimal clinically important difference (MCID) that would distinguish one group from another is unknown. In an evaluative setting, little information is available on the MCID in any of the five instruments.

In summary, all five instruments have similar properties when they are used in a discriminative setting. In an evaluative setting, most of the instruments have not demonstrated good responsiveness among patients with COPD. Therefore, in a clinical trial involving patients with COPD, we would recommend a combination of a generic health profile (to broadly reflect quality of life) and a disease-specific instrument (to detect small changes over time).

Utility Measures

Utility measures use a preference-based or value-based approach to express the HRQL of an individual in a single number. This number incorporates the overall assessment of HRQL and the values attached to it. This number is usually between 0 and 1. The two extreme values are anchored to specific states, most commonly death at 0 and full health at 1.

There are two different approaches to obtaining the preference weight, which can come either directly from the patient or from other people. In two common measures, the Standard Gamble (49) and the Time Trade-Off (49), the preference comes from the patient. In these measures, the patient trades a specific health state for full health by risking death or by shortening his or her life span.

In the second approach, the preference weight is obtained from other people, most commonly through the use of a multi-attribute questionnaire. A series of health states of increasing severity is compiled based on limitations in different dimensions of HRQL. Either people of the general population or specific population groups are asked to rate these states on a scale. Based on the responses, preference weights are assigned to the different states. A patient's utility value is determined from the preference weight assigned to the combination of limitations identified by the patient. This is the basis of the Quality of Well-Being scale (48) and the Health Utilities Index—MarkIII (50). The advantage of utility measures is that they allow comparison among different diseases. In addition, a single value summarizing the overall state of health facilitates economic analyses.

In a discriminative setting, only the Quality of Well-Being scale was validated in patients with COPD and showed good discriminative power (80). Neither the

Standard Gamble nor the Rating Scale demonstrated strong discriminative ability in asthmatic patients (81). The Health Utilities Index is a relatively new instrument with only one study showing discriminative power () among adolescents. In the evaluative setting, the Standard Gamble (81), Rating Scale (81), and Quality of Well-Being (80) have all been validated against other measures. However, only weak correlations were seen when they were compared to physiological measures such as the FEV_1 and the forced vital capacity (FVC) (80,81).

All five measures demonstrated good reliability except for some attributes of the Health Utilities Index (50,81,83). The responsiveness of the Standard Gamble was disappointing. Although it could detect changes before and after a treatment in pulmonary patients, it was unable to detect differences among groups even though these differences were noted in physiological measures and in disease-specific quality-of-life instruments (81). The Rating Scale (81) and the Quality of Well-Being scale (84,85) showed better responsiveness. Responsiveness data for pulmonary patients were not available for the Time Trade-Off and Health Utilities Index. Little information was available for any of the five instruments regarding MCID in either a discriminative or an evaluative setting.

In summary, information on the measurement properties of the utility measures was limited. These instruments demonstrated weak discriminative ability and poor responsiveness to change. Although it is very attractive to use these instruments as part of an economic analysis, caution must be exercised in their interpretation. We recommend that utility measures be used in conjunction with other measures of quality of life.

Discussion

Finally, our findings suggest several topics that should be discussed.

Selection of a Questionnaire for Clinical Research

In order to use a questionnaire most appropriately, it is important to consider whether it is to be discriminative or evaluative or both (86). A discriminative instrument is one that can distinguish among groups of patients. Accordingly, the most important properties of a discriminative instrument are its validity, its reliability, and its interpretability. An evaluative instrument is one that measures changes in individuals or groups over time. Accordingly, the most important properties of an evaluative instrument are its validity, its responsiveness, and its interpretability. The requirement for maximizing one of these functions (discrimination or evaluation) may influence the choice of questionnaire (86). A disease-specific questionnaire is more likely to be responsive to change than a generic instrument because the former focuses on specific areas of HRQL, whereas the latter is designed to measure all important aspects of HRQL (18).

In selecting a questionnaire to be used in clinical research, the investigator should first answer the following questions:

1. Do I want to evaluate an intervention or discriminate among patients?
2. Which of the domains am I most interested in measuring (symptoms, function, emotion, etc.)?
3. What is the time frame of the study?

These questions will direct the investigator toward identifying the most appropriate questionnaire(s) for the study. In a rehabilitation trial, a generic questionnaire can help to characterize the patients at baseline, whereas a disease-specific (and responsive) questionnaire can be used to evaluate the effect of the intervention on symptoms, for example the Baseline and Transition Dyspnea Index (1) or the Chronic Respiratory Questionnaire (30); or on the impact of the disease, for example the St. George's Respiratory Questionnaire (3,36). In selecting a questionnaire, it is also important to consider the mode, ease, and duration of administration (18). In addition, if an economic evaluation is to be included in the trial, it is useful to add a utility measure.

Exercise Capacity or Health-Related Quality of Life?

Whereas exercise capacity testing is intended to measure impairment, such as the reduction of organ function (87), quality of life has more to do with disability, such as the inability to engage in substantial gainful activities (88) and handicap, for example, the disadvantage for a given individual, resulting from impairment or disability, that limits or prevents fulfillment of a role that is normal for that individual (88). Therefore, although exercise capacity testing constitutes an invaluable tool in many respects, it serves different purposes in measuring different constructs (see table 19.1).

Laboratory exercise testing can be helpful for diagnosis and management (89). An initial exercise test is useful in describing the physiological consequences of the disease and may reveal coronary or peripheral arterial disease as limiting vigorous training in some patients with COPD. Exercise testing is also useful in assisting with the prescription of an appropriate level of exercise training (90,91). Retesting provides physiological evidence that a training response has occurred and may be useful in the adjustment of intensity levels during the program (89). Exercise testing may also be useful in motivating the patient to continue the activities (89). Thus, measurements of health status and exercise capacity are complementary. Given that they measure different constructs, each should be evaluated separately.

Future Directions

Health status measurement has become important in identifying the impact of a management strategy in patients with COPD and is likely to become of further interest as rehabilitation professionals (physicians as well as nonphysicians) continue clinical research aimed at improving the comprehensive and integrative care of patients with COPD. Future research should include validation and a more precise understanding of the interpretability of existing instruments rather than the development of more questionnaires.

References

1. Mahler, D.A., D.H. Weinberg, C.K. Wells, and A.R. Feinstein. 1984. The measurement of dyspnea. Contents, interobserver agreement, and physiologic correlates of two new clinical indexes. *Chest* 85:751-758.
2. Guyatt, G.H., P.J. Thompson, and L.B. Berman, et al. 1985. How should we measure function in patients with chronic heart and lung disease? *J Chron Dis* 38:517-524.
3. Jones, P.W., F.H. Quirk, C.M. Baveystock, and P. Littlejohns. 1992. A self-complete measure of health status for chronic airflow limitation. The St. George's Respiratory Questionnaire. *Am Rev Respir Dis* 145:1321-1327.
4. McCord, M., and D. Cronin-Stubbs. 1992. Operationalizing dyspnea: focus on measurement. *Heart Lung* 21:167-179.
5. Eakin, A.G., R.M. Kaplan, and A.L. Ries. 1993. Measurement of dyspnoea in chronic obstructive pulmonary disease. *Qual Life Res* 2:181-191.
6. Lareau, S.C., E.H. Breslin, and P.M. Meek. 1996. Functional status instruments: outcome measure in the evaluation of patients with chronic obstructive pulmonary disease. *Heart Lung* 25:212-224.
7. Lacasse, Y., E. Wong, G.H. Guyatt, and R.S.Goldstein. 1997. Health-status measure instruments in chronic obstructive pulmonary disease. *Can Respir J* 4:152-164.
8. Guyatt, G.H. 1995. A taxonomy of health status instruments. *J Rheumatol* 22:1188-1190.
9. Killian, K.J., P. Leblanc, D.H. Martin, E. Summers, N.L. Jones, and E.J.M. Campbell. 1992. Exercise capacity and ventilatory, circulatory, and symptom limitation in patients with chronic airflow limitation. *Am Rev Respir Dis* 146:935-940.
10. Jones, N.L., G. Jones, and R.H.T. Edwards. 1971. Exercise tolerance in chronic airway obstruction. *Am Rev Respir Dis* 103:477-491.

11. Kinsman, R.A., R.A. Yaroush, E. Fernandez, J.F. Dirks, M. Schocket, and J. Fukuhara. 1983. Symptoms and experiences in chronic bronchitis and emphysema. *Chest* 83:755-761.

12. Guyatt, G.H., M. Townsend, L.B. Berman, and S.O. Pugsley. 1987. Quality of life in patients with chronic airflow limitation. *Br J Dis Chest* 81:45-54.

13. Casaburi, R. 1993. Exercise training in chronic obstructive lung disease. In *Principles and Practice of Pulmonary Rehabilitation,* ed. R. Casaburi and T.L. Petty. Philadelphia: W.B. Saunders.

14. Light, R.W., E.J. Merrill, J.A. Despars, G.H. Gordon, and L.R. Mutalipassi. 1985. Prevalence of depression and anxiety in patients with COPD. Relationship to functional capacity. *Chest* 87:35-38.

15. Lacasse, Y., E. Wong, G.H. Guyatt, D. King, D.J. Cook, and R.S. Goldstein. 1996. Meta-analysis of respiratory rehabilitation in chronic obstructive pulmonary disease. *Lancet* 348:1115-1119.

16. McGavin, C.R., S.P. Gupta, E.L. Lloyd, and G.J.R. McHardy. 1977. Physical rehabilitation for the chronic bronchitis: results of a controlled trial of exercises in the home. *Thorax* 32:307-311.

17. Cockroft, A.E., M.J. Saunders, and G. Berry. 1981. Randomised controlled trial of rehabilitation in chronic respiratory disability. *Thorax* 36:200-203.

18. Guyatt G.H., D.H. Feeny, D.L. Patrick. 1993. Measuring health-related quality of life. *Ann Intern Med* 118:622-629.

19. Alexander, M.R., W.L. Dull, and J.E. Kasik. 1980. Treatment of chronic obstructive pulmonary disease with orally administered theophylline: a double-blind, controlled study. *JAMA* 244:2286-2290.

20. Jaeschke, R., G.H. Guyatt, J. Singer, J. Keller, and M.T. Newhouse. 1991. Mechanism of bronchodilator effect in chronic airflow limitation. *Can Med Assoc J* 144:35-39.

21. Jaeschke, R., G.H. Guyatt, A. Willan, D. Cook, S. Harper, and J. Morris, et al. 1994. Effect of increasing dose of beta-agonists on spirometric parameters, exercise capacity, and quality of life in patients with chronic airflow limitation. *Thorax* 49:479-484.

22. McKay, S.E., C.A. Howie, A.H. Thomson, B. Whiting, and G.J. Addis. 1993. Value of theophylline treatment in patients handicapped by chronic obstructive lung disease. *Thorax* 48:227-232.

23. McSweeny, A.J., and T.L. Creer. 1995. Health-related quality-of-life assessment in medical care. *Dis Month* 41:1-71.

24. Shipper, H., J. Clinch, and V. Powell. 1990. Definition and conceptual issues. In *Quality of Life Assessment in Clinical Trials,* ed. B. Spilker. New York: Raven Press Ltd.

25. Fletcher, C.M., P.C. Elmes, A.S. Fairbairn, and C.H. Wood. 1959. The significance of respiratory symptoms and the diagnosis of chronic bronchitis in a working population. *Br Med J* 2:257-266.

26. American Thoracic Society. 1978. Recommended respiratory disease questionnaire for use with adults and children in epidemiological research. *Am Rev Respir Dis* 118 (suppl.):7-53.

27. McGavin, C.R., M. Artvinli, H. Naoe, and G.J.R. McHardy. 1978. Dyspnea, disability, and distance walked: comparison of estimates of exercise performance in respiratory disease. *Br Med J* 2:241-243.

28. Daughton, D.M., A.J. Fix, I. Kass, C.W. Bell, and K.D. Patil. 1992. Maximum oxygen consumption and the ADAPT quality-of-life scale. *Arch Phys Med Rehabil* 63:620-622.

29. Stoller, J.K., R. Ferranti, and A.R. Feinstein. 1986. Further specification and evaluation of a new clinical index for dyspnea. *Am Rev Respir Dis* 134:1129-1134.

30. Guyatt, G.H., L.B. Berman, M. Townsend, S.O. Pugsley, and L.W. Chambers. 1987. A measure of quality of life for clinical trials in chronic lung disease. *Thorax* 42:773-778.

31. Weaver, T., and G. Narsavage. 1989. Reliability and validity of Pulmonary Impact Profile Scale. *Am Rev Respir Dis* 139:A244.

32. Weaver, T.E., G.L. Narsavage, and M.J. Guilfoyle. 1998. The development and psychometric evaluation of the Pulmonary Functional Status Scale: an instrument to assess functional status in pulmonary disease. *J Cardiopulm Rehabil* 18:105-111.

33. Moody, L.E. 1990. Measurement of psychophysiologic response variables in chronic bronchitis and emphysema. *Appl Nurs Res* 3:36-38.

34. Wigal, J.K., T.L. Creer, and H. Kotses. 1991. The COPD Self-Efficacy Scale. *Chest* 99:1193-1196.

35. Cox, N.J.M., J.C.M. Hendriks, R. Dijkhuizen, R.A. Binkhorst, and C.L.A. van Herwaarden. 1991. Usefulness of a medicopsychological questionnaire for lung patients. *Int J Rehab Res* 14:267-272.

36. Jones, P.W., F.H. Quirk, and C.M. Baveystock. 1991. The St. George's Respiratory Questionnaire. *Respir Med* 85 (suppl. B):25-31.

37. Lareau, S.C., V. Carrieri-Kohlman, S. Janson-Bjerklie, and P.J. Ross. 1994. Development and testing of the Pulmonary Functional Status and Dyspnea Questionnaire (PFSDQ). *Heart Lung* 23:242-250.

38. Lareau, S.C., P.M. Meek, and P.J. Roos. 1998. Development and testing of the modified version of the Pulmonary Functional Status and Dyspnea Questionnaire (PFSDQ-M). *Heart Lung* 27:159-168.

39. Eakin, E.G., D.E. Sassi-Dambron, A.L. Ries, and R.M. Kaplan. 1995. Reliability and validity of dyspnea measures in patients with obstructive lung diseases. *Int J Behav Med* 2:118-134.

40. Eakin, E.G., P.M. Resnikoff, L.M. Prewitt, A.L. Ries, and R.M. Kaplan. 1998. Validation of a new dyspnea measure: the UCSD Shortness of Breath Questionnaire. *Chest* 113:619-624.

41. Tu, S.P., M.B. McDonnell, J.A. Spertus, B.G. Steele, and S.D. Fihn. 1997. A new self-administered questionnaire to monitor health-related quality of life in patients with COPD. *Chest* 112:614-622.

42. Morrow, G.R., R.J. Chiarello, and L.R. Derogatis. 1978. A new scale for assessing patient's psychosocial adjustment to medical illness. *Psychol Med* 8:605-610.

43. Derogatis, L.R. 1977. *Psychological Adjustment to Illness Scale*. Baltimore, MD: Clinical Psychometric Research.

44. Hunt, S.M., S.P. McKenna, J. McEwen, E.M. Backett, J. Williams, and E. Papp. 1980. A quantitative approach to perceived health status: a validation study. *J Epidemiol Comm Health* 34:281-286.

45. Bergner, M., R.A. Bobbitt, W.B. Carter, and B.S. Gilson. 1981. The Sickness Impact Profile: development and final revision of a health status measure. *Med Care* 19:878-885.

46. Ware, J.E., Jr., and C.D. Sherbourne. 1992. The MOS 36-item short form health survey (SF-36): I. Conceptual framework and item selection. *Med Care* 30:473-483.

47. McHorney, C.A., J.E. Ware Jr., and A.E. Raczek. 1993. The MOS 36-item short form health survey (SF-36): II. Psychometric and clinical tests of validity in measuring physical and mental health constructs. *Med Care* 31:247-263.

48. Kaplan, R.M., J.W. Bush, and C.C. Berry. 1976. Health status: types of validity and the Index of Well-Being. *Health Serv Res* 11:478-507.

49. Torrance, G.W. 1976. Social preferences for health states: an empirical evaluation of three measurement techniques. *Socio Econ Plan Sci* 10:129-136.

50. Boyle, M.H., W. Furlong, D. Feeny, G.W. Torrance, and J. Hatcher. 1995. Reliability of the Health Utilities Index—Mark III used in the 1991 cycle 6 Canadian General Social Survey Health Questionnaire. *Qual Life Res* 4:249-257.

51. Killian, K.J. 1985. The objective measurement of breathlessness. *Chest* 88:84S-90S.

52. Gift, A.G., and S.H. McCrone. 1993. Depression in patients with COPD. *Heart Lung* 22:289-297.

53. Agle, D.P., G.L. Baum, E.H. Chester, and M. Wendt. 1973. Multidiscipline treatment of chronic pulmonary insufficiency: psychologic aspects of rehabilitation. *Psychosom Med* 35:41-49.

54. Karajgi, B., A. Rifkin, S. Doddi, R. Kolli, and L.R. Mutalipassi. 1990. The prevalence of anxiety disorders in patients with chronic obstructive pulmonary disease. *Am J Psychiatr* 147:200-201.

55. Yellowlees, P.M., J.H. Alpers, J.J. Bowden, G.D. Bryant, and R.E. Ruffin. 1987. Psychiatric morbidity in patients with chronic airflow limitation. *Med J Aust* 146:305-307.

56. McSweeny, A.J., I. Grant, R.K. Heaton, K.M. Adams, and R.M. Timms. 1982. Life quality of patients with chronic obstructive pulmonary disease. *Arch Intern Med* 142:473-478.

57. Radloff, L.S. 1977. The CES-D Scale: a self-report depressive scale for research in the general population. *J Appl Psychol Meas* 1:385-401.

58. Beck, A.T., C.H. Ward, M. Mendelson, J. Mock, and J. Erbaugh. 1961. An inventory for measuring depression. *Arch Gen Psychiatr* 4:561-571.

59. Zung, W.W.K. 1974. The measurement of affects: depression and anxiety. *Mod Probl Pharmacopsychiatr* 7:170-188.

60. Spielberger, C.D., R.L. Gorsuch, R.E. Lushene, P.R. Vagg, and G.A. Jacobs. 1983. *STAI: Manual for the State-Trait Anxiety Inventory (Form Y)*. Palo Alto, CA: Consulting Psychologists Press.

61. Lader, M. 1981. The clinical assessment of depression. *Br J Clin Pharm* 1:5-14.

62. Mulrow, C.D., J.W. Williams, and M.B. Gerety, et al. 1995. Case-finding instruments for depression in primary care settings. *Ann Intern Med* 122:913.

63. Morgan, A.D., D.F. Peck, and D. Buchanan, et al. 1983. Effect of attitudes and beliefs on exercise tolerance in chronic bronchitis. *Br Med J* 286:171-173.

64. Bandura, A. 1982. Self-efficacy mechanism in human agency. *Am Psychol* 37:122-147.

65. Kaplan, R.M., C.J. Atkins, and S. Reinsch. 1984. Specific efficacy expectations mediate exercise compliance in patients with COPD. *Health Psychol* 3:223-242.

66. Scherer, Y.K., and L.E. Schmieder. 1997. The effect of a pulmonary rehabilitation program on self-efficacy, perception of dyspnea, and physical endurance. *Heart Lung* 26:15-22.

67. Harper, R., J.E. Brazier, J.C. Waterhouse, S.J. Walters, N.M.B. Jones, and P. Howard. 1997. Comparison of outcome measures for patients with chronic obstructive pulmonary disease (COPD) in an outpatient setting. *Thorax* 52:879-887.

68. Hajiro, T., K. Nishimura, M. Tsukino, A. Ikeda, H. Koyama, and T. Izumi. 1998. Comparison of discriminative properties among disease-specific questionnaires for measuring health-related quality of life in patients with chronic obstructive pulmonary disease. *Am J Respir Crit Care Med* 157: 785-790.

69. Kind, P., and R. Carr-Hill. 1987. The Nottingham Health Profile: A useful tool for epidemiologists. *Soc Sci Med* 25:905-910.

70. Hunt, S.M., J. McEwen, and S.P. McKenna. 1985. Measuring health status: a new tool for clinicians and epidemiologists. *J Roy Coll Gen Pract* 1985:185-188.

71. Brazier, J.E., R. Harper, N.M.B. Jones, A. O'Cathain, K.J. Thomas, and T. Usherwood, et al. 1992. Validating the SF-36 health survey questionnaire: new outcome measure for primary care. *BMJ* 305:160-164.

72. Van Schayck, C.P., E. Dompeling, M.P.M.H. Rutten, H. Folgering, G. Van den Boom, and C. Van Weel. 1995. The influence of an inhaled steroid on quality of life in patients with asthma or COPD. *Chest* 107:1199-1205.

73. Van Schayck, C.P., M.P.M.H. Rutten-van Mölken, E.K.A. Van Doorslaer, H. Folgering, and C. Van Weel. 1992. Two-year bronchodilator treatment in patients with mild airflow obstruction. *Chest* 102:1384-1391.

74. The Intermittent Positive Pressure Breathing Trial Group. 1983. Intermittent positive pressure breathing therapy of chronic obstructive pulmonary disease: a clinical trial. *Ann Intern Med* 99:612-620.

75. Ware, J.E. Jr., M. Kosinski, M.S. Bayliss, C.A. McHorney, W.H. Rogers, and A. Raczek. 1995. Comparison of methods for the scoring and statistical analysis of SF-36 health profile and summary measures: summary of results from the Medical Outcomes Study. *Med Care* 33:AS264-AS279.

76. Katz, J.N., M.G. Larson, C.B. Phillips, A.H. Fossel, and M.H. Liang. 1992. Comparative measurement sensitivity of short and longer health status instruments. *Med Care* 30:917-925.

77. Wilhelmsen, I., and A. Berstad. 1994. Quality of life and relapse of duodenal ulcer before and after eradication of *Helicobacter pylori*. *Scand J Gastroenterol* 29:874-879.

78. Schrier, A.C., F.W. Dekker, A.A. Kaptein, and J.H. Dijkman. 1990. Quality of life in elderly patients with chronic nonspecific lung disease seen in family practice. *Chest* 98:894-899.

79. Viramontes, J.L., and B. O'Brien. 1994. Relationship between symptoms and health-related quality of life in chronic lung disease. *J Gen Intern Med* 9:46-48.

80. Kaplan, R.M., C.J. Aitkins, and R. Timms. 1984. Validity of a quality of well-being scale as an outcome measure in chronic obstructive pulmonary disease. *J Chron Dis* 37:85-95.

81. Rutten-van Mölken, M.P.M.H., F. Custers, E.K.A. Van Doorslaer, C.C.M. Jansen, L. Heurman, and F.P.V. Maesen, et al. 1995. Comparison of performance of four instruments in evaluating the effects of salmeterol on asthma quality of life. *Eur Respir J* 8:888-898.

82. Torrance, G.W. 1987. Utility approach to measuring health-related quality of life. *J Chron Dis* 40:593-603.

83. Anderson, J.P., R.M. Kaplan, C.C. Berry, J.W. Bush, and R.G. Rumbaut. 1989. Interday reliability of function assessment for a health status measure: the quality of well-being scale. *Med Care* 27:1076-1084.

84. Ries, A.L., R.M. Kaplan, T.M. Limberg, and L.M. Prewitt. 1995. Effects of pulmonary rehabilitation on physiologic and psychological outcomes in patients with chronic obstructive pulmonary disease. *Ann Intern Med* 122:823-832.

85. Manzetti, J.D., L.A. Hoffman, S.M. Sereika, F.C. Sciurba, and B.P. Griffith. 1994. Exercise, education, and quality of life in lung transplant candidates. *J Heart Lung Transpl* 13:297-305.

86. Kirshner, B., and G. Guyatt. 1985. A methodological framework for assessing health indices. *J Chron Dis* 38:27-36.

87. Richman, S.I. 1980. Meanings of impairment and disability. *Chest* 79 (suppl.):367-371.

88. American Thoracic Society. 1986. Evaluation of impairment/disability secondary to respiratory disorders. *Am Rev Respir Dis* 133:1205-1209.

89. Jones, N.L. 1988. Approaches to clinical exercise testing. *In Clinical Exercise Testing*, ed. N.L. Jones. Philadelphia: W.B. Saunders.

90. Casaburi, R., A. Patessio, and F. Ioli, et al. 1991. Reductions in exercise lactic acidosis and ventilation as a result of exercise training in patients with obstructive lung disease. *Am Rev Respir Dis* 143:9-18.

91. Vallet, G., S. Ahmaïdi, and I. Serres, et al. 1997. Comparison of two training programs in CAL patients: standardized versus individualized method. *Eur Respir J* 10:114-122.

CHAPTER 20

Measurement of Quality of Life in Cardiac Rehabilitation

Gilles Dupuis[1,2], Marie Christine Taillefer[1,2], Anne Marie Étienne[3], Ovide Fontaine[3], Sonia Boivin[1,2], and Alexandra Von Turk[4]
[1]Université du Québec à Montréal, Montréal, Québec, Canada
[2]Institut de Cardiologie de Montréal, Montréal, Québec, Canada
[3]Université de Liège, Liege, Belgium
[4]Université de Lausanne, Lausanne, Switzerland

> "Il est difficile de rester un empereur en présence d'un médecin, et difficile aussi de garder sa qualité d'homme. L'œil du praticien ne voyait en moi qu'un monceau d'humeurs, triste amalgame de lymphe et de sang."

This citation, from Marguerite Yourcenar (1), described how the Roman Emperor Hadrian felt when consulting his personal doctor. In substance, he found it difficult to remain an emperor in front of his doctor, or even just to preserve his human nature. To the practitioner, he felt but an aggregate of humors, a sad combination of blood and lymph. Nearly 2000 years later, Leplège and Hunt deplored this mechanistic view, which modern medicine applied to the concept of quality of life (QL), noting, "This component approach may well be appropriate for the assessment of health status, but whether it can reasonably evaluate quality of life remains, at best, equivocal"(2).

Gill and Feinstein (3) emphasized the point that QL must not only be refined to a statistically elegant measure of health, but also improve its face validity by addressing the right issue: the way one feels about one's health status as well as nonmedical aspects of life.

This problem is one of several affecting current opinion on the validity of the concept of quality of life. Kinney, in 1995, suggested that the quality-of-life concept is in a state of emergency and mentioned that it is time to "move forward in conceptual and operational clarity, methodological sophistication, and theoretical inspiration. It is important that we make this happen before we become disillusioned and abandon our goal of finding the harmony of which Bacon spoke so long ago"(4). She was referring to Bacon's statement that "The office of medicine is but to tune this curious harp of man's body and reduce it to harmony" (4).

This chapter first describes some of the actual problems in the field. Current definitions of QL are then presented and analyzed in light of their background theoretical model. Finally, a theoretical model based on the system control approach is described. This model helps to clarify the concept and provides one possible answer to a central question in quality-of-life evaluation: "What makes life worth living?" Some preliminary results are described in order to illustrate the strategy of evaluation put forward by the model. It will be useful for readers to keep the following questions in mind:

1. Do you have a goal in reading this article?
2. If you do not reach your goal, how will you feel?
3. Would you prefer
   a. to be a millionaire,
   b. to have glory and fame,
   c. to be loved, or
   d. to be perfectly happy?

Problems

In 1989, Dupuis et al. (5) presented a table summarizing four of the main problems of the field at that time. This table has been reorganized into six categories that are discussed on the following pages: objective versus subjective measures; QL and the notions of health status, performance, well-being, happiness, and satisfaction; multidimensionality and specificity of the concept; measuring the patient's life plan and goals attainment; lack of theoretical and conceptual bases for QL; and measuring alpha, beta, and gamma changes.

Objective Versus Subjective Measures and Confusion Between Factors Influencing QL

The dilemma of objective versus subjective is no longer a major issue. No one objects to the importance of measuring both aspects. Objective measures are those describing the patient's medical (e.g., number of stenosed vessels, treadmill test, etc.), demographic, and neuropsychological (performance on cognitive tests) condition. Questions measuring presence or absence of a symptom (or problem) can also be included in the category of objective information. The cognitive demand placed by this type of question is less complex than that needed for estimating the intensity or severity of a symptom. Except under particular circumstances, the reliability of this information is good. It represents a fact reported by the patient. Now, the question is: Should this objective information be considered as part of QL?

Strictly speaking, if we considered QL as being more than simply a health-related phenomenon (3,6), the answer is no. This information describes a person's global condition (physical, social condition, etc.). These indicators may surely influence an individual's QL but should not be part of the concept (7-9). Just as age, gender, and level of education describe someone's social condition, the number of stenosed vessels and physical capacity describe a person's medical condition. If someone says he or she is 50 years old, has a high school education, and has a treadmill of 5 METs, that does not provide information about his or her actual quality of life. For the sake of concept specificity, these factors should be considered as dimensions of a person's life that may influence his or her QL.

Subjective information is obtained by asking patients to evaluate the intensity or severity of symptoms on a variety of dimensions: physical, psychological, cognitive, social, and so forth. Providing such information is more cognitively complex because the patient has to think about a referent to estimate the severity of the symptoms. Nonetheless, this type of information is frequently used, and the reliability and validity of such measurements have proven to be adequate in many fields of research (anxiety, depression, etc.). However, in the QL area, the use of psychometry and clinimetry approaches has not always been successful (2,3). Not only are the face validity and the psychometric validity of many questionnaires unsatisfactory, but almost anything is considered as being QL: depression, anxiety, self-esteem, optimism, capacity to do activities of daily living, and so on. This maintains confusion and lack of specificity in the concept (10).

QL and the Notions of Health Status, Performance, Well-Being, Happiness, and Satisfaction

The following are concepts frequently used to define QL: health, well-being, satisfaction with life, functioning or performance, and happiness. The following are some generally accepted definitions of each.

Health Status and Performance The foundation of health status evaluation relies on the WHO definition of health: "a state of complete physical, mental and social well-being and not merely the absence of disease" (11). Bergner (12) presented a framework for dimensions of health status and commented that it had been defined with better clarity many years before the concept of QL became popular. It includes genetic foundation; biological, physiological, and anatomic conditions (disease state, disability or handicap state); functional condition (social role performance, physical performance, and cognitive performance); mental condition (mood or feeling state, affective state); and health potential (longevity, functioning, disease, disability, and disadvantage). These factors are measured using inventories that assess functioning and status in the different domains.

Well-Being and Satisfaction Well-being is a concept that has driven many studies. Diener (13) emphasized the fact that studies of well-being should be more concerned with life satisfaction and affect balance. He deplored the use of the term "happiness" in the study of well-being because of its loose definition. He defined three characteristics of well-being:

1. subjectivity, with potential influence of objective living conditions but not inherent to the notion,
2. positive aspects and not only the absence of negative aspects,
3. inclusion of global assessment of all aspects of an individual's life.

Happiness and Satisfaction Packa (14) and Campbell et al. (15) have suggested that happiness is an affective and transient state compared to satisfaction, which is a more long-term cognitive appraisal of someone's global condition. Packa (14) also stated that well-being reflects satisfaction and happiness and that the construct of well-being is closely tied to global QL. McCall (16), on the other hand, viewed happiness as a state close to life enhancement. This view is closer to Aristotle's (17). However, if we limit the definition of happiness to the restricted notion of "an activity of soul in accordance with perfect virtue" (17), it is not very clear how it can be useful in defining QL. The first important characteristic of happiness is that it is an end. In fact, it is the ultimate end. In every goal we set, we seek it in order to be happy. "Happiness, then, is something final and self-sufficient and is the end of action."(17).

The second characteristic of happiness is that it is: "the best, noblest, and the most pleasant thing in the world."(17). Third, happiness is not something transient such as pleasure. It has a more permanent meaning. The state of happiness is something that is not easily changed by temporary life events or misfortunes. Because happiness comes mainly from virtuous activity (someone's capacity to behave in the mean between extremes; e.g., "with regard to honour and dishonour, the mean is proper pride, the excess is known as a sort of 'empty vanity' and the deficiency is undue humility" [17]), the person who has a "disposition to choose the mean" (17) in all his or her activities will more easily reach happiness. However, Aristotle also conceded that external factors may influence someone's happiness: "Why then should we not say that he is happy who is active in accordance with complete virtue and is sufficiently equipped with external goods, not for some chance period but throughout a complete life?"(17).

In summary, happiness (not as pleasure or joy, but as existential plenitude) is a relatively steady state that continuously drives our behaviors (we seek it) in every life domain and is influenced by external factors and by our way of coping (searching for the mean between extremes).

Summary This confusion between terms or their use as QL synonyms contributes to QL concept vagueness. The model proposed in this paper integrates the pursuit of happiness as the basic mechanism of QL, but does not equal QL and happiness, as it will be demonstrated in the section on system control analysis and QL.

Multidimensionality and Specificity of the Concept

The scientific community now agrees that QL is a multidimensional construct. However, there is less agreement about how many dimensions should be measured and how they should be measured. Table 20.1 presents the most frequently cited dimensions in the literature in the last 15 years. Note that, despite the diversity of dimensions and subdimensions assessed, the authors tend to converge toward 3-8 main dimensions. However, these dimensions are constituted from a variety of subdimensions that may differ among authors. Further, this exhaustive list of dimensions appears to be overinclusive. Factors influencing QL are confused with QL dimensions. Here again, the specificity of the concept is unclear.

Another important point to raise is the use of dimensions to define QL. The similarity of the dimensions listed in table 20.1 and Bergner's (12) definition of health status is troubling. How can we arrive at a definition of QL that is unique and separate from health status? It is suggested that we turn away from dimensions. The only consensus that has been reached concerns the existence of 3-8 global domains. It will be impossible to arrive at conceptual clarity if the concept continues to be defined by dimensions. Anyone can add an important dimension or rearrange dimensions to fit a particular conception of human life. A final point raised by Stewart (10) about dimensions is that, by defining QL by its dimensions, one does not necessarily describe an operational way of measuring them. Should we use performance, incapacity, well-being, or other factors? At this level, there is no consensus. The old gestalt principle that the whole is greater than the sum of its parts takes its full sense in defining QL.

QL must be defined without reference to dimensions. Dimensions are accessories, epiphenomena. Once QL is defined without reference to dimensions, then the operational definition can be applied to dimensions. The focus on dimensions has led the field to a dead end. We must now reconsider the basic question, "What makes life worth living?" to better capture the concept.

Measuring the Patient's Life Plan and Goal Attainment

In 1982, Cohen noted that the patient's life plan is ignored in the evaluation of his or her QL (35). McCullough, two years later, underlined the fact that there is a lack of a hierarchical conception of the patient's values and belief system (36). More recently, Gill and Feinstein added that the values of individual patients could be captured by asking them about their preferences (3). Consequently, the evaluation of patients' QL should be improved by comparing their ratings to nonweighted ratings based on a standardized instrument. In 1997, Leplège and Hunt reemphasized this point: "Each consciousness is different from every other consciousness and the preferences and values of the one will not be the same as those of the other. Moreover, these preferences and values evolve according to the subject's experiences over time as a consequence of the multiple (free) decisions that the subject has

Table 20.1 Dimensions Used in the Conceptualization of Quality of Life in the Last 15 Years

Authors	Dimensions	# of dimensions
Wenger et al. (1984) (18)	*Functional capacity:* daily routine, social, intellectual, emotional, economic. *Perceptions:* health status, well-being, life satisfaction. *Symptoms:* disease under study, other illnesses.	3 majors 8 subdomains
Ware (1984) (19)	Disease, personal functioning, psychological distress, health perception, social role functioning.	5
Evans et al. (1985) (20)	*General well-being:* material well-being, physical well-being, personal growth. *Interpersonal relations:* marital relations, parent-child relations, extended relations, familial relations. *Organization activity:* altruistic behavior, political behavior. *Occupational activity:* job characteristics, occupational relations, job satisfiers. *Leisure and recreational activity:* creative/aesthetic behavior, sport activity, vacation behavior.	5 majors >10 subdomains
Calman (1987) (21)	*Physical problems:* pain, nausea, immobility, etc.; toxicity of the treatment. *Psychological, social, and spiritual problems:* psychological (coping, anxiety, depression, etc.); interpersonal dimension (family, friends, medical staff, etc.); happiness, spiritual, financial. *Wider dimensions:* individual ambitions, priorities, work, hobbies, accomplishments, cultural, political, philosophical, time.	3 majors >10 subdomains
Aaronson (1989) (22)	*Physical functioning, disease-related and treatment symptoms, psychological functioning, social functioning.* Other domains may be added for specific population (e.g., self-image, sexual functioning).	4 majors
Consensus from NHLBI meeting held in 1988. Cited by Croog (1993) (23)	*Physical status:* symptoms, sleep and rest, sexual functioning. *Functional status:* physical activity. *Emotional status:* anxiety, depression, irritability and anger, stress, spiritual well-being. *Cognitive function:* attention and concentration, clarity of thinking, psychomotor functioning. *Performance of social roles:* family membership roles (spouse, parent, sibling, etc.), work performance (household management), community activities. *General well-being:* life satisfaction, energy and vitality.	6 majors >10 subdomains
Bergner (1989) (12)	*Symptoms, functional status:* self-care, mobility, physical activity. *Role activity:* work, household management. *Social functioning:* personal inter-	10 majors >10 subdomains

Authors	Dimensions	# of dimensions
Bergner (1989) (12) *(continued)*	action, intimacy. *Emotional functioning:* anxiety, depression, locus of control, spiritual well-being. *Cognition, sleep and rest, energy and vitality, perceptions, general life satisfaction.*	
Schipper et al. (1990) (24)	Physical and occupational function, psychological state, social interaction, somatic sensation.	4
Schumaker et al. (1990) (25)	Cognitive, social, physical, emotional, personal productivity, intimacy.	6
Cella (1992) (26)	Physical well-being, functional well-being, emotional well-being, social well-being.	4
Ware and Sherbourne (1992) (27)	Physical functioning, role-physical, bodily pain, general health, vitality, social functioning, role-emotional, mental health (SF-36).	8
Dazord et al. (1993) (28)	*Functions:* cognitive, sexual, work, etc. *Relational life:* social, familial, etc. *Interior life:* meditation, artistic satisfaction, etc. *Socioeconimic context, global QL and humor, unpredictable life domains important for a given person.*	6 majors >10 subdomains
WHOQOL (1995) (29)	Physical, psychological, level of independence, social relationships, environment, spirituality/religion/personal beliefs.	6 majors divided into many facets
Cohen et al. (1995) (30)	Physical symptoms, psychological symptoms, outlook on life, meaningful existence.	4
Ferrans (1996) (31)	*Health and functioning domain:* usefulness to others, physical independence, ability to meet family responsibilities, own health, pain, energy (fatigue), stress or worries, control over own life, leisure-time activities, potential for happy old age/retirement, ability to travel on vacations, potential for a long life, sex life, health care. *Psychological/spiritual domain:* satisfaction with life, happiness in general, satisfaction with self, achievement of personal goals, peace of mind, personal appearance, faith in God. *Social and economic domain:* standard of living, financial independence, home (house, apartment), neighborhood, job/unemployment, friends, emotional support from others, education. *Family domain:* family happiness, children, relationship with spouse, family health.	4 majors >10 subdomains
Oldridge et al. (1998) (32)	*Limitations domain:* physical symptoms and restriction. *Emotions domain:* emotional functioning,	4 majors 9 subdomains

(continued)

Table 20.1 *(continued)*

Authors	Dimensions	# of dimensions
Oldridge et al. (1998) (32) *(continued)*	confidence, self-esteem. *Global score, well-being:* mobility, physical activity, social activity. *Time trade-off global preference for health states score, exercise tolerance.*	
Davidson et al. (1999) (33)	Physical functioning, role-physical, bodily pain, general health, vitality, social functioning, role-emotional, mental health (SF-36). Symptoms, activity, impacts (St. George's Respiratory Questionnaire).	11
Weintraub et al. (1999) (34)	Functional status, emotional function, symptom frequency and distress, global health perception, treatment satisfaction.	5

made in the various circumstances he or she has lived through" (2). Very few attempts have been made to consider the patient's priorities and life plan (5,28,37,38).

In 1986, Feinstein, Josephy, and Wells (39) mentioned three important and clinically relevant advantages of using patients' preferences:

1. It gives to the components of an index values that are the patient's and not the clinician's or the health practitioner's. The patient is therefore the primary focus.
2. It may help the practitioner better target the intervention toward what the patient values.
3. It may help to better detect changes because the important dimension scores will not be masked or diluted by scores from other less important ones.

Among authors that have defined QL in terms of goal achievement, few have conceived an operational way of measurement (see table 20.2) that avoids falling back to the "satisfaction with" type of question. This likely reflects the lack of a theoretical model of goal attainment as the general way of human functioning.

Lack of Theoretical and Conceptual Bases for QL

In 1984, Levine and Croog reported that there was a lack of integrated models in the field (40). Quality of life is a patchwork of dimensions with poor theoretical connections between them. Eleven years later, Kinney reemphasized the need for sound theoretical models because models are necessary for progress in science (4).

Table 20.2 Current Definitions of QL

Definitions based on satisfaction of needs, happiness, or performance	1	2	3	4	5	6	7
A person's sense of well-being, satisfaction or dissatisfaction with life, or happiness or unhappiness. (Dalkey and Rourke 1973 [45])	1	N	N	Y	13	Y	N
Quality of life, as we have defined it, consists in the fulfillment of General Happiness Requisites (GHR). Because the presence or absence of unsatisfied wants is a mental phenomenon, fulfillment of the GHRs cannot lie in the satisfaction of human wants. If anything, it must lie in the satisfaction of human needs. (McCall 1975 [16])	0	N	N	N	na	na	na
Satisfaction of needs. (Campbell et al. 1976 [15])	2	N	Y	N	18	Y	N
The degree of satisfaction that an individual feels with his or her life and surroundings. (Vetter et al. 1988 [46])	1	N	N	Y	6	N	N
The quality of an individual's life comprises (a) general happiness or satisfaction of his or her needs, and (b) performance or actualization of his or her abilities. (Bigelow et al. 1982 [47])	2	N	Y	N	17	Y	Y
The degree of need satisfaction within the areas of the physical, psychological, social, activity, material, and structural needs. (Hörnquist 1982 [48])	2	N	N	Y	6	N	N
Quality of life could be defined as fulfillment of one's values, goals, aspirations, and needs. (Milbrath 1982 [49])	2	N	N	N	na	Y	N
The subjective satisfaction expressed or experienced by an individual in his or her physical, mental, and social situation. (Jonsen et al. 1986 [50])	0	N	N	Y	3	na	na
A person's sense of well-being that stems from satisfaction or dissatisfaction with the areas of life that are important to him/her. (Ferrans 1990 [51], 1996 [31])	1	N	Y	Y	4	N	N
Quality of life is the patient's perception of performance in four areas: physical and occupational function, psychological state, social interaction, and somatic sensation. (Schipperet et al. 1990 [24])	1	N	N	Y	4	N	N
Quality of life is defined as an individual's overall satisfaction with life and general sense of personal well-being. Six dimensions that determine quality of life are proposed: cognitive, social, physical and emotional functioning, personal productivity, and intimacy. (Schumaker et al. 1990 [25])	1	N	N	Y	6	N	N
Thus, whilst the notion of "well-being" refers mostly to emotional states, the term "quality of life" includes a cognitive	1	N	N	Y	3	N	N

(continued)

Table 20.2 *(continued)*

Definitions based on satisfaction of needs, happiness, or performance	1	2	3	4	5	6	7
dimension and involves the relationship between objective living conditions and subject's assessment of them. (Corten et al. 1994 [52])							
We mean by objective quality of life, the objective life conditions in the person's different life domains. On the other hand, subjective quality of life is the person's satisfaction about his life conditions. (Chambon and Marie-Cardine 1994 [53])	2	N	N	N	3	Y	N
Quality of life is defined as an overall general well-being that comprises objective descriptors and subjective evaluations of physical, material, social and emotional well-being together with the extent of personal development and purposeful activity, all weighted by a personal set of values. (Felce and Perry 1995 [54])	2	N	N	Y	5	Y	N
The terms "quality of life" and more specifically "health related quality of life" refer to the physical, psychological, and social domains of health, seen as distinct areas that are influenced by a person's experiences, beliefs, expectations and perceptions. (Testa and Simonson 1996 [55])	1	N	N	Y	3	N	N

Definitions based on goal attainment	1	2	3	4	5	6	7
QL results from a negotiation between individuals and society. It is defined in terms of outcomes of these negotiations. At a given moment in time, these negotiation outcomes are called sovereignties of individuals and settings. Sovereignties consist of patterns of commitment made by the individuals among settings and conversely. These patterns are measured by joint allocation of money, time, skill, and sentiment from both parts. (Gerson 1976 [56])	1	Y	N	N	4	Y	N
The extent to which an individual is able to achieve security, self-esteem and the opportunity to use intellectual and physical capabilities in pursuit of personal goals. (Engquist 1979 [57])	0	N	N	na	na	na	na
Satisfaction, contentment, happiness, fulfillment, and the ability to cope. Quality of life therefore measures the difference, at a particular period of time, between the hopes and expectation of the individual and the individual's present experience. It is concerned with the difference between perceived goals and the	0	Y	N	N	13	N	N

Definitions based on goal attainment	1	2	3	4	5	6	7
actual goals. It is the assessment of the potential for growth. (Calman 1987 [21])							
Distance between a person's position and his goals, within the framework set by vital needs of communities and societies. Satisfaction refers to the achievement of a goal (or to the sense of approaching it). QL is the individual's feeling about his distance from his goals that should have a preference or greater weight than judgment of his peers of how well or how badly he fares, and both of these groups of judgments are preferred to the judgments of an assessor. (Sartorius 1987 [58])	0	N	N	na	na	N	N
QL refers to patients' appraisal of and satisfaction with their current level of functioning compared to what they perceive to be possible or ideal. (Cella and Cherin 1988 [59])	0	N	N	na	na	N	N
(a) The discrepancy between a person's achieved and unmet needs and desire. This refers to the subjective, or perceived, and objective assessment of an individual's domains. The greater the discrepancy the poorer the QL; and (b) the extent to which an individual increasingly controls aspects of life regardless of original baseline. (Brown et al. 1989 [60])	1	N	N	N	6	N	N
Quality of life, at a given time, is a state that corresponds to the level attained by a person in his continuing pursuit of hierarchically organized goals. (Dupuis et al. 1989 [5])	4	Y	Y	N	7	Y	Y
Quality of life corresponds to the distance between the subject's position and his goals, the ensemble modulated by: the importance of the goal for the subject, the subject's tolerance to the distance between the goals and their attainment, and at last, the subject's capacity to find compensations or to displace investments or to modify his values hierarchy. (Gérin et al. 1989 [61])	3	Y	Y	N	6	Y	N
Each of us has a picture, however vague, of what we would like to accomplish before we die. How close we get to attaining this goal becomes the measure for the quality of our lives. If it remains beyond reach, we grow resentful or resigned; if it is at least in part achieved, we experience a sense of happiness and satisfaction. (Csikszentmihalyi 1990 [62])	3	Y	N	N	na	na	Y
QL is best understood as representing the gap between one's actual functional level and one's ideal standard. It is composed of four domains: physical well-being, functional well-being, emotional well-being, and social well-being. (Cella 1992 [26])	0	N	N	Y	4	N	N

(continued)

Table 20.2 *(continued)*

Definitions based goal attainment	1	2	3	4	5	6	7
Quality of life is the individual's perception of their position in life in the context of the culture and value systems in which they live and in relation to their goals, expectations, standards, and concerns. (WHOQOL 1995 [29])	1	N	Y	N	6	N	N

1 = Theoretical model (0 = no, 1 = conceptual model, 2 = conceptual framework, 3 = theoretical framework, 4 = model for causes of behavior), 2 = Specific (Y/N), 3 = Operational measurement (Y/N), 4 = Dimension-driven (Y/N), 5 = Number of dimensions, 6 = Does the model distinguish between antecedents and consequences?, 7 = Does it capture notion of happiness?, na = nonapplicable.

However, what type of model do we need? Before answering this question, we must define what is meant by models because, in the field, terms such as "models," "theoretical models," "conceptual models," and "theoretical framework" are frequently used without distinction. Akinsanya presents a distinction that may be useful (41). A conceptual model consists of a descriptive representation of a concept without necessarily specifying the relationships between the elements of the concept. In a conceptual framework, relationships between elements (represented schematically by blocks) are described with directional arrows. Finally, a theoretical framework contains structure and functions. Powers made another interesting distinction (42). There are "abstract generalizations" (the previous types can be of this sort), models for consequences of organization, and models for causes of behavior. Most of the "models" encountered in the field of QL are actually abstract generalizations. Some address social or individual observable factors (symptoms, physical functioning, psychological status, etc.), others, hidden dimensions (self-esteem, potential for growth, happiness, satisfaction, etc.) revealed by measurement instruments. Both can be useful, in schematic models, to capture various dimensions of QL or dimensions associated with QL. However, they are schematic representations of dimensions (directly observable or not) that are consequences of the individual's inner organization.

Even though these kinds of models are useful in understanding QL, they do not fully capture the nature of QL. "As long as one is only dividing observed behavior into units that seem to hang together in some way, he has the problem that many different ways of subdividing the same whole will result in a self-consistent description"(42). Powers suggested that we think about a model for causes of behaviors, by looking at some internal mechanism that makes human beings behave. Quality of life is mainly defined by dimensions that represent consequences or results of human functioning, such as health status or physical capacity, affective condition, and so on. In order to truly capture QL, we must look at what makes us move and live, at what makes life worth living, which is the pursuit of happiness through goal setting in different life domains, the whole, within the system control analysis approach inspired from cybernetic models. Table 20.2 presents a brief analysis of some frequently cited definitions in the field with a note about the degree of theoretical deepness of their associated models.

Measuring Alpha, Beta, and Gamma Changes

Allison, Locker, and Feine (43) have pointed out a very important problem in the evaluation of QL, which is that most of the existing instruments measure what Golembiewski, Billingsley, and Yeager (44) called "alpha" change: a variation in an existing state over time. However, this measurement assumed that the construct being assessed is constant over time (for example, blood pressure). Beta change is a change in state (like alpha) but the process is complicated by the fact that the referring point changes over time. For example, a man may mention that before the treatment, the pain he felt was the most terrible he has ever felt. Now, suppose that the treatment has induced, for a short time, an even more terrible pain. The fact that the pain reported after treatment is "less" may be a result of treatment but also because of the fact that the referring point for the "most terrible pain ever felt" has changed. Gamma change consists of a major shift in the person's perspective. For example, a woman who has lived with chronic pain may feel that to be totally free of pain is not so important. Therefore, the rating she will give to her actual pain will be less than the one she would have given at the beginning of her problem. This shift, due to adaptation, makes her evaluate her state of pain as less intolerable. Allison, Locker, and Feine (43) suggest that it is very important to capture these three levels of change when assessing QL. We are dealing with human beings, and human beings are living organisms that are organized toward adaptation, and the process of adaptation frequently implies changes in an individual's priorities and goal setting. One possible way to account for this is to measure the person's priorities, referring point, and status before and after treatment. If a change occurs in the status, it will be possible to verify whether this is due to the two other parameters or not. Very few instruments do this.

Definition and Theoretical Models

This section examines a set of definitions and related models. Table 20.2 presents definitions classified in two broad categories: definitions based on satisfaction, happiness, performance, and well-being, and those using the goal attainment principle. The table is not an exhaustive repertoire of definitions and models.

However, it is a representative sample of what exists in the field. The first column provides definitions. The second column assesses the type of model, if any, behind the definition according to categories proposed by Akinsanya (41) and Powers (42). To be specific (column 2), a definition must not borrow from a concept such as well-being, satisfaction, or health status. It must stand on its own. A definition and a model received a "Yes" in column 3 if the strategy of measurement directly followed from the model. For example, if a model specifies that QL is well-being in different domains, there are two possibilities:

1. instruments that already exist are used, or
2. an instrument is designed directly from the elements of the model.

Only in the second case does the model receive a "Yes." Many QL definitions and models are based on dimensions. They are called "dimension-driven" (column 4). Column 5 gives the number of dimensions in the models. Distinctions between antecedents and consequences (column 6) pertain to the ability of the model to separate what influences QL from QL itself. For example, initial physical and psychological health, as well as posttreatment physical and psychological health, are not QL. These conditions may influence QL to a certain degree, but to be specific, a definition of QL must not include the concept of health. Otherwise, we should use the concept of health instead of the concept of QL. Finally, column 7 provides answers to the question of whether to include happiness in the measurement of QL.

As can be seen, six of the models whose definitions are based on satisfaction, happiness, and so forth consist of conceptual frameworks, seven are conceptual models, and one has no model behind the definition. None of the definitions are specific because, in essence, they consider QL to be a global term for performance, satisfaction, well-being, and so forth. The table does not include definitions that equate QL and health status. The notion of health is of great importance but should be evaluated by itself and not confounded with QL. Three of the models have driven the design of measurement instruments. Most of the definitions are dimension-driven. Seven of the models make a clear distinction between QL and what influences QL. Finally, only one measures happiness.

Of the definitions based on goal attainment, five have no underlying model, three are conceptual models, two are theoretical frameworks, and one is a model for causes of behavior. Four definitions are specific, whereas some, despite using the notion of gap between state and goals, employed well-being or satisfaction as an estimate of the gap. Only three models have an instrument directly derived from their characteristics, and few are dimension-driven. Only one distinguishes QL from antecedents and consequences, and three measure happiness.

In addition to the models presented in table 20.2, there are others that do not provide a definition of QL but rather specify what factors (medical, psychological, etc.) may influence QL. Cowan, Young-Graham, and Cochrane (9) and Wilson and Cleary (63) are good examples.

System Control Analysis and Quality of Life: Convergence With Other Human Behavior Theories

Dupuis (64); Dupuis et al. (5); and Duquette, Dupuis, and Perreault (38) have presented in detail the main components of the system control analysis approach applied to QL assessment. These components are goals, control, negative and positive feedback loop, and hierarchical order. Goals are the essence of our behaviors. They organize, orient, and give sense to our behaviors; they make life worth living. "Control is the attainment and maintenance of the desirable preselected state through actions on the environment" (42). Control is best achieved under a negative feedback loop. This loop constantly reduces the gap between the actual state and the preselected goal (or maintains it at a steady-state acceptable level) through actions. Under a positive feedback loop, the gap constantly increases. Therefore, the measurement of the gap must take into account this dynamic situation. The measured gap must be weighted by the speed of the positive or the negative loop. In order to avoid conflict between goals, they must be hierarchically organized. Some life domains are very important and others less important. The subjective effect on global QL of a gap in a very important life domain will be heavier than the effect of one in a less important domain. Consequently, in addition to being weighted by the speed of the loop, the gap must also be weighted by the importance the individual gives to each life domain.

Therefore, the strategy of measurement used in the Quality of Life Systemic Inventory (QLSI) is directly linked to these notions (38). The gap between the actual state and the desired goal is measured on a dial (38). The desired goal and the actual state are indicated in reference to a general ideal situation worded identically for each item and as follows: "to be perfectly happy . . ." This absolute reference point has been chosen in accordance with what we said earlier about the Aristotelian notion of happiness. Happiness is what we search for. To be perfectly happy is the ultimate goal, though not necessarily attainable. Each of us has a certain idea of what could be a state of perfect happiness, even though the way to reach it may vary among individuals. The person also indicates whether his or her situation is improving or deteriorating (negative or positive feedback loop) and at which speed. Finally, the importance of each item is also rated on a 1 (essential to my life) to 7 (completely useless) Likert scale. Details of this measurement strategy have been presented elsewhere (38). The QLSI gives four scores: the gap score, which is the QL score; the goal score, which provides information about level of goal settings; the rank score, which illustrates the degree of prioritization among life domains; and the state score, which gives information about the patient's current condition. Finally an impact score (not reported here) can also be calculated to evaluate the impact of the disease on QL, reflecting what part of the gap the patient attributes to the disease. Each of these scores can be calculated for the nine subscales and for a global score.

Levels of factors influencing quality of life and a global model of quality of life are presented in figure 20.1. The complete model was presented in 1989 (5); a slightly modified version is presented in figure 20.1b. Each life domain is considered a feedback loop for which three conditions are possible: no change (nc), negative feedback (–f), and positive feedback (+f). The immediate consequence of no change and negative feedback is satisfaction. From positive feedback, a state of anxiety-depression-anger is generated, combined with a feeling of inefficacy for the domain in such a loop. On the contrary, in a negative feedback loop, a sense of efficacy is developed. If there are more domains in negative loops, the person has a global sense of personal efficacy. On the other hand, if there are more positive loops, the person feels a global sense of personal inefficacy and helplessness. This model is very close to that of Bandura (65), who noted that human self-motivation is based on discrepancy production and reduction through feedback control loops. People set goals, and, when they reach them, they reset new goals at higher levels.

Csikszentmihalyi (62), in his theory of flow, which has an Aristotelian conception of happiness, presents principles that converge with those of Bandura (65) and Duquette, Dupuis, and Perreault (38). The experience of flow is possible when there is an equilibrium between skills and challenges. Challenges that are too high induce anxiety, and those that are too low, boredom. The autotelic person is one who sets goals not only for external reinforcement but for the pleasure of performing the actions leading toward the goal. This person monitors his progress through feedback and increases the level of the goal when it is reached. Happiness occurs through action toward the goal, and a sense of control over personal life is felt when the individual behaves toward consciously chosen goals.

Antonovsky's (66) theory about the "sense of coherence" mentioned that the feeling of life coherence for a person is based on three parameters: comprehensibility (life experiences and events are organized, predictable, and explainable); manageability (personal resources are available to meet environmental demands); and meaningfulness (the demands are worthy enough to engage actions). Sense of coherence has been associated with better adaptation to disease.

Finally, Kuhl and Beckman's (67) theory identifies two types of personality: oriented toward action or toward state. Action-oriented people focus attention on the means to reduce the gap between their current state and the anticipated goal. Cognition and emotion are mobilized toward this desired future and help the process of gap reduction. State-oriented people focus attention on their actual condition. Affective and cognitive processes are mobilized by this analysis and cannot push toward action because the analysis of the actual condition is overwhelming. People in this state become passive as well as cognitively and emotionally disturbed. Their efficacy in managing their lives is greatly reduced.

QL is a global concept that attempts to capture the person as a whole. As such, considerations about human functioning must be incorporated in the concept. The proposed model provides possible answers to some of the problems cited in the first section of this chapter. It distinguishes QL measurement from objective and

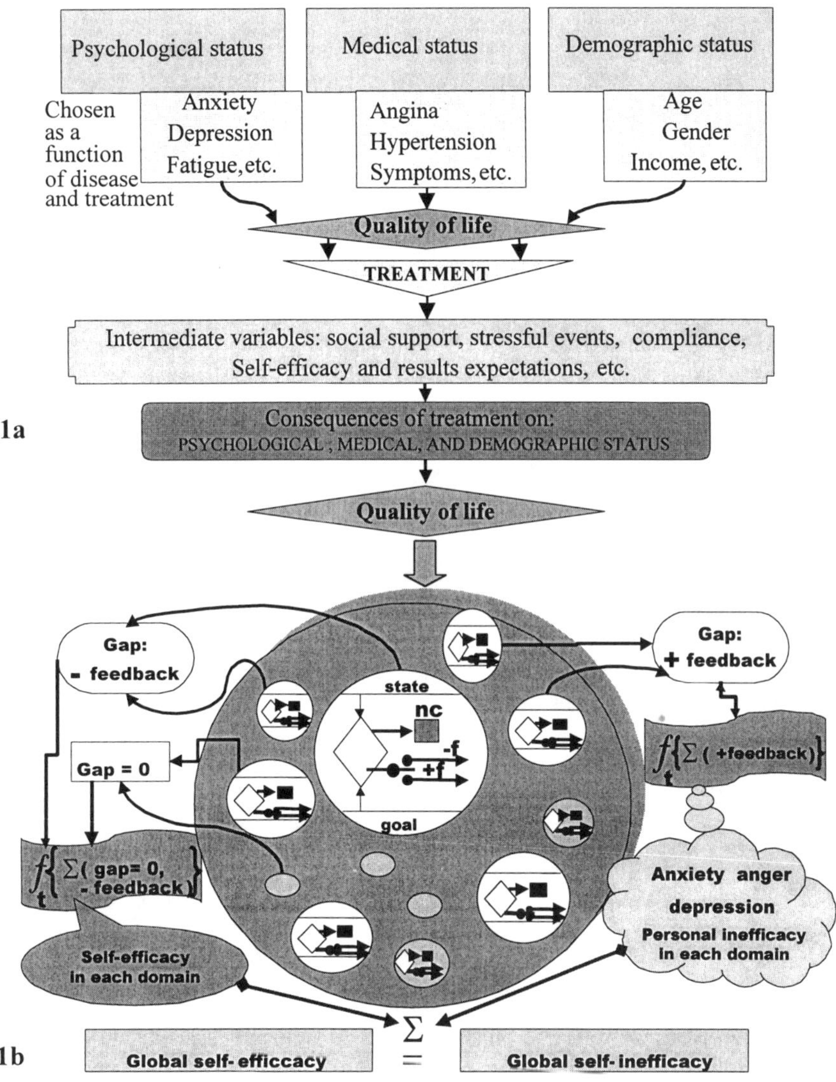

Figure 20.1 Levels of factors influencing quality of life (a) and global model of quality of life (b). Each life domain is represented as a circle with a feedback loop inside. The gap generated by the comparison (lozenge) loop between state and goal has three possibilities: no change (nc), positive feedback (+f), and negative feedback (–f). The size of the circle represents the relative importance of each domain. The gap between the state and the goal represents QL. The cognitive integration ($\int_T$) by the person over a certain period of time (t) of stable loops (no change with gap = 0) and negative loops creates domain-specific self-efficacy. The same process for positive feedback loop creates the trilogy of anxiety-anger-depression with domain-specific self-inefficacy. If the summation of the two is in favor of stable and negative loops, the person develops a global sense of self-efficacy. Otherwise, he or she may feel inefficient and helpless.

subjective measures of health (physical or psychological). It incorporates the notion of happiness. The patient's life plan is considered. The model is based on a comprehensive theoretical model that generates a specific definition that is not based on dimensions and for which an operational method of measurement has been designed, through goal settings and prioritization. Medical, psychological, and social status are considered as dimensions that may influence QL but are not part of its definition (see figure 20.1a). Instruments already exist to measure these dimensions and should be used as descriptors of the patient's condition. Finally, by looking at states, gaps, and goal settings and prioritization, one can interpret improvement in QL (reduction of the gap) as resulting from an alpha, beta, or gamma change, and consequently better target areas of intervention.

Quality of Life in Two Different Settings: (A) Comparison of Rehab and Nonrehab Groups and (B) Gender Differences 5 Years After CABG

Table 20.3 presents results from two studies. The first study was done in Liege (Belgium)(68) and compared QL in two groups of patients: a rehab group and a nonrehab group. The program started 6 weeks after coronary artery bypass graft (CABG) and lasted for 6 weeks at a rate of five sessions per week. Results presented here concern two periods of measurement: before surgery and after the rehab program at the 24-week follow-up. The nonrehab group was evaluated with the same schedule. Only results concerning the QLSI global scores are reported here. The other study involved a 5-year follow-up of CABG patients. Seventy-five men and 39 women participated in the study. Only results from the Duke Activity Survey (69), the Functional Status Questionnaire (70), Cantril's QL scale (71), the Profile of Mood States, Bi-Polar Form (POMS-BI) (72), and the QLSI are presented. From the initial sample of 114 (75 men, 39 women), only 61 men and 31 women completed the QLSI. Here, too, only global score results are presented.

Interestingly, both Belgian groups showed an improvement in the state and gap scores. Because there were no major changes in the goal scores and in the rank scores, the improvement observed on the gap score was interpreted as a true alpha change, since the two other dimensions did not change over time. In the rehab group, however, there was a trend for higher goal settings at follow-up (eta square = 0.24) combined with an improvement in the gap and state scores. This suggests that although the patients' actual conditions improved (from 31.7 to 21.2), they also raised their goal setting (from 16.5 to 12.6); nevertheless, the resulting gap (2.0) was smaller than prior to surgery (5.6). The fact that change in goal score is weaker (eta square = 0.10) in the nonrehab group is likely a result of better initial goal scores (13.5 compared to 16.5), leaving less room for improvement.

There were no gender differences between the two groups on QLSI scores, nor on anxiety, depression, basic and social functional status, or global QL. However,

Table 20.3 Comparisons of Cardiac Patients in Different Settings on QL, Physical, and Psychological Status

	No rehab (19)			Rehab (14)			Gender (M: 61, W: 31)		
	Pre	Post	Anova	Pre	Post	Anova	Men	Women	Anova
QLSI			df (1,18)			df (1,13)			df (1,90)
State *M*	26.4	20.2	$p = 0.047$	31.7	21.2	$p = 0.014$	21.8	22.7	$p = 0.80$
SD	11.2	18.3	$F = 4.50$	12.3	14.2	$F = 8.00$	17.3	13.5	$F = 0.07$
			$\eta^2 = 0.20$			$\eta^2 = 0.38$			$\eta^2 = 0.00$
Goal *M*	13.5	10.7	$p = 0.177$	16.5	12.6	$p = 0.061$	10.6	11.1	$p = 0.71$
SD	8.2	9.1	$F = 1.97$	7.2	7.4	$F = 4.20$	6.3	7.6	$F = 0.14$
			$\eta^2 = 0.10$			$\eta^2 = 0.24$			$\eta^2 = 0.00$
Gap *M*	5.1	2.4	$p = 0.039$	5.6	2.0	$p = 0.003$	3.3	4.0	$p = 0.59$
SD	5.0	3.4	$F = 4.98$	3.9	3.4	$F = 12.77$	5.0	6.8	$F = 0.29$
			$\eta^2 = 0.22$			$\eta^2 = 0.50$			$\eta^2 = 0.00$
Rank *M*	1.5	1.5	$p = 0.630$	1.4	1.5	$p = 0.184$	1.5	1.5	$p = 0.38$
SD	0.2	0.2	$F = 0.241$	0.2	0.2	$F = 1.97$	0.2	0.2	$F = 0.79$
			$\eta^2 = 0.13$			$\eta^2 = 0.13$			$\eta^2 = 0.00$

(continued)

Table 20.3 *(continued)*

Measures		Men (75)	Women (39)	Anova (df = 1114)		
DAS	*M* (SD)	45.3 (12.7)	31.3 (13.9)	p = 0.000	F = 31.19	$\eta^2 = 0.21$
FSQ Basic	*M* (SD)	96.6 (10.4)	92.6 (14.2)	p = 0.090	F = 3.00	$\eta^2 = 0.02$
FSQ inter.	*M* (SD)	84.8 (16.9)	67.3 (24.6)	p = 0.000	F = 20.69	$\eta^2 = 0.15$
FSQ social;	*M* (SD)	93.0 (16.8)	88.0 (20.3)	p = 0.160	F = 2.00	$\eta^2 = 0.01$
Anxiety	*M* (SD)	24.5 (7.2)	23.3 (6.6)	p = 0.360	F = 0.81	$\eta^2 = 0.00$
Depression	*M* (SD)	24.8 (5.7)	24.6 (6.5)	p = 0.860	F = 0.03	$\eta^2 = 0.00$
Global QL	*M* (SD)	6.8 (2.0)	7.1 (1.6)	p = 0.330	F = 0.94	$\eta^2 = 0.00$

QLSI = Quality of Life Systemic Inventory; DAS = Duke Activity Survey; FSQ = Functional Status Questionnaire (inter. = intermediate functioning); η^2 = coefficient eta square (the strength of association: of % of variance); df = degree of freedom; numbers in parentheses = sample size for rehab, no rehab, men, and women; *M* (SD) = Mean and standard deviation. Smaller values on QLSI gap and state scores mean a better situation. For goal scores, it means being closer to the ideal. For the rank or priorities scores, it means better hierarchy. If someone gets a score closer to 2, this means that all his or her life domains received the rank number 1, reflecting therefore a bad hierarchy and a high potential for conflict among life domains. For DAS, FSQ, and global QL, higher scores reveal a better situation. For anxiety and depression, higher scores indicate a poorer condition.

on the Duke Activity Survey (DAS) and the intermediate functional status, men had better scores than women. This fact illustrates the importance of distinguishing QL from physical and psychological functioning. Here, one must conclude that even though women rated their physical status as poorer than the men rated theirs, it did not seem to affect their QL. They presented state, goal, gap, and rank scores that were similar to those of the men. The following two factors may explain this phenomenon. First, it is congruent with many studies reporting that subjective well-being, happiness, and global subjective QL are weakly correlated with objective measures of economical and physical status. Second, it is difficult to determine if lower scores on a self-administered questionnaire reflect women's poorer status compared to men, different response styles to such questionnaires, or a combination of the two. Some researchers (73-77) have shown that women have a tendency to report emotions and symptoms of different kinds more easily than men because of cultural and social factors. Therefore, in order to control for this effect in gender comparisons, one could use the effect size of the gender difference on a given questionnaire in a group of persons having no health problem and use it as a referring point to better interpret the observed gender differences in the clinical population, before and after treatment. The problem is that for many of the existing QL questionnaires there is no reference group because most of the instruments have been designed for clinical populations. This fact also creates another puzzling situation. When a clinical group improves, it is difficult to know whether it is approaching (or not approaching) the functional status of healthy individuals. This aspect is also of great importance when the research question is whether the subjective QL of a clinical group has improved sufficiently to be comparable to a nonclinical group. This situation makes it impossible to use strategies described by Jacobson, Follette, and Revenstorf (78) to evaluate clinical significance, based on the distance between the mean of the treated group and the mean of a "normal" referent group. On the QLSI global gap score, the effect size of the gender difference is small ($r = 0.17$) (79). Therefore, given the absence of differences in male and female CABG patients, we can conclude that this absence of differences reflects a true similarity in QL between men and women 5 years after surgery.

Conclusion

We have proposed a model that provides interesting solutions to problems encountered in the field of QL over the last 40 years. Although it is probably not the ideal model, it has the advantage of giving a specific definition to the QL concept. Whether this model is applicable to many different settings is currently unknown. However, preliminary data have been presented (79) for diabetics and AIDS patients, and the actual version of the QLSI is used with valve replacement patients, angioplasty patients, and cancer patients. Psychometric characteristics of the QLSI first version have also been presented elsewhere (38). The validation process of the second version is currently under way.

The drawback of this approach, however, is that, in order to study QL in a given setting, one must measure QL, physical and psychological health, and other aspects that may influence QL (figure 20.1a).

In light of the prior considerations, we strongly suggest bypassing the term "health-related quality of life" because it is misleading and meaningless. Some authors (80) presented a taxonomy of QL in which they suggested two types of QL (health-related QL and non-health-related QL). However, dimensions such as physical and psychological functioning (health-related quality of life), coping strategies, social support, and personality, as well as those such as air pollution, safety of a given area, quality of water (non-health-related QL) are undoubtedly factors that may influence QL but are not necessarily part of it. This split of the QL concept into health-related and non-health-related dimensions maintains confusion and adds nothing more to the QL construct than the preexisting concepts (some already well defined) that already serve to describe the patient's biopsychosocial profile. The concept of health-related QL must undergo a major surgery because the cholesterol of confusion has so obstructed the arteries of knowledge that the heart of the field is in a state of acute MI. As a rehabilitation program, we suggest that future studies clarify whether they measure physical and psychological health or functioning in a specific way and in a given setting, or whether they measure QL, or whether they measure both. It is far more scientifically healthy to be specific about what we measure and how we name what we measure than to measure a nonspecific concept with nonspecific instruments for a specific purpose.

In statistics, there are two well-known types of error: type I and type II. Two other types of errors were described in 1977 in *Futures Research: New Directions.* In this book, Mitroff (81) and Loveridge (82) described two more errors that researchers should avoid. As Mitroff noted, "The most general error is not just that of solving the wrong problem but that of solving the wrong problem at the wrong time in the wrong organization or institutional context by the wrong person"(81). Another error is "asking questions to reveal an unstructured problem, as the 'rightness' or the 'wrongness' of the questions is indeterminate in any absolute sense"(82).

The field of QL has had its share of errors of every kind. The approach proposed here may also suffer from another type of error that is yet to be identified. On the other hand, this approach has the advantage of providing a specific definition of QL and of considering global human functioning and the question of what makes life worth living. For the rest, we all know that science progresses from error to error. The important thing is to avoid repeating the same ones!

References

1. Yourcenar, M. 1972. *Mémoires d'Hadrien*. Paris: Gallimard.
2. Leplège, A., and S. Hunt. 1997. The problem of quality of life in medicine. *JAMA* 278:47-50.

3. Gill, T.M., and A.R. Feinstein. 1994. A critical appraisal of the quality of life measurements. *JAMA* 272:619-626.
4. Kinney, M.R. 1995. Quality of life research: rigor or rigor mortis. *Cardiovasc Nurs* 31:25-28.
5. Dupuis, G., J. Perrault, M.C. Lambany, E. Kennedy, and P. David. 1989. A new tool to assess quality of life: the Quality of Life Systemic Inventory. *Qual Life Cardiovasc Care* 5(suppl. 1):36-45.
6. Offerhaus, L. 1991. Measurement of the quality of life in clinical trials: in pursuit of the unapproachable? *Eur J Pharmacol* 40:205-208.
7. Tatossian, A. 1994. La notion de qualité de vie subjective: Évidences et illusions. In *Qualité de vie subjective et santé mentale: Aspects conceptuels et méthodologiques,* ed. J.L. Terra. Paris: Marketing.
8. Mercier, C., and J. Filion. 1987. La qualité de vie: perspectives théoriques et empiriques. *Santé Mentale au Québec* XII:135-143.
9. Cowan, M.J., K. Young-Graham, and B.L. Cochrane. 1992. Comparison of a theory of quality of life between myocardial infarction and malignant melanoma: a pilot study. *Prog Cardiovasc Nurs* 7:18-28.
10. Stewart, A.L. 1992. Conceptual and methodologic issues in defining quality of life: state of the art. *Prog Cardiovasc Nurs* 7:3-11.
11. World Health Organization. 1948. *Constitution in Basic Documents.* Geneva: World Health Organization.
12. Bergner, M. 1989. Quality of life, health status, and clinical research. *Med Care* 27(suppl.):S148-S156.
13. Diener, E. 1984. Subjective well-being. *Psychol Bull* 95:542-575.
14. Packa, D. 1989. Quality of life of cardiac patients: a review. *J Cardiovasc Nurs* 3:1-11.
15. Campbell, A., P.E. Converse, and W.L. Rodgers. 1976. *The Quality of American Life: Perceptions, Evaluations, and Satisfactions.* New York: Russell Sage Foundation.
16. McCall, S. 1975. Quality of life. *Soc Indicators Res* 2:229-248.
17. Aristotle. 1987. *The Nichomachean Ethics.* New York: Oxford University Press.
18. Wenger, N., M. Mattson, C. Furberg, and J. Elinson, eds. 1984. *Assessment of Quality of Life in Clinical Trials of Cardiovascular Therapies.* New York: Le Jacq.
19. Ware, J.E., Jr. 1984. Conceptualizing disease impact and treatment outcomes. *Cancer* 53:2316-2326.
20. Evans, D.R., J.E. Burns, W.E. Robinson, and O. Garrett. 1985. The Quality of Life Questionnaire: a multidimensional measure. *Am J Commun Psychol* 13:305-322.

21. Calman, K.C. 1987. Definitions and dimensions of quality of life. In *Quality of Life of Cancer Patients,* ed. N.K. Aaronson and J. Beckmann. New York: Raven Press.

22. Aaronson, N.K. 1989. Quality of life assessment in clinical trials: methodologic issues. *Control Clin Trials* 10(suppl.):195-208.

23. Croog, S.H. 1993. Current issues in conceptualizing and measuring quality of life. In *Quality of Life Assessment: Practice, Problems and Promises,* ed. J.A. Schuttinger and C.D. Furberg. Washington, DC: Department of Health and Human Resources.

24. Schipper, H., J. Clinch, and V. Powell. 1990. Definitions and conceptual issues. In *Quality of Life Assessment in Clinical Trials,* ed. B. Spilker. New York: Raven Press.

25. Schumaker, S.A., R.T. Anderson, and S.M. Czajkowski. 1990. Psychological tests and scales. In *Quality of Life Assessment in Clinical Trials,* ed. B. Spilker. New York: Raven Press.

26. Cella, D.F. 1992. Quality of life: the concept. *J Palliat Care* 8:8-13.

27. Ware, J.E., Jr., and C.D. Sherbourne. 1992. The MOS 36-item Short-Form Health Survey (SF-36): conceptual framework and item selection. *Med Care* 30:473-483.

28. Dazord, A., P. Gérin, C. Brochier, M. Cluse, J.L. Terra, and C. Seulin. 1993. Un modèle de qualité de vie subjective adapté aux essais thérapeutiques: Intérêt chez les patients dépressifs. *Santé Mentale au Québec* XVIII:49-74.

29. The WHOQOL Group. 1995. The World Health Organization quality of life assessment: position paper from the World Health Organization. *Soc Sci Med* 41:1403-1409.

30. Cohen, S.R., B.M. Mount, M.G. Strobel, and F. Bui. 1995. The McGill Pain Questionnaire: a measure of quality of life appropriate for people with advanced disease. A preliminary study. *Palliat Med* 5:207-219.

31. Ferrans, C.E. 1996. Development of a conceptual model of quality of life. *Sch Inq Nurs Pract* 10:293-304.

32. Oldridge, N., M. Gottlieb, G. Guyatt, N. Jones, D. Steiner, and D. Feeny. 1998. Predictors of health related quality of life with cardiac rehabilitation after acute myocardial infarction. *J Cardiopulm Rehabil* 18:95-103.

33. Davidson, T.A., E.S. Caldwell, J.R. Curtis, L.D. Hudson, and K.P. Steinberg. 1999. Reduced quality of life in survivors of acute respiratory distress syndrome compared with critically ill control patients. *JAMA* 281:354-360.

34. Weintraub, W.S., S.D. Culler, and A. Kosinski, et al. 1999. Economics, health related quality of life, and cost effectiveness methods for the TACTICS (treat angina with aggrastat (tirofiban) and determine cost of therapy with invasive or conservative strategy)-TIMI 18 trial. *Am J Cardiol* 83:317-322.

35. Cohen, C. 1982. On the quality of life: some philosophical reflections. *Circulation* 65(suppl. III):29-33.

36. McCullough, L.B. 1984. Concept of the quality of life: a philosophical analysis. In *Assessment of Quality of Life in Clinical Trials of Cardiovascular Therapies,* ed. N.K. Wenger, M.E. Mattson, C.D. Furberg, and J. Elinson. New York: Le Jacq.

37. Ferrans, C.E., and M.J. Powers. 1985. Quality of Life Index: development and psychometric properties. *Adv Nurs Sci* 1985:15-24.

38. Duquette, R.L., G. Dupuis, and J. Perreault. 1994. A new approach for quality of life assessment in cardiac patients: rationale and validation of the Quality of Life Systemic Inventory (QLSI). *Can J Cardiol* 10:106-112.

39. Feinstein, A.R., B.R. Josephy, and A.K. Wells. 1986. Scientific and clinical problems in indexes of functional disability. *Ann Intern Med* 105:413-420.

40. Levine, S., and S.H. Croog. 1984. What constitutes quality of life? A conceptualization of the dimensions of life quality in healthy populations and patients with cardiovascular disease. In *Assessment of Quality of Life in Clinical Trials of Cardiovascular Therapies,* ed. N.K. Wenger, M.E. Mattson, C.D. Furberg, and J. Elinson. New York: Le Jacq.

41. Akinsanya, J. 1994. General introduction. In *The Roy Adaptation Model in Action,* ed. J. Akinsanya, G. Cox, C. Crouch, and L. Fletcher. New York: Macmillan.

42. Powers, W.T. 1973. *Behavior: The Control of Perception.* Chicago: Aldine.

43. Allison, P.J., D. Locker, and J.S. Feine. 1997. Quality of life: a dynamic construct. *Soc Sci Med* 45:221-230.

44. Golembiewski, R.T., K. Billingsley, and S. Yeager. 1976. Measuring change and persistence in human affairs: types of change generated by OD designs. *J Appl Behav Sci* 1976:133-157.

45. Dalkey, N., and D. Rourke. 1973. *The Delphi Procedure and Rating Quality of Life Factors. The Quality of Life Concept.* Washington, DC: Environmental Protection Agency.

46. Vetter, N.J., D.A. Jones, and C.R. Victor. 1988. The quality of life of the over 70's in the community. *Health Visitor* 61:10-13.

47. Bigelow, D.A., G. Brodsky, L. Stewart, and M. Olson. 1982. The concept and measurement of quality of life as a dependent variable in evaluation of mental health services. In *Innovative Approaches to Mental Health Evaluation,* ed. G.J. Stahler and W.B. Tash. New York: Academic Press.

48. Hörnquist, J.O. 1982. The concept of quality of life. *Scand J Soc Med* 10:57-61.

49. Milbrath, L.W. 1982. A conceptualization and research strategy for the study of ecological aspects of the quality of life. *Soc Indicators Res* 10:133-157.

50. Jonsen, A.R., M. Siegler, and W.J. Winslade. 1986. Quality of life. In *Clinical Ethics,* ed. A.R. Jonsen, M. Siegler, and W.J. Winslade. New York: Macmillan.

51. Ferrans, C.E. 1990. Development of a quality of life index for cancer patients. *Oncol Nurs Forum* 17(suppl.):15-21.

52. Corten, P., C. Mercier, and I. Pelc. 1994. Subjective quality of life: clinical model for assessment of rehabilitation treatment in psychiatry. *Soc Psychiatr Psychiatr Epidemiol* 29:178-183.

53. Chambon, O., and M. Marie-Cardine. 1994. Qualité de vie subjective et fonctionnement mental: le point de vue cognitiviste. In *Qualité de vie subjective et santé mentale: Aspects conceptuels et méthodologiques,* ed. J.L. Terra. Paris: Marketing.

54. Felce, D., and J. Perry. 1995. Quality of life: its definition and measurement. *Res Dev Disabil* 16:51-74.

55. Testa, M.A., and D.C. Simonson. 1996. Assessment of quality-of-life outcomes. *N Engl J Med* 334:835-840.

56. Gerson, E.M. 1976. On "quality of life." *Am Soc Rev* 41:793-806.

57. Engquist, C.L. 1979. Can quality of life be evaluated? *Hospitals* 16:97-100.

58. Sartorius, N. 1987. Cross-cultural comparisons of data about quality of life: a sample of issues. In *The Quality of Life of Cancer Patients,* ed. N.K. Aaronson and J. Beckmanns. New York: Raven Press.

59. Cella, D.F., and E.A. Cherin. 1988. Quality of life during and after cancer treatment. *Compr Ther* 14:69-75.

60. Brown, R.I., M.B. Bayer, and C. MacFarlane. 1989. Rehabilitation programmes: performance and quality of life of adults with developmental handicaps. Toronto: Lugus.

61. Gérin, P., A. Dazord, J. Boissel, M. Hanauer, P. Moleur, and F. Chauvin. 1989. L'évaluation de la qualité de vie dans les essais thérapeutiques: aspects conceptuels et présentation d'un questionnaire. *Thérapie* 44:355-364.

62. Csikszentmihalyi, M. 1990. *Flow: The Psychology of Optimal Experience.* New York: Harper Collins.

63. Wilson, I.B., and P.D. Cleary. 1995. Linking clinical variables with health-related quality of life. *JAMA* 273:59-65.

64. Dupuis, G. 1987. Quality of life: a new concept for an old problem. *Cardiology* 3:73-84.

65. Bandura, A. 1989. Human agency in social cognitive theory. *Am Psychol* 44:1175-1184.

66. Antonovsky, A. 1987. *Unraveling the Mystery of Health: How People Manage Stress and Stay Well.* San Francisco: Jossey-Bass.

67. Kuhl, J., and J. Beckman. 1994. *Volition and Personality: Action Versus State Orientation.* Seattle: Hogrefe & Huber.

68. Étienne, A.M. 1997. *Impact de la réadaptation cardiaque sur la qualité de vie chez des patients ayant subi un pontage aorto-coronaire.* Liège, Belgium: Université de Liège.

69. Hlatky, M.A., R.E. Boineau, M.B. Higginbotham, K.L. Lee, D.B. Mark, and R.M. Califf, et al. 1989. A brief self-administered questionnaire to determine functional capacity (The Duke Activity Status Index). *Am J Cardiol* 64:651-654.

70. Jette, A.M., and P.D. Cleary. 1987. Functional disability assessment. *Phys Ther* 67:1854-1859.

71. Cantril, H. 1965. Discovering people's aspirations: the method used. In *The Pattern of Human Concerns,* ed. H. Cantril. New Brunswick, NJ: Rutgers University Press.

72. Lorr, M., and D.M. McNair. 1988. *Profile of Mood States, Bi-Polar Form (POMS-BI).* San Diego, CA: Educational and Industrial Testing Services.

73. Lips, H.M., ed. 1997. *Sex and Gender: An Introduction,* 3rd ed. Mountain View, CA: Mayfield.

74. Nathanson, C.A.1975. Illness and the feminine role: a theoretical review. *Soc Sci Med* 9:57-62.

75. Kandrack, M.A., K.R. Grant, and A. Segall. 1991. Gender differences in health related behaviour: some unanswered questions. *Soc Sci Med* 32:579-590.

76. Kring, A.M., and A.H. Gordon. 1998. Sex differences in emotion: expression, experience, and physiology. *J Pers Soc Psychol* 74:686-703.

77. Gross, J.J., and O.P. John. 1998. Mapping the domain of expressivity: multimethod evidence for a hierarchical model. *J Pers Soc Psychol* 74:170-191.

78. Jacobson, N.S., W.C. Follette, and D. Revenstorf. 1984. Psychotherapy outcome research: methods for reporting variability and evaluating clinical significance. *Behav Ther* 15:336-352.

79. Dupuis, G., R. Duquette, F. Mathieu, M.-E. Taggart, and M. Reidy. 1994. Quality of life: conceptual model, psychometric and descriptive data of the Quality of Life Systemic Inventory (QLSI) for normal, diabetic and AIDS subjects. *Proc Soc Behav Med Conv*: 16:S91.

80. Spilker, B., and D.A. Revecki. 1996. Taxonomy of quality of life. In *Quality of Life and Pharmacoeconomics in Clinical Trials,* ed. B. Spilker. 2nd ed. New York: Lippincott-Raven.

81. Mitroff, I.I. 1977. On the error of the third kind: toward a generalized methodology for future studies. In *Futures Research: New Directions,* ed. H.A. Linstone and W.H.C. Simmonds. London: Addison-Wesley.

82. Loveridge, D.J. 1977. Values and futures. In *Futures Research: New Directions,* ed. H.A. Linstone and W.H.C. Simmonds. London: Addison-Wesley.

PART VIII

Cardiopulmonary Rehabilitation in the Third Millennium

CHAPTER 21

Horizons in Pulmonary Rehabilitation

Andrew L. Ries
Professor of Medicine, University of California, San Diego, California, USA

Origins of Pulmonary Rehabilitation

Rehabilitation programs for patients with chronic lung diseases are well established as a means of enhancing standard therapy in order to control and alleviate symptoms and optimize functional capacity (1-8).

The origins of comprehensive pulmonary rehabilitation programs parallel the epidemic rise in morbidity and mortality resulting from chronic obstructive pulmonary diseases (COPD) over the last 50 years. In 1996, it was estimated that 106,146 people in the United States died of COPD (9). This represents an age-adjusted death rate of 21 per 100,000 in the population. COPD is the fourth most common cause of death in the United States. In persons 55-74 years of age, COPD ranks third among men and fourth among women (10). More than 95% of deaths from COPD occur after the age of 55 years (11). However, epidemiological surveys indicate that COPD is listed in multiple-cause coding on less than 50% of death certificates for individuals with COPD (12). In contrast to other major diseases (e.g., heart disease deaths, which have declined), death rates from COPD have increased rapidly in recent years—47% between 1979 and 1993 (13-15).

Morbidity from COPD is even more significant than mortality, but estimates are inadequate and incomplete (16). COPD develops insidiously, and, because of the large reserve in lung function, many patients with significant disease have few symptoms and are undiagnosed. In a population survey in Tucson, Burrows reported that only 34% of persons with COPD had ever consulted a physician for the condition, 36% denied any respiratory symptoms, and 30% denied shortness of breath with exertion, the primary symptom (17). On the other hand, when COPD is recognized later in life, lung function is severely compromised and the disease process is largely irreversible.

Definitions and Goals

Pulmonary rehabilitation programs enhance standard therapy and may help control and alleviate symptoms, optimize functional capacity, and reduce the medical and economic burdens of patients with disabling diseases (1,5,6,8,14,15,18). Such programs typically include education, instruction in respiratory and chest physiotherapy techniques, psychosocial support, and exercise training (7,14,15). The primary goal of any rehabilitation program is to restore the patient to the highest possible level of independent function. This goal is accomplished by helping patients and significant others learn more about their disease, treatment options, and coping strategies. Patients are encouraged to become actively involved in providing their own health care, more independent in daily activities, and less dependent on health professionals and expensive medical resources. Rather than focusing solely on reversing the disease process, rehabilitation attempts to improve disability from disease.

The Rehabilitation Team

A key element of the practice of rehabilitation medicine is the use of an interdisciplinary team of health care professionals (19). The team in pulmonary rehabilitation may include physicians, nurses, respiratory and physical therapists, psychologists, exercise specialists, and/or others with appropriate expertise. The use of the term "interdisciplinary," as opposed to "multidisciplinary," relates to the extent of team collaboration and coordination in planning and carrying out patient treatment goals. In a multidisciplinary approach, team members work independently in their own areas of expertise in parallel with other team members. Information is typically shared during regular team meetings. The interdisciplinary team model emphasizes a more integrated team approach to decision making and goal setting. Team members may conduct separate assessments, but they come together to develop common goals and treatment plans. In the future, rehabilitation may move toward the development of "transdisciplinary" teams, the most integrated model, in which team members work across boundaries of their professional disciplines. In this model, although team members may bring professional training from various disciplines, they tend to work more interchangeably as "pulmonary rehabilitation specialists."

Established Benefits

Benefits of pulmonary rehabilitation include improved exercise tolerance and symptoms, decreased health care expenditures, and reduced use of expensive medical resources. Published results provide a sound scientific basis for the overall intervention as well as for specific components of it (5,8,14,15). Several studies have demonstrated the cost effectiveness of a decrease in hospital days and in the use of medical resources (6,14,15,20). After rehabilitation, patients report improved quality of life with a reduction in respiratory symptoms, increase in exercise tolerance and ability to perform physical activities of daily living, more independence, and improvement in psychological function with less anxiety and depression and increased feelings of hope, control, and self-esteem. Studies that have examined individual program components have shown that even patients with severe disease can learn to understand their disease better, increase their activity levels, and improve their exercise tolerance as a result of training. Pulmonary rehabilitation for patients with COPD has not resulted in significant changes in lung function. Studies of survival have shown variable results. Vocational benefits may be difficult to achieve in the presence of severe, disabling disease. However, patients with less severe disease may return to work and increase vocational and recreational activities considerably.

Given the weight of evidence supporting the use of pulmonary rehabilitation as a standard of care for patients with chronic lung diseases, future additional randomized trials to demonstrate the effectiveness of rehabilitation may not be needed. Rather, future investigation should concentrate on better delineation of the optimal models and methods to incorporate into such programs to maximize benefits, reduce costs, and optimize the cost effectiveness of such programs.

Future Challenges in Pulmonary Rehabilitation

Several factors will influence the future of pulmonary rehabilitation and are discussed below.

Maintenance of Long-Term Behavior Change

Previous clinical trials have demonstrated substantial benefits of pulmonary rehabilitation in exercise tolerance, symptoms (e.g., dyspnea), psychosocial measures such as self-efficacy, and quality of life (8,14,15,21,22). Some have suggested substantial long-term benefits of rehabilitation in patients with COPD (6). However, a recently published systematic review (14,15) and a meta-analysis (8) of the COPD rehabilitation literature reveal little evidence for lasting, long-term benefits from pulmonary rehabilitation. The evidence-based tables in the review list the length of follow-up for each of the published trials. Most trials report benefits at 6 months, but trials rarely follow patients longer than 1 year. Studies with longer-term follow-up indicate that these benefits last approximately 12 to 18 months. Such changes in health behavior over this period of time are reasonable for a short-term intervention such as that provided in a typical pulmonary rehabilitation program.

One reason that programs may not be effective over a longer term is that we have the wrong conceptual model. Behavioral intervention programs have followed an acute disease model. According to the acute disease model, a health problem is treated and the treatment is expected to alleviate the problem. However, diseases such as COPD are chronic problems. The acute disease approach may not be well suited to enduring problems. Chronic problems may require chronic treatment. For example, the treatment of hypertension, diabetes mellitus, and congestive heart failure all require continuing intervention. The rationale for behavioral interventions has been that they provide skills for coping with illness. However, the challenges of chronic illness create a series of new and different problems. Not only are there continuing problems associated with progressive illness and associated complications, but the aging process and deteriorating health create continuous streams of new challenges. Patients with chronic disease need ongoing reassessment and changes in their treatment regimen. Further, social contacts for older patients often change. Death of spouse or friends is common and these create major disruptions in behavior patterns.

In the future, it may be appropriate to examine the use of pulmonary rehabilitation as part of a model for chronic disease management. Programs may need to be modified to incorporate intermittent, repeated evaluations and treatments, rather than one-time interventions, in order to assist patients with coping with the life changes associated with a chronic, progressive disease process.

Funding

In the future, securing appropriate funding for pulmonary rehabilitation programs is a high priority. If, in fact, pulmonary rehabilitation is a cost-effective preventive health care strategy, then it should be possible to convince payers and policy makers to provide the necessary support. As more and better-designed studies are conducted that document the benefits and cost savings of pulmonary rehabilitation, it will be easier to make convincing arguments. Currently, program structure is too often dictated by the funding available—e.g., paying for a fixed number of sessions puts the emphasis on short-term programs; paying for "procedures" and "monitoring" rather than education, training, or psychosocial counseling may require programs to include certain types of activities to cover expenses for others.

What one thinks about a particular medical treatment depends a lot on one's point of view. Fortunately, in pulmonary rehabilitation, there is often a "win-win" situation with benefits for all involved. Patients are concerned with how they feel and function. Health professionals are concerned with how their patients feel, but also with how difficult they are to care for—particularly difficult patients with chronic diseases with limited therapeutic options. Providers are happy if their patients are satisfied with their care and don't overutilize services. Funders are interested in bottom-line issues of how much a treatment costs—or saves. Patients with chronic lung disease are heavy users of health care systems and difficult to care for.

Effective pulmonary rehabilitation as part of a disease management program for such patients can help them feel and function better, become more self-reliant and less dependent on health care professionals, improve their satisfaction with health care providers, reduce their use of unnecessary services, and save money.

Beyond COPD

Many rehabilitation strategies have been developed for patients with chronic obstructive pulmonary disease (COPD). Pulmonary rehabilitation has also been applied successfully to patients with other chronic lung conditions such as interstitial diseases, cystic fibrosis, bronchiectasis, and thoracic cage abnormalities (23,24). In addition, it has been used successfully as part of the evaluation and preparation for surgical treatments such as lung volume reduction surgery and lung transplantation as well as in maximizing recovery after surgery (25-27). Pulmonary rehabilitation is appropriate for any patient with stable chronic lung disease who is disabled by respiratory symptoms.

Recently, the resurgence of interest in lung volume reduction surgery in the treatment of patients with severe emphysema has highlighted the role of pulmonary rehabilitation in the management of such patients (28-32). Pulmonary rehabilitation has been recommended as an important modality in the evaluation for and preparation of patients for this procedure as well as in the postoperative recovery phase (24,33). In the National Emphysema Treatment Trial (sponsored by the National Institutes of Health and Health Care Finance Administration), designed to evaluate the role of lung volume reduction surgery in addition to maximal medical therapy in the management of patients with emphysema, all subjects are required to complete a comprehensive pulmonary rehabilitation program as part of their maximum medical care program prior to the decision to enroll in the randomized trial.

The use of rehabilitation for patients with lung cancer is another new and innovative application of sound principles. As pointed out by Bernhard and Ganz (34), lung cancer is associated with both physical and psychosocial symptoms, not all of which result from the cancer. In particular, dyspnea is common, present in up to 65% of patients. It can be related to the tumor, treatment, complications, underlying lung or heart disease, or a combination of factors. Psychological disturbances are common, including depression and anxiety. Social problems are also frequent, as cancer patients have a tendency to withdraw and become socially isolated. Normal family and social interactions are disturbed as patients are forced to change roles and become more dependent on others. In these situations, rehabilitation may be used to help patients cope with disabling symptoms and improve functional status and quality of life.

Cardiac Versus Pulmonary Rehabilitation

There are similarities, but also distinct differences, between the application of rehabilitation principles to patients with pulmonary versus cardiac diseases. Many rehabilitation programs in one area are expanding their services to accommodate other types of patients. The facilities needed for components of the programs are similar, including exercise training, education, and psychosocial support. However, the functional status and specific issues for the various types of patients are quite different. Patients with COPD, for instance, typically present at an older age and at a more advanced stage of disease when their level of function is considerably less than many cardiac patients. Also, not all lung diseases are the same. The important rehabilitation issues for an older individual with COPD may be quite different from those for the typical younger patient with interstitial lung disease, asthma, cystic fibrosis, or lung cancer. Principles of exercise training are also different for pulmonary and cardiac patients. For instance, for many patients with chronic lung disease, lactic acidosis does not develop during maximum exercise, heart rate targets are less helpful in prescribing exercise training levels, variable changes in arterial oxygenation are common with exercise, and training targets can approach or even exceed maximum levels reached during initial exercise tests. It is important to recognize the differences among these types of patients and ensure that appropriate experience and expertise are available in the rehabilitation programs.

Documenting Health Outcomes

In the new world of medical practice and finance, it is critically important to document outcomes of treatments. In pulmonary medicine, much needs to be learned about the most appropriate methods to evaluate health outcomes such as symptoms (e.g., dyspnea, depression), quality of life, and costs. Well-designed studies in both research and clinical settings will be necessary to establish that pulmonary rehabilitation does, in fact, contribute to improved health outcomes and reduced costs. Investigators and health policy makers will be challenged to make rational decisions based on scientifically sound evidence.

Conclusion

The third millennium is an exciting time for pulmonary rehabilitation. The application of rehabilitation principles to the management of patients with chronic lung disease has become a well-accepted practice and recommended as a standard of care for such patients (2,3). We must now accept the challenge of determining the optimal structure of such programs and ensure that they are based on sound scientific principles, while, at the same time, paying attention to and optimizing cost effectiveness. There are many patients and other lung diseases for whom pulmonary rehabilitation may play an important role in improving their function and quality of life and helping to control health care costs in disease management. Opportunities abound in this field. We need to seize the day.

References

1. American Thoracic Society. 1981. Pulmonary rehabilitation. *Am Rev Respir Dis* 124:663-666.
2. American Thoracic Society. 1995. Standards for the diagnosis and care of patients with chronic obstructive pulmonary disease (COPD) and asthma. *Am Rev Respir Dis* 152:S78-S121.
3. Siafakas, N.M., P. Vermeire, and N.B. Pride, et al. 1995. Optimal assessment and management of chronic obstructive pulmonary disease (COPD). *Eur Respir J* 8:1398-1420.
4. Cotes, J.E., J.M. Bishop, and L.H. Capel, et al. 1981. Disabling chest disease: prevention and care: a report of the Royal College of Physicians by the College Committee on Thoracic Medicine. *J R Coll Phys* 15:69-87.
5. Ries, A.L. 1990. Position paper of the American Association of Cardiovascular and Pulmonary Rehabilitation: scientific basis of pulmonary rehabilitation. *J Cardiopulm Rehabil* 10:418-441.
6. Hodgkin, J.E., G.L. Connors, and C.W. Bell. 1993. *Pulmonary Rehabilitation: Guidelines to Success.* 2nd ed. Philadelphia: J.B. Lippincott.
7. American Association of Cardiovascular and Pulmonary Rehabilitation. 1998. *Guidelines for Pulmonary Rehabilitation Programs*. 2nd ed. Champaign, IL: Human Kinetics.
8. Lacasse, Y., E. Wong, G.H. Guyatt, D. King, D.J. Cook, and R.S. Goldstein. 1996. Meta-analysis of respiratory rehabilitation in chronic obstructive pulmonary disease. *Lancet* 348:1115-1119.
9. Monthly Vital Statistics. 1997. *Monthly Vital Statistics Report* 46 (suppl 1).
10. American Cancer Society. 1989. Cancer statistics, 1989. *CA* 39:6-11.
11. Feinleib, M., H.M. Rosenberg, J.G. Collins, J.E. Delozier, R. Pokras, and F.M. Chevarley. 1989. Trends in COPD morbidity and mortality in the United States. *Am Rev Respir Dis* 140:S9-S18.
12. Sherrill, D.L., M.D. Lebowitz, and B. Burrows. 1990. Epidemiology of chronic obstructive pulmonary disease. *Clin Chest Med* 11:375-387.
13. Massachusetts Medical Society. 1993. Mortality patterns—United States, 1993. *MMWR* 45:161-164.

14. American College of Chest Physicians/American Association of Cardiovascular and Pulmonary Rehabilitation. 1997. Pulmonary Rehabilitation Guidelines Panel. Pulmonary rehabilitation: joint ACCP/AACVPR evidence based guidelines. *Chest* 112:1363-1396.

15. ACCP/AACVPR Pulmonary Rehabilitation Guidelines Panel. 1997. Pulmonary rehabilitation: joint ACCP/AACVPR evidence based guidelines. *J Cardiopulmonary Rehabil* 17:371-405.

16. Higgins, M.W., and T.J. Thom. 1989. Incidence, prevalence and mortality: intra- and intercountry differences. In *Clinical Epidemiology of Chronic Obstructive Pulmonary Disease,* ed. M.J. Hensley and N.A. Saunders. New York: Marcel Dekker.

17. Burrows, B. 1991. Epidemiologic evidence for different types of chronic airflow obstruction. *Am Rev Respir Dis* 143:1452-1455.

18. Casaburi, R. 1993. *Principles and Practice of Pulmonary Rehabilitation.* Philadelphia: W.B. Saunders.

19. Ries, A.L., and H.C. Squier. 1996. The team concept in pulmonary rehabilitation. In *Pulmonary Rehabilitation,* ed. A.P. Fishman. New York: Marcel Dekker.

20. Hudson, L.D., M.L. Tyler, and T.L. Petty. 1976. Hospitalization needs during an outpatient rehabilitation program for severe chronic airway obstruction. *Chest* 70:606-610.

21. Ries, A.L., R.M. Kaplan, T.M. Limberg, and L.M. Prewitt. 1995. Effects of pulmonary rehabilitation on physiologic and psychosocial outcomes in patients with chronic obstructive pulmonary disease. *Ann Intern Med* 122:823-832.

22. Toshima, M.T., R.M. Kaplan, and A.L. Ries. 1990. Experimental evaluation of rehabilitation in chronic obstructive pulmonary disease: short-term effects on exercise endurance and health status. *Health Psychol* 9:237-252.

23. Foster, S., and H.M. Thomas. 1990. Pulmonary rehabilitation in lung disease other than chronic obstructive pulmonary disease. *Am Rev Respir Dis* 141:601-604.

24. Crouch, R., and N.R. MacIntyre. 1998. Pulmonary rehabilitation of the patient with nonobstructive lung disease. *Respir Care Clin N Am* 4:59-67.

25. Craven, J.L., J. Bright, and C.L. Dear. 1990. Psychiatric, psychosocial, and rehabilitative aspects of lung transplantation. *Clin Chest Med* 11:247-257.

26. Biggar, D.G., J.F. Malen, E.P. Trulock, and J.D. Cooper. 1993. Pulmonary rehabilitation before and after lung transplantation. In *Principles and Practice of Pulmonary Rehabilitation,* ed. R. Casaburi and T.L. Petty. 1st ed. Philadelphia: W.B. Saunders.

27. Palmer, S.M., and V.F. Tapson. 1998. Pulmonary rehabilitation in the surgical patient: lung transplantation and lung volume reduction surgery. *Respir Care Clin N Am* 4:71-83.

28. Weinmann, G.C., and R. Hyatt. 1996. Evaluation and research in lung volume reduction surgery. *Am J Respir Crit Care Med* 154:1913-1918.

29. Sciurba, F.C. 1997. Early and long-term functional outcomes following lung volume reduction surgery. *Clin Chest Med* 18:259-276.

30. Benditt, J.O., and R.K. Albert. 1995. Lung reduction surgery: great expectations and a cautionary note. *Chest* 107:297-298.

31. Fein, A.M. 1998. Lung volume reduction surgery: answering the crucial questions. *Chest* 113:277S-282S.

32. Cooper, J.D., E.P. Trulock, and A.N. Triantafillou, et al. 1995. Bilateral pneumectomy (volume reduction) for chronic obstructive pulmonary disease. *J Thorac Cardiovasc Surg* 109:106-119.

33. Moser, K.M., K.M. Kerr, H.G. Colt, and A.L. Ries. 1996. Lung reduction surgery: what role in emphysema? *J Respir Dis* 17:351-358.

34. Bernhard, J., and P.A. Ganz. 1991. Psychosocial issues in lung cancer patients (parts 1 and 2). *Chest* 99:216-223, 480-485.

CHAPTER 22

Integrating Technology and Self-Care in Cardiology: Challenge for the Future

Martin J. Sullivan
Department of Medicine, Duke University Medical Center, Durham, North Carolina, USA

Lifestyle interventions in patients with coronary artery disease have been proven to significantly reduce future coronary events and delay underlying disease progression (1-11). Although these interventions should be the cornerstone of therapy in this disorder, and evidence supporting this approach continues to accumulate, the vast majority of patients with coronary artery disease receive no lifestyle prevention or rehabilitation services (12,13). Why is this so? The answer here lies not solely in the data on outcomes, but in the basic conceptual framework of our current medical system and in how medicine interacts with society. Our current difficulty with implementing lifestyle-based therapies provides an important avenue of inquiry about the evolution of medicine in the next century.

Medicine has made impressive scientific strides in the last century. By the 1960s, major advances in the fields of microbiology, pharmacology, and laboratory medicine led to the ability to effectively treat many infectious diseases that had previously posed major health risks, especially for children. In the last 40 years, technological advances in surgery, medical devices, and clinical informatics have led to an impressive ability to cure or palliate a number of conditions that were previously untreatable. For example, pacemaker therapy can now easily treat bradyarrhythmias and, in many cases, can treat tachyarrhythmias. These advances have led to the "magic bullet" approach to medicine: a specific physician-directed therapy to eradicate a specific ailment. At present, we are pursuing new advances in genetics, biomedical engineering, and transplantation that offer exciting new horizons in therapy. Yet, when we view medicine from the practitioner's office, it is apparent that technology alone does not hold all the answers, especially for patients with chronic illnesses that are closely related to lifestyle choices. At present, it appears that we can more easily insert a coronary artery stent or an insulin pump in a patient with severe adult onset diabetes and coronary artery disease than we can facilitate lifestyle changes that we know can have major benefits on long-term outcome.

How will medicine advance in the next 100 years? Certainly we will see major advances in gene therapy, biomedical engineering, and transplantation. However, at present it appears that we are getting smaller and more marginal returns from increasingly expensive technological and pharmacological interventions. There are clear limits to how far we can advance health care with more technology. Our efforts to develop effective models to better connect with patients and engage them in their own health care in a way that will change their lifestyles will be a very important development in medicine of the future. This new paradigm in medicine offers a chance for implementation of effective cardiac rehabilitation and prevention service networks that can have major effects on health care outcomes. Our current management of coronary artery disease is a prime example of how our current medical paradigm is not optimal in engaging patients in their own health care through lifestyle changes.

Lifestyle and Health

At least half of what influences the health status of the population is rooted in the lifestyle of individuals and in the environments in which they live (14). It is estimated that only 10% of health determinants are linked to specific medical treatment interventions. This is illustrated in table 22.1, which estimates the contributions of various lifestyle factors on mortality in the United States. Although we typically view heart disease, cancer, stroke, pulmonary disease, accidents, and diabetes as causes of death, the "real causes" are rooted in lifestyle and behaviors. This concept is supported by the Cornell China project (15). This study examined health records in 220 localities in China over a 3-year period and found a very low incidence of coronary artery disease (CAD) in Chinese men (risk ratio of 0.06 compared to contemporary norms for U.S. men) in their survey. They examined several geographic locations in which evidence of CAD could not be found in populations of several hundred thousand individuals. These results, when combined with those of the Honolulu Heart Program (16) and others (17-19), demonstrate the critical role of cultural factors in the genesis of CAD.

It has long been established that diet and smoking are related to CAD. More recent studies have refined the components of diet that are related to the incidence of CAD (20-28). Although early studies focused on total fat and saturated fat, more recent studies have explored the protective roles of monounsaturated fatty acids, vegetable and cereal intake, and dietary vitamins (23,25,26). Over the last decade, more information linking sedentary lifestyle to CAD has accumulated (29,30). It now appears that even short intervals of regular exertion at low levels of aerobic activity confer significant health benefits when compared to a completely sedentary lifestyle.

Only recently has the weight of evidence clearly pointed to psychosocial factors as causative for CAD (31-37). Although early studies demonstrated a link between CAD and Type A behavior, more recent studies have not shown that all people manifesting Type A behavior are at risk (33). It now appears that hostility is an important risk-conferring behavior in Type A individuals (33). Numerous articles have demonstrated that social isolation is linked to CAD (32,33). Over the last 5 years, several well-done

Table 22.1 Estimates of Mortality Contributions of Specific Lifestyle Factors

	Deaths	
Cause	Estimated no. *	Percentage of total deaths
Tobacco	400,000	19
Diet/activity patterns	300,000	14
Alcohol	100,000	5
Microbial agents	90,000	4
Toxic agents	60,000	3
Firearms	35,000	2
Sexual behavior	25,000	1
Illicit use of drugs	20,000	<1
Total	1,060,000	50

*Composite approximation drawn from studies that use different approaches to derive estimates, ranging from actual counts (e.g., firearms) to population attributable risk calculations (e.g., tobacco). Numbers over 100,000 rounded to the nearest 100,000; over 50,000, rounded to the nearest 10,000; below 50,000, rounded to the nearest 5000.

McGinnis and Foege 1993 (14). Reprinted with permission, *JAMA*.

studies have shown a clear link between depression and CAD (33-37), often with risk ratios for CAD of 3-4 for those who have major depression. This hazard ratio would be equal to or greater than that conferred by any other single risk factor.

Studies in high-risk westernized populations clearly demonstrate strong relationships between lifestyle and CAD. Diet, physical inactivity, and psychosocial factors, including social isolation, depression, and hostility are dependent on culture, and may possibly be changed significantly over time in a given population. The finding in cross-cultural studies that some populations have very low incidences of CAD supports the concept that atherosclerosis may be largely an unintended result of our current culture. Although public health initiatives have improved many of these factors (diet and toxic exposures), there have been significant limitations in advancing others (weight, exercise, stress, and smoking).

Lifestyle Interventions in Patients With CAD

From the 1960s to the early 1980s, lifestyle changes in patients with CAD focused primarily on exercise training of patients after myocardial infarction. This is supported by numerous studies demonstrating reduced mortality after exercise training in this population (37-39). Until the late 1980s, most investigators thought atherosclerosis was a relentlessly progressive process that could not be altered by modifying risk factors. As stated in the *British Medical Journal* in 1977, "Only the optimists among us believe that obstructive atheroma in the coronary arteries of our patients with angina might regress if we could persuade them to reduce the load of adverse factors in their lifestyle." The first indication of coronary lesion regression came from case studies in the 1970s and the early 1980s. In these studies, patients who underwent serial angiography had less than 6% regression with standard medical therapy (41,42).

At present, numerous studies have examined the effect of lifestyle interventions in patients with CAD, demonstrating important reductions in symptoms and recurrent events (1-10). In addition, at least four dozen clinical trials (43-65), many using serial angiography, have demonstrated that pharmacological lipid-lowering intervention programs can improve coronary luminal diameter, improve myocardial blood flow, reduce myocardial ischemia and infarction, and reduce coronary events in patients with coronary artery disease. Even though the changes in coronary lesions are small, they translate into significant improvement in outcome. This is likely a result of prevention of plaque rupture, which is known to cause most acute cardiac events. Although pharmacological management of lipids is an important therapeutic focus in managing patients with CAD, it should be viewed as part of a comprehensive risk reduction program. Pharmacotherapy can have major effects on LDL-cholesterol (LDL-C), and yet is not more effective (and in some comparisons is less effective) in reducing coronary events or angiographic disease progression when compared to lifestyle interventions. In addition, pharmacological therapy is often more costly than lifestyle management.

The St. Thomas' Atherosclerosis Regression Study (STARS) (7) examined the effects of dietary changes with or without cholestyramine versus usual care in men with angina or previous myocardial infarction. By decreasing total cholesterol and LDL-C more than control subjects, the progression of coronary atherosclerosis declined from almost half (46%) in those receiving usual care to only 12% in those receiving diet and cholestyramine and 15% in those receiving diet alone. Regression was seen in 4% of the usual care group and in 33% and 38% of the diet plus cholestyramine and diet alone groups, respectively. Although the addition of cholestyramine further reduced LDL-C when compared to diet alone, it did not improve angiographic or clinical outcomes. As in previous studies, lesions with greater than 50% stenosis demonstrated the most improvement. In addition to demonstrating anatomic effects of these diet-based therapies, the two treatment groups had fewer clinical cardiac events than the usual care group ($p < 0.05$) and had less angina compared to baseline ($p < 0.05$), whereas angina in controls did not change.

The blinded, randomized, controlled Lifestyle Heart Trial (1,2) examined symptoms, risk factors, and coronary anatomy before and at 1 and 5 years after a comprehensive set of diet, exercise, and behavioral interventions in the treatment group. All participants in this study had significant coronary atherosclerosis, a left ventricular ejection fraction greater than 25%, and were not taking lipid-lowering medications. The treatment group (N = 22) was assigned to a low-fat (10% of calories from fat) vegetarian diet, 1 hour a day of stress management, and 3 hours or more of aerobic exercise per week. Controls (N = 19) were given usual care and were counseled to follow a 30% fat diet and to perform three hours per week of aerobic exercise. At 1 and 5 years, compliance was quite good in treated patients for diet (~9% calories from fat), aerobic exercise (3-4 hours/week), and stress management (5-8 hours/week). By 5 years, nine of the control and no treatment patients were taking lipid-lowering medications. Of note, at 5 years, controls also exercised (~3 hours/week) and modified diet (~25% of calories from fat), while not participating in stress reduction to any significant degree. Although LDL-C was much lower in treated patients at 1 year (86 + 9 vs. 141 + 15 mg/dl; $p < 0.05$), there was no difference in LDL-C at year 5.

At 1 year, the incidence of angina dropped 91% in the treatment group and increased 165% in controls (1). At 5-year follow-up, there were 25 events in 108 person-years of observation in treated patients versus 45 events in 78 person-years in control patients ($p < 0.001$); 10 of 28 treatment patients and 19 of 20 controls underwent percutaneous transluminal coronary angioplasty (PTCA) or coronary artery bypass graft (CABG) procedures ($p < 0.01$). The change in average stenosis severity in CAD lesions mirrored the clinical improvements, as illustrated in figure 22.1. The average percent diameter of stenosis decreased from 41% to 37% in treated patients, whereas an increase was seen in the control group, from 41% to 52% ($p = 0.001$). It is interesting to note that there was significant disease progression in controls despite their risk factor changes, which would be considered average for clinical populations with CAD. The Lifestyle Heart Trial was the first study to demonstrate that lesion progression could be slowed using lifestyle changes alone and, although small in size, has important ramifications for treatment of this disorder.

Compliance with the treatment program correlated with lesion changes in a dose-response fashion as illustrated in figure 22.2, and yet changes in LDL-C or in trial LDL-C did not correlate with angiographic changes. This finding serves to emphasize the concept that factors other than serum lipids may have a major role in the atherosclerotic process. Also of note is the finding that although serum LDL and exercise levels were not different in the two groups at 5 years, treated patients had marked reductions in both events and atherosclerosis progression compared to controls. Although this is very likely at least partly a result of lower LDL-cholesterol levels at 1 year, it is interesting to consider the role of the psychosocial arm of the Lifestyle Heart Trial intervention. A recent study by Blumenthal et al. (8) raises the possibility that stress reduction alone may have powerful effects on reducing morbidity. In this study, patients with CAD and angina were randomized to exercise or stress management interventions and compared with a matched control group that received usual care only. As illustrated in figure 22.3, there was a 70% reduction in events in the stress management group as compared to controls. In the psycho-

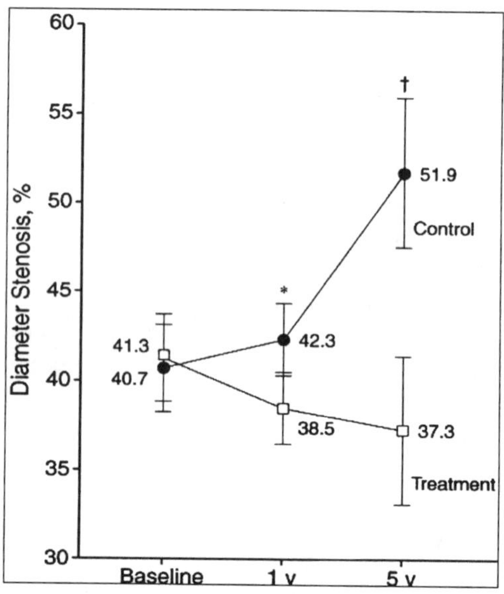

Figure 22.1 Average percent diameter stenosis for index lesions at baseline and 1- and 5-year follow-ups in control and treatment patients in the Lifestyle Heart Trial. Ornish et al. 1998 (2). Reprinted with permission, *JAMA*.

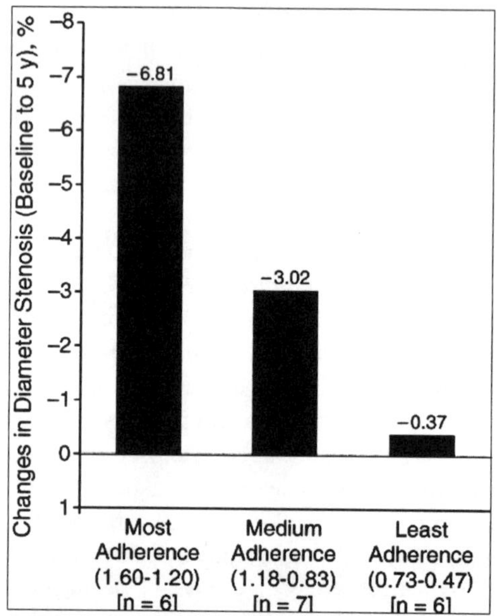

Figure 22.2 Relationship of change in diameter stenosis with program adherence in the treatment group at 5 years' follow-up in the Lifestyle Heart Trial. Ornish et al. 1998 (2). Reprinted with permission, *JAMA*.

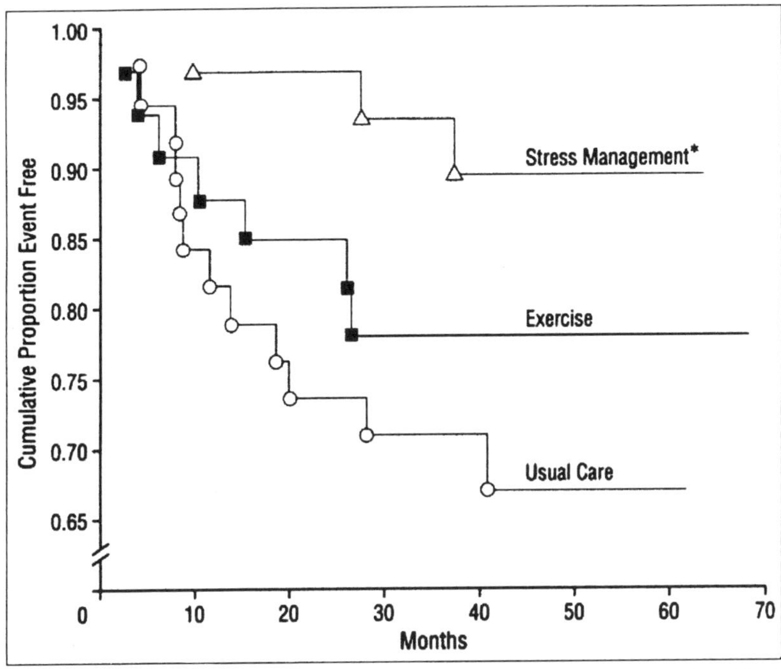

Figure 22.3 Five-year cumulative event-free survival in patients with CAD and angina randomized to stress management or exercise interventions compared with a usual care control group. Blumenthal et al. 1997 (8). Reprinted with permission, *Arch Int Med.*

social intervention group, this event reduction was accompanied by reductions in ischemia as measured by ambulatory Holter monitor and by radionuclide angiography during laboratory-induced mental stress. These results suggest that psychosocial interventions may play an important role in the management of CAD and certainly deserve careful study and consideration in the future.

The Stanford Coronary Risk Intervention Project (SCRIP) (10) also demonstrated the beneficial impact that a multidisciplinary approach could have on CAD. This study randomized 300 men and woman to usual care of their own physician or to multifactor risk reduction that included diet education, exercise, weight loss, smoking cessation, and lipid-lowering medical therapy. A significant increase in the use of lipid-lowering therapy was seen in the treatment group when compared to controls. In the intervention group, significant changes versus the usual care patients occurred in LDL-C and apolipoprotein B (–22%), HDL-cholesterol (HDL-C) (+12%), plasma triglycerides (–20%), body weight (–4%), and exercise capacity (+20%). The rate of coronary artery narrowing was 47% less than that for usual-care subjects ($p < 0.02$). Further analysis of the coronary lesions found that new lesions tended to occur in the usual-care patients rather than the risk reduction patients (new lesions/patient 0.47 vs. 0.30, $p = 0.06$). Although there was no significant difference between groups in overall mortality or cardiac death, there was a significant difference when comparing the combined end point of cardiac deaths and hospitalizations for nonfatal myocardial infarction, PTCA, and CABG (25% vs. 44%, $p = 0.05$).

Schuler et al. (4) have examined the effects of intensive exercise and a 20% fat diet in patients with coronary artery disease. The study design gave controls a 1-week hospitalization for instructions about the need for regular exercise and low-fat diet (American Heart Association [AHA] phase 1 diet) and then discharged them to the care of their private physicians. The intervention group received 3 weeks of in-hospital instruction on a diet with less than 20% of calories from fat and less than 200 mg cholesterol per day. In addition, they were asked to exercise at home on a bicycle ergometer for a minimum of 30 minutes a day with two 60-minute group exercise sessions per week. Patients were seen at the clinic at least four times a year. In the Heidelberg study (4), 111 male patients were randomized to these two arms. In the intervention, arm lesion progression was delayed, as shown by quantitative coronary angiography at 1 year. When total cholesterol was decreased by 11% and LDL-C by 9% with no change in HDL-C in treated patients, there was an increase in regression when compared to controls (32% vs. 17%, $p < 0.05$) and a decrease in progression (23% vs. 48%, $p < 0.05$) of coronary lesions. In addition, myocardial ischemia (as measured by quantitative thallium scanning after the intervention) improved while there was no change in controls. These investigators also reported that exercise may have increased collateral formation in treated patients (5).

Another important dietary intervention was examined in the Lyon Diet Heart Study (6,23), which randomized patients after myocardial infarction to a Step I AHA diet or a Mediterranean diet that emphasized use of monounsaturated fats and increases in fruits and vegetables. Both groups consumed 30% of calories from fat. There was no difference in serum LDL-C or HDL-C in the two groups at baseline or at 1-year follow-up. Of note, serum tocopherol levels were higher in the Mediterranean diet group during follow-up, suggesting higher dietary vitamin E and therefore higher antioxidant intake. Despite no differences in blood cholesterol levels, there was a 70% reduction in events in patients in the treatment group when compared to controls during long-term follow-up (figure 22.4). This study clearly delineates the importance of diet in treating patients with CAD independently of changes in serum lipids. The magnitude of event reduction in this study exceeds that seen with lipid-lowering pharmacotherapy (~30%-40%) and highlights the concept that the goal in the treatment of CAD is not just manipulation of serum lipids but the reduction of events and delayed progression of disease. These results indicate that major event reduction can occur in CAD with diet alone without changes in LDL-C or HDL-C.

Implementing Secondary Prevention in CAD

The data at this point are clear and compelling: lifestyle interventions are effective therapies in patients with coronary artery disease. They increase quality of life,

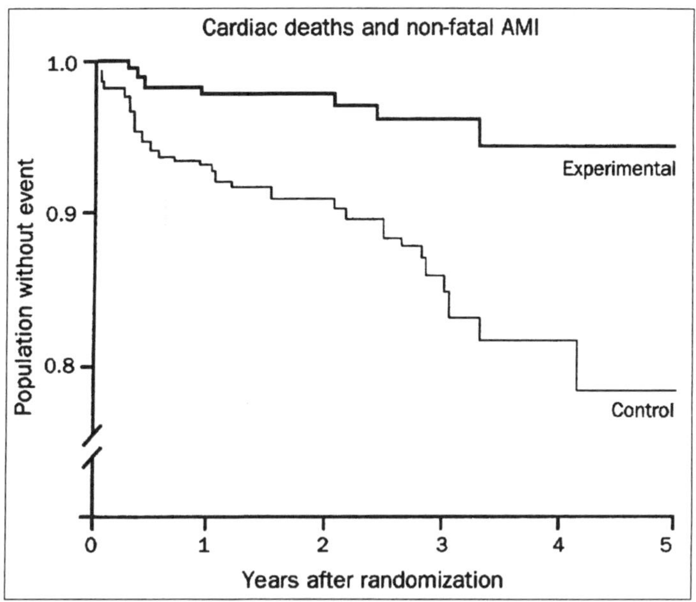

Figure 22.4 Event-free survival in patients randomized to Mediterranean diet versus usual care. de Lorgeril et al. 1994 (6). Reprinted with permission, *Lancet*.

reduce symptoms and objective evidence of ischemia, reduce morbidity, and delay progression of atherosclerosis (1-11). Although meta-analysis in this area is subject to difficulties in interpretation, one such analysis found that treatment reduced the odds for coronary lesion progression by 49%, increased the odds for no change by 33%, and increased the odds for coronary artery regression by 219%. Cardiovascular events declined by 47% (66).

Whereas 10 years ago, the role of secondary prevention in CAD was unclear, intensive risk factor reduction has now emerged as important therapy in this disorder. The evidence for secondary prevention as a means of limiting coronary artery atherosclerosis, decreasing recurrent myocardial infarction, and improving survival has grown to the point that the current standard of care dictates that cardiologists incorporate these interventions into their practice. In 1994, the AHA recommended that patients with known coronary artery disease undergo a comprehensive risk factor reduction program centered on lipid-lowering therapy, blood pressure control, smoking cessation, diet, exercise, weight reduction, and stress reduction (67). Although the guidelines here are clear, medicine has been slow to respond in implementing effective strategies to meet these goals.

Several studies have examined the current implementation rates of secondary prevention strategies in patients with CAD (11,12,68). Across geographic locations and practice types, the results are consistent in showing very low implementation rates. In 1991, Cohen et al. (12) reported that only 25% of patients with CAD had either pharmacological or dietary therapy for hyperlipidemia 1 month after catheterization. Less than 20% of eligible patients participate in cardiac rehabilitation, largely as a result of low physician referral rates (12). A 1998 study of hospitalized patients with CAD showed that less than 15% of patients had received any formalized lifestyle intervention (stop smoking consult, cardiac rehabilitation, nutrition consult, or psychological referral) (12). There was a 1% rate of referral for exercise therapy with less than 50% of patients receiving appropriate lipid-lowering therapy.

Roadblocks to Change

The efficacy data for lifestyle changes in CAD are compelling, and the interventions are cost effective. Why are these treatment rates so low when we have clearly identified safe and cost-effective lifestyle interventions for CAD? Several factors are making progress difficult:

1. inherent delays in implementing research,
2. the "medical nemesis" (see discussion of this concept in the following section),
3. treatment versus prevention paradigms,
4. reimbursement and economic lobbies, and
5. limited models for care.

Our medical system has inherent inefficiencies that prevent well-proven therapies from being used. This is well documented in the use of aspirin or β-blocker therapy in patients after myocardial infarction. Physicians generally do not change practices overnight on the basis of a few studies. Although these factors are operative in this area, they do not explain the extremely low use of lifestyle interventions in CAD. This is supported by the perception that utilization rates do not seem to be increasing over the last 5 years, even though the published evidence is growing.

In 1976, Illich published *Limits to Medicine: Medical Nemesis: The Expropriation of Health* (69), which outlined the concept that the medical establishment, through its very success in technology, was promulgating the idea that "magic bullet" therapy was or would soon be available for our medical problems. This idea, in essence, significantly decreases patient participation and responsibility in health care. This phenomenon is reflected by patients who want the health care system to alleviate their problems without their own participation. I recently saw a patient who had undergone a three-vessel CABG procedure. Without his medical records, the following conversation ensued:

Dr. Sullivan: "What brings you here today?"

Patient: "I am here for a checkup."

Dr. Sullivan: "Do you have heart disease?"
Patient: "No."
Dr. Sullivan: "Who exactly sent you?"
Patient: "My surgeon."
Dr. Sullivan: "What kind of surgery did you have?"
Patient: "A heart bypass operation."
Dr. Sullivan: "I thought you said you didn't have any heart disease."
Patient: "I don't. My surgeon fixed my heart."

This phenomenon is clearly related to both what we as physicians say to patients and what they choose to hear. However, it illustrates the "medical nemesis" at work in our current system. With the information given, this patient would not be likely to pursue risk factor interventions, even though he would have a 10-year recurrent event rate of 50%-65%. This is a clear example of the subtle ways in which active treatment is more highly valued than prevention and self-care. This bias toward treatment is evident in medical education and clinical practice. The very fact that most of what we define as medical practice occurs only in clinics or hospitals reflects this bias and leads to the medical system in which we currently practice. This bias is reflected by our current reimbursement policies in medicine. At present it is very difficult to obtain third-party reimbursement for outpatient nutrition counseling, risk factor education, or psychological interventions in patients with CAD. This situation has persisted over the last decade, even in the face of growing evidence of the cost effectiveness of lifestyle interventions. It seems that our existing medical systems act to narrowly define health care and limit our creativity in exploring new ways to solve problems. The question is: could we design a better system to improve cardiovascular health care with the expenditures that we currently have in this area?

Economic lobbies play an important role in shaping health care. Each year, millions of dollars are spent promoting the use of drugs, devices, and health systems. Over time, these factors play a major role in shaping the agendas in health care delivery and standards of care. Although these lobbies may have positive benefits in certain areas, these interests do not generally promote the kind of thinking that would lead to the advancement of major reforms in prevention or rehabilitation. It is also important to note that there is no significant lobbying effort for self-care to balance these interests.

Self-care is an important issue in medicine. In our current culture, with our current mind-set and education, many individuals have difficulty grasping the self-care concept. This difficulty is most likely a matter of education and can be significantly improved over time. It is interesting that ongoing cultural changes may improve the outlook for self-care in the coming century. Ray (70) has reported that American culture is currently undergoing a major transformation. Whereas now modernism dominates the culture (a reliance on science, technology, and organization to solve problems), Ray suggests that in the future the cultural-creative culture may be predominant. These individuals are more interested in eclectic world views, psychospiritual factors in life, and holistic thinking. As demonstrated by Astin (71), individuals identifying with this latter cultural stream are more likely to use holistic or alternative medical services and are more likely to emphasize self-care. It is likely that, as this cultural mind-set becomes more predominant, interest in self-care will increase markedly in the general public.

Although there have been overall improvements in general preventive health in the last 20 years, it seems that as we enter the 21st century, we are poised to make important headway in this area. Comprehensive lifestyle interventions for patients with CAD are effective in reducing disease progression and are cost effective. These programs can be delivered by modifying our existing exercise-based cardiac rehabilitation programs (72). Even though this would seem to be a first-line therapy in all patients, in practice, only a small minority receive any kind of formalized lifestyle intervention. It seems that many of the barriers to higher utilization of lifestyle interventions lie in the very foundations of how we practice medicine, how we design medical systems, and how we relate to patients. Therapy for patients with CAD could be improved significantly if

- patients were given the correct information about CAD prevention in a clear and consistent manner from all of their health care contacts,
- lifestyle programs were reimbursed by third-party payers,
- patients became more interested in self-care, and
- health care policy was focused solely on optimal patient care.

The challenge of medicine in the future lies not only in advancing technology, but also in combining the best of technology with improvements in patient-centered self-care to practice the best medicine. At this juncture it appears that moving ahead in patient self-care will require not only additional outcomes research but also a careful look at the basic paradigms of care delivery that shaped medicine in the last century.

Summary

Coronary artery disease incidence and outcomes are closely related to culture and lifestyle. At present, rehabilitation and secondary prevention efforts are underutilized and generally insufficient in scope to produce optimal results. For example, cardiac rehabilitation has focused primarily on exercise training. Recent studies clearly demonstrate that long-term lifestyle interventions, especially those that contain mind-body components, can have a more profound impact on risk factors and outcomes than our current therapeutic paradigms.

The challenge for the future in rehabilitation will be to develop cost-effective long-term models that maintain cultural congruence in patient care in order to effect greater long-term risk factor modification. As culture in North America shifts, and our patients embrace an increased emphasis on self-care, it is likely that these models will be more applicable. Our challenge in the future is to transform our current acute illness care model to one that truly embraces health care and wellness and facilitates optimal functioning in all aspects—mind, body, and spirit—of our patients' lives.

References

1. Ornish, D., S.E. Brown, and L.W. Scherwitz. 1990. Can lifestyle changes reverse coronary heart disease? The Lifestyle Heart Trial. *Lancet* 336:129-133.
2. Ornish, D., L. Scherwitz, J. Billings, K. Gould, T. Merritt, S. Sparler, W. Armstrong, T. Ports, R. Kirkeeide, C. Hogeboom, and R. Brand. 1998. Intensive lifestyle changes for reversal of coronary artery disease. *JAMA* 280(23):2001-2007.
3. Levy, R.I., J.F. Brensike, S.E. Eptstein, S.F. Kelsey, and E.R. Passamani, et al. 1984. The influence of changes in lipid values induced by cholestyramine and diet on progression of coronary artery disease: results of the NHLBI Type II Coronary Intervention Study. *Circulation* 69:325-337.
4. Schuler, G., R. Hambrecht, and G. Schlierf. 1992. Myocardial perfusion and regression of coronary artery disease in patients on a regimen of intensive physical exercise and low fat diet. *J Am Coll Cardiol* 19:34-42.
5. Niebauer, J., R. Hambrecht, C. Marburger, and K. Hauer, et al. 1995. Impact of intensive physical exercise and low-fat diet on collateral vessel formation in stable angina pectoris and angiographically confirmed coronary artery disease. *Am J Cardiol* 76:771-775.
6. de Lorgeril, M., S. Renaud, N. Mamelle, P. Salen, J.L. Matin, I. Monjaud, J. Guidollet, P. Touboul, and J. Delaye. 1994. Mediterranean alpha-linolenic acid-rich diet in secondary prevention of coronary heart disease. *Lancet* 343(8911):1454-1459.
7. Watts, G.F., B. Lewis, and J.N.H. Brunt. 1992. Effects on coronary artery disease of lipid-lowering diet, or diet plus cholestyramine, in the St. Thomas' Atherosclerosis Regression Study (STARS). *Lancet* 339:563-569.
8. Blumenthal, J.A., W. Jiang, M.A. Babyak, D.S. Krantz, D.J. Frid, R.E. Coleman, R. Waugh, M. Hanson, M. Appelbaum, C. O'Connor, and J.J. Morris. 1997. Stress management and exercise training in cardiac patients with myocardial ischemia. Effects on prognosis and evaluation of mechanisms. *Arch Med* 157(19):2213-2223.
9. Esselstyn, C.B. Jr., S.G. Ellis, S.V. Medendorp, and T.D. Crowe. 1995. A strategy to arrest and reverse coronary artery disease: a 5-year longitudinal study of a single physician's practice. *J Fam Pract* 41(6):560-568.

10. Haskell, W.L., E.L. Alderman, J.M. Fair, D.J. Maron, S.F. Mackey, H.R. Superko, P.T. Williams, I.M. Johnstone, M.A. Champagne, R.M. Krauss, and J.W. Farquhar. 1994. Effects of intensive multiple risk factor reduction on coronary atherosclerosis and clinical cardiac events in men and women with coronary artery disease: the Stanford Coronary Risk Intervention Project (SCRIP). *Circulation* 89:975-990.

11. Connor, W.E., S.L. Connor, M.B. Katan, S.M. Grundy, and W.C. Willett. 1997. Should a low-fat, high-carbohydrate diet be recommended for everyone? *NEJM* 337(8):562-563.

12. Cohen, M.V., M. Byrne, B. Levine, T. Gutowski, and R. Adelson.1991. Low rate of treatment of hypercholesterolemia by cardiologists in patients with suspected and proven coronary artery disease. *Circulation* 83:1294-1304.

13. Frolkis, J., S. Zyzanski, J. Schwartz, and P. Suhan. 1998. Physician noncompliance with the 1993 national cholesterol education program (NCEP-ATPII) guidelines. *Circulation* 98(9):851-855.

14. McGinnis, J.M., and W.H. Foege. 1993. Actual causes of death in the United States. *J Am Med Assoc* 270(18):2207-2212.

15. Campbell, T.C., B. Parpia, and J. Chen. 1998. Diet, lifestyle, and the etiology of coronary artery disease: the China study. *Am J Cardiol* 82(10B):18T-21T.

16. Reed, D., and K. Yano. 1991. Predictors of arteriographically defined coronary stenosis in the Honolulu Heart Program. Comparisons of cohort and arteriography series analyses. *Am J Epidemiol* 134(2):111-122.

17. Marmot, M.G., S.L. Syme, and A. Kagan, et al. 1975. Epidemiologic studies of coronary heart disease and stroke in Japanese men living in Japan, Hawaii and California: prevalence of coronary and hypertensive heart disease and associated risk factors. *Am J Epidemiol* 102:514-525.

18. Shaper, A.G. 1974. Communities without hypertension. In *Cardiovascular Disease in the Tropics,* ed. A.G. Shaper, M.S.R. Hutt, and Z. Fejfar. London: British Medical Association.

19. Malmros, H. 1950. The relation of nutrition to health. A statistical study of the effect of wartime on arteriosclerosis, cardiosclerosis, tuberculosis and diabetes. *Acta Med Scand* (suppl)246:137-150.

20. Neaton, J.D., L.H. Kuller, D. Wentworth, and N.O. Borhani. 1984. Total and cardiovascular mortality in relation to cigarette smoking, serum cholesterol concentration, and diastolic blood pressure among black and white males followed up for five years. *Am Heart J* 108(3 pt.2):759-769.

21. Keys, A., ed. 1970. Coronary heart disease in seven countries. *Circulation* 41(suppl 1):I1-I198.

22. Keys, A., C. Aravanis, and F.S.P. Van Buchem. 1981. The diet and all-causes death rate in the Seven Countries Study. *Lancet* 2:58-61.

23. de Lorgeril, M., P. Salen, E. Caillat-Vallet, M.T. Hanauer, J.C. Barthelemy, and N. Mamelle. 1997. Control of bias in dietary trial to prevent coronary recurrences: the Lyon Diet Heart Study. *Eur J Clinl Nutr* 51(2):116-122.

24. Carlson, L.A., and L.E. Bottiger. 1972. Ischaemic heart-disease in relation to fasting values of plasma triglycerides and cholesterol: Stockholm Prospective Study. *Lancet* 1:865-868.

25. Rimm, E., A. Ascherio, E. Giovannucci, D. Spiegelman, M. Stampfer, and W. Willett. 1996. Vegetable, fruit, and cereal fiber intake and risk of coronary heart disease among men. *JAMA* 275(6):447-451.

26. Hu, F.B., M.J. Stampfer, and J.E. Manson, et al. 1997. Dietary fat intake and the risk of coronary artery disease in women. *N Engl J Med* 337:1491-1499.

27. Rosenman, R.H., R.J. Brand, and D. Jenkins, et al. 1975. Coronary heart disease in the Western Collaborative Group Study. *JAMA* 233(8):872-877.

28. Hubert, H.B., M. Feinleib, P.M. McNamara, and W.P. Castelli. 1983. Obesity as an independent risk factor for cardiovascular disease: a 26-year follow-up of participants in the Framingham Heart Study. *Circulation* 67:968-977.

29. Ekelund, L.-G., W.L. Haskell, S.L. Johnson, F.S. Whaley, M.H. Criqul, and D.S. Sheps. 1988. Physical fitness as a predictor of cardiovascular mortality in asymptomatic North American men. *N Engl J Med* 319:1379-1384.

30. Haskell, W.L. 1994. Health consequences of physical activity: understanding and challenges regarding dose response. *Med Sci Sports Exerc* 26:649-660.

31. Reed, D., D. McGee, K. Yano, and M. Feinleib. 1983. Social networks and coronary heart disease among Japanese men in Hawaii. *Am J Epidemiol* 117(4):384-396.

32. Williams, R.B., J.C. Barefoot, and R.M. Califf, et al. 1992. Prognostic importance of social and economic resources among medically treated patients with angiography documented coronary artery disease. *JAMA* 267(4):520-524.

33. Pandya, D. 1998. Psychological stress, emotional behaviour and coronary artery disease. (Review) *Comp Ther* 24(5):265-271.

34. Brezinska, V., and F. Kittel. 1996. Psychosocial factors of coronary heart disease in women: a review. *Soc Sci Med* 42(10):1351-1365.

35. Barefoot, J.C., and M. Schroll. 1996. Symptoms of depression, acute myocardial infarction, and total mortality in a community sample. *Circulation* 93:1976-1980.

36. Ford, D.E., L.A. Mead, P.P. Chang, L. Cooper-Patrick, N.Y. Wang, and J. Klag. 1998. Depression is a risk factor for coronary artery disease in men: the precursors study. *Arch Intern Med* 158(13):1422-1426.

37. Carney, R.M., M. W. Rich, and A. S. Jaffee. 1995. Depression as a risk factor for cardiac events in established coronary heart disease: a review of possible mechanisms. *Ann Behav Med* 17:142-129.

38. O'Connor, G.T. 1989. An overview of randomized trials of rehabilitation with exercise after myocardial infarction. *Circulation* 80:235-244.

39. Miller, T.D., G.J. Balady, and G.F. Fletcher. 1997. Exercise and its role in the prevention and rehabilitation of cardiovascular disease. *Ann Behav Med* 19(3):220-229.

40. British Medical Journal. Regression of atheroma. 1977. *Br Med J* 2:1-2.

41. Gensini, G.G., P. Esente, and A. Kelly. 1974. Natural history of coronary disease in patients with and without bypass graft surgery. *Circulation* 49(suppl.2):II98-II102.

42. Landmann, J., W. Kolster, A.V.G. Bruschke. 1976. Regression of coronary artery obstructions demonstrated by coronary arteriography. *Eur J Cardiol* 4:475-479.

43. Sacks, F.M., M.A. Pfeffer, L.A. Moyé, J.L. Rouleau, J.D. Rutherford, T.G. Cole, L. Brown, J. Warnica, J.M.O. Arnold, C.-C. Wun, B.R. Davis, and E. Braunwald, for the Cholesterol and Recurrent Events Trial Investigators. 1996. The effect of pravastatin on coronary events after myocardial infarction in patients with average cholesterol levels. *N Engl J Med* 335:1001-1009.

44. Cashin-Hemphill, L., W.J. Mack, and J.M. Pogoda. 1990. Beneficial effects of colestipol-niacin on coronary atherosclerosis: a 4-year follow-up. *JAMA* 264:3013-3017.

45. Brown, G., J.J. Albers, and L.D. Fisher. 1990. Regression of coronary artery disease as a result of intensive lipid-lowering therapy in men with high levels of apolipoprotein B. *N Engl J Med* 323:1289-1298.

46. Kane, J.P., M.J. Malloy, and T.A. Ports. 1990. Regression of coronary atherosclerosis during treatment of familial hypercholesterolemia with combined drug regimens. *JAMA* 264:3007-3012.

47. Buchwald, H., R.L. Varco, and J.P. Matts. 1990. Effect of partial ileal bypass surgery on mortality and morbidity from coronary heart disease in patients with hypercholesterolemia: report of the Program on the Surgical Control of the Hyperlipidemias (POSCH). *N Engl J Med* 323:946-955.

48. Waters, D., L. Higginson, P. Gladstone, B. Kimball, M. LeMay, S.J. Boccuzzi, and J. Lesperance: the CCAIT Study Group. 1994. Effects of monotherapy with an HMG-CoA reductase inhibitor on the progression of coronary atherosclerosis as assessed by serial quantitative arteriography: The Canadian Coronary Atherosclerosis Intervention Trial. *Circulation* 89:959-968.

49. Waters, D., L. Higginson, P. Gladstone, B. Kimball, M. LeMay, and J. Lesperance. 1993. Design features of a controlled clinical trial to assess the effect of an HMG CoA reductase inhibitor on the progression of coronary artery disease. *Control Clin Trials* 14:45-74.

50. Pitt, B., G.B.J. Mancini, and S.G. Ellis, et al., for the PLAC-I Investigators. 1995. Pravastatin limitation of atherosclerosis in the coronary arteries (PLAC-I): reduction in atherosclerosis progression and clinical events. *J Am Coll Cardiol* 26:1133-1139.

51. Jukema, J.W., A.V.G. Bruschke, A.J. van Boven, and J.H.C. Reiber et al. 1995. Coronary artery disease/myocardial infarction: effects of lipid lowering by pravastatin on progression and regression of coronary artery disease in symptomatic men with normal to moderately elevated serum cholesterol levels: the regression growth evaluation statin study (REGRESS). *Circulation* 91:2528-2540.

52. Rossouw, J.E. 1995. Lipid-lowering interventions in angiographic trials. *Am J Cardiol* 76:86C-92C.

53. Scandinavian Simvastatin Survival Study Group. 1994. Randomised trial of cholesterol lowering in 4444 patients with coronary heart disease: the Scandinavian Simvastatin Survival Study (4S). *Lancet* 344:1383-1389.

54. Scandinavian Simvastatin Survival Study Group. 1993. Design and baseline results of the Scandinavian Simvastatin Survival Study of patients with stable angina and/or previous myocardial infarction. *Am J Cardiol* 71:393-400.

55. Kjekshus, J., and T.R. Pedersen, for the Scandinavian Simvastatin Survival Study Group. 1995. Reducing the risk of coronary events: evidence from the Scandinavian Simvastatin Survival Study (4S). *Am J Cardiol* 76:64C-68C.

56. Pearson, T.A., and H.J.C. Swan. 1996. Lipid lowering: the case for identifying and treating the high-risk patients. *Cardiol Clin* 14:117-130.

57. Scandinavian Simvastatin Survival Study Group. 1995. Baseline serum cholesterol and treatment effect in the Scandinavian Simvastatin Survival Study (4S). *Lancet* 345:1274-1275.

58. Sacks, F.M., M.A. Pfeffer, L.A. Moyé, and J.L. Rouleau, et al., for the Cholesterol and Recurrent Events Trial Investigators. 1996. The effect of pravastatin on coronary events after myocardial infarction in patients with average cholesterol levels. *N Engl J Med* 335:1001-1009.

59. Sacks, F.M., M.A. Pfeffer, and L. Moyé, et al. 1991. Rationale and design of a secondary prevention trial of lowering normal plasma cholesterol levels after acute myocardial infarction: the Cholesterol and Recurrent Events trial (CARE). *Am J Cardiol* 68:1436-1446.

60. Tonkin, A.M., for the LIPID Study Group. 1995. Management of the Long-Term Intervention with Pravastatin in Ischaemic Disease (LIPID) study after the Scandinavian Simvastatin Survival Study (4S). *Am J Cardiol* 76:107C-112C.

61. Treasure, C.B., J.L. Klein, W.S. Weintraub, and D.J. Talley, et al. 1995. Beneficial effects of cholesterol-lowering therapy on the coronary endothelium in patients with coronary artery disease. *N Engl J Med* 332:481-487.

62. Anderson, T.J., I.T. Meredith, A.C. Yeung, B. Frei, A.P. Selwyn, and P. Ganz. 1995. The effect of cholesterol-lowering and antioxidant therapy on endothelium-dependent coronary vasomotion. *N Engl J Med* 332:488-493.

63. Leung, W.H., C.P. Lau, and C.K. Wong. 1993. Beneficial effect of cholesterol-lowering therapy on coronary endothelium-dependent relaxation in hypercholesterlaemic patients. *Lancet* 341:1496-1500.

64. Pearson, T.A. 1998. Primary and secondary prevention of coronary artery disease: trials of lipid lowering with statins. *Am J Cardiol* 82(10A):28S-30S.

65. Gould, A.L., J.E. Rossouw, N.C. Santanello, J.F. Heyse, and C.D. Furberg. 1998. Cholesterol reduction yields clinical benefit: impact of statin trials. *Circulation* 97:946-952.

66. Whellan, D.J., M. Molloy, R. Quillian, J. Norris, and M.J. Sullivan. In press. Coronary artery disease: the basis for secondary prevention. In *Interventional Cardiovascular Medicine: Principles and Practices,* ed. R. Stack, W. Oneil, and G. Roubin. 2nd ed. New York: Churchill-Livingstone.

67. Pearson, T., E. Rapaport, M. Criqui, and C. Furberg, et al. 1994. Optimal risk factor management in the patients after coronary revascularization: a statement for healthcare professionals from an American Heart Association writing group. *Circulation* 90:3125-3133.

68. Marcelino, J.J., and K.R. Feingold. 1996. Inadequate treatment with HMG-CoA reductase inhibitors by health care providers. *Am J Med* 100(6):605-610.

69. Illich, I. 1976. *Limits to Medicine: Medical Nemesis: The Expropriation of Health.* London: Boyars.

70. Ray, P.H. 1996. The rise of integral culture. *Noetic Sci Rev* (spring):4-15.

71. Astin, J.A. 1998. Why patients use alternative medicine: results of a national study. *JAMA* 279(19):1548-1553.

72. Merz, C.N.B., and A. Rozanski. 1996. Remodeling cardiac rehabilitation into secondary prevention programs. *Am Heart J* 132(2):418-427.

Conclusion: Cardiopulmonary Rehabilitation in Clinical Practice—the Underused Intervention

François Maltais, Jean Jobin, Clermont Simard, and Pierre LeBlanc

The increasing incidence of coronary artery disease (CAD) and chronic obstructive pulmonary disease (COPD) is closely linked to lifestyle, and it is now well established that proper habits such as quitting smoking, eating well, and exercising regularly are most effective in preventing the development and progression of these disorders. In contrast to pharmacological approaches, smoking cessation is the only intervention that has been shown to slow the deterioration of lung function in patients with chronic obstructive pulmonary disease (1). Similarly, nutritional intervention is extremely effective in reducing the occurrence of subsequent ischemic events (2) in patients with coronary artery disease. Despite these observations, most health resources are still used for treatment of the acute phase of disease, and relatively little is invested in changing the lifestyle habits that have contributed in part, if not totally, to the development of the disease. This situation is one of the interesting paradoxes of medicine at the end of this century.

As their life expectancy improves through better medical care, patients with chronic heart failure (CHF) or COPD are likely to develop systemic complications such as peripheral muscle wasting and weakness (3,4), osteoporosis (5), and depression. Despite documented evidence indicating that these problems adversely influence exercise tolerance, quality of life, and survival independent of the impairment caused by the primary diseased organ (4,6,7,8), their potential impact is largely unrecognized and often neglected in overall therapeutic strategies. Their clinical significance and management should also be addressed in order to provide more comprehensive disease management and to provide patients with a better chance to improve their quality of life.

Cardiopulmonary rehabilitation is advocated as an important therapeutic modality for patients with heart or lung disorders, its objectives being to optimize functional status and quality of life and to prevent further deterioration and disease through education, psychosocial support, and exercise training. In essence, cardiopulmonary rehabilitation promotes the use of a healthy lifestyle to improve global patient status. It is likely that changing lifestyle is one of the better methods of having a long-term impact on the lives of patients with CAD and COPD. Because of its comprehensive nature, cardiopulmonary rehabilitation also provides a unique opportunity to address all the systemic consequences of chronic heart or lung diseases. As discussed in section IV of this volume, it is the most effective therapeutic strategy to improve peripheral muscle dysfunction in patients with CHF and in those with COPD. Despite this, cardiopulmonary rehabilitation remains largely underused, at least in North America (9,10).

Several factors may explain the apparent contrast between the efficacy of rehabilitation and the fact that very few patients seem to make use of it. The low availability or lack of availability of pulmonary rehabilitation programs certainly appears to be one of these factors. In Canada, for instance, a recent study has shown that there are 36 pulmonary rehabilitation programs that can accept 4000-5000 patients per year, a number that represents less than 1% of all patients with COPD in the entire country (10). A second factor, at least in North America, is the long distances that patients often have to travel in order to come to the nearest program. We should increase the availability of cardiopulmonary rehabilitation programs and, for selected patients, home-based rehabilitation is currently under evaluation to improve accessibility of service (11).

A third factor is the skepticism of the medical community toward the efficacy of cardiopulmonary rehabilitation. This skepticism results from an incomplete understanding of the mechanisms of action of cardiopulmonary rehabilitation. More specifically, physicians wonder how rehabilitation can be effective if it does not improve lung or heart function (12), or why there are no well-documented long-term benefits of this approach (13). These issues have been partly resolved because research efforts over the past 10-15 years have provided significant data demonstrating the efficacy of cardiopulmonary rehabilitation in improving patients' clinical status (14). Exercise training is also perceived by many as being dangerous for patients with advanced disease. As indicated in recent literature and in papers included in this volume (see section V), cardiopulmonary rehabilitation is safe and effective even in patients with advanced lung (15) or heart diseases (16) providing that there is appropriate clinical evaluation and that the patient is supervised by well-trained health professionals. As discussed by Juneau in chapter 13, exposure to extreme climatic conditions is safer for patients than once thought.

Another factor that may explain the low popularity of rehabilitation is the lack of patient motivation. From the patient's point of view, it is less appealing to make an effort and adopt a different and healthier lifestyle than to accept a "magic cure" through pharmacological or surgical interventions. Patients are too often passive witnesses of their treatment, and it is important to have them understand the critical and active role they must play in the maintenance of their health. In this regard, education will need to be more extensive if patients are to be directly involved in their treatment. As discussed in chapter 22, interventions on lifestyle should become an even more important feature of cardiopulmonary rehabilitation programs of the next century.

In this era, when high technology and expensive drugs are the most valued aspects of medical care, cardiopulmonary rehabilitation should be promoted within the medical community and the general population because it offers the best chance, not only to prevent further deterioration of heart and lung diseases, but also to optimize the quality of life of those already affected by these chronic disorders. This is our greatest challenge for the future.

References

1. Anthonisen, N.R., J.E. Connett, J.P. Kiley, and M.D. Altose et al. 1994. Effects of smoking intervention and the use of an inhaled anticholinergic bronchodilator on the rate of decline of FEV1. The Lung Health Study. *JAMA* 272:1497-1505.
2. DeLorgeril, M., S. Renaud, and N. Mamelle, et al. 1994. Mediterranean alpha-linolenic acid-rich diet in secondary prevention of coronary heart disease. *Lancet* 343:1454-1459.
3. Bernard, S., P. LeBlanc, and F. Whittom, et al. 1998. Peripheral muscle weakness in patients with chronic obstructive pulmonary disease. *Am J Respir Crit Care Med* 158:629-634.
4. Mancini, D.M., G. Walter, and N. Reichek, et al. 1992. Contribution of skeletal muscle atrophy to exercise intolerance and altered muscle metabolism in heart failure. *Circulation* 85:1364-1373.
5. McEvoy, C.E., K.E. Ensrud, and E. Bender, et al. 1998. Association between corticosteroid use and vertebral fractures in older men with chronic obstructive pulmonary disease. *Am J Respir Crit Care Med* 157:704-709.
6. Gosselink, R., T. Troosters, and M. Decramer. 1996. Peripheral muscle weakness contributes to exercise limitation in COPD. *Am J Respir Crit Care Med* 153:976-980.
7. Simpson, K., K. Killian, N. McCartney, D.G. Stubbing, and N.L. Jones. 1992. Randomised controlled trial of weightlifting exercise in patients with chronic airflow limitation. *Thorax* 47:70-75.
8. Wilson, D.O., R.M. Rogers, E.C. Wright, and N.R. Anthonisen. 1989. Body weight in chronic obstructive pulmonary disease. The National Institutes of Health Intermittent Positive-Pressure Breathing Trial. *Am Rev Respir Dis* 139:1435-1438.
9. Armstrong, K.L., L.A. Wolfe, and M.C. Amey. 1994. Cardiovascular rehabilitation in Canada. A national survey. *J Cardiopulm Rehabil* 14:262-272.
10. Brooks, D., Y. Lacasse, and R.S. Goldstein. 1999. Pulmonary rehabilitation programs in Canada: national survey. *Can Respir J* 6:55-63.
11. Debigaré, R., F. Maltais, F. Whittom, J. Deslauriers, and P. LeBlanc. 1999. Feasibility and efficacy of home exercise training before lung volume reduction. *J Cardiopulm Rehabil* 19:235-241.

12. Celli, B.R. 1995. Pulmonary rehabilitation in patients with COPD. *Am J Respir Crit Care Med* 152:861-864.

13. American Thoracic Society. 1994. Pulmonary rehabilitation research. NIH workshop summary. *Am Rev Respir Dis* 49:825-833.

14. Lacasse, Y., E. Wong, G.H. Guyatt, D. King, D.J. Cook, and R.S. Goldstein. 1996. Meta-analysis of respiratory rehabilitation in chronic obstructive pulmonary disease. *Lancet* 348:1115-1119.

15. Maltais, F., P. LeBlanc, and J. Jobin, et al. 1997. Intensity of training and physiologic adaptation in patients with chronic obstructive pulmonary disease. *Am J Respir Crit Care Med* 155:555-561.

16. Giannuzzi, P., P.L. Temporelli, U. Corrà, M. Gattone, A. Giordano, and L. Tavazzi. 1997. Attenuation of unfavorable remodeling by exercise training in postinfarction patients with left ventricular dysfunction (ELVD) trial. *Circulation* 96:1790-1797.

Index

Note: Page numbers followed by *f* or *t* refer to the figure or table on that page.

— N

— T

About the Editors

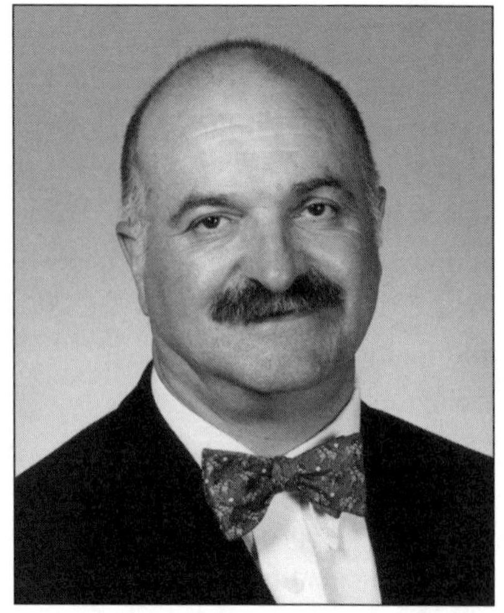

Jean Jobin

Jean Jobin, PhD, professor of medicine at Laval University in Québec, is director of the Cardiopulmonary Rehabilitation Research Laboratory at the Institut de Cardiologie et de Pneumologie de l'Université Laval at Laval Hospital.

Dr. Jobin is a certified program director of the American College of Sports Medicine's (ACSM) Certification for Exercise Specialists in French at Laval University; he is a fellow of the ACSM and of the American Association of Cardiovascular and Pulmonary Rehabilitation, a member of the Canadian Association of Cardiac Rehabilitation and the Canadian Cardiovascular Society. He was president of the scientific committee of the First Québec International Symposium on Cardiopulmonary Rehabilitation in May 1999.

Dr. Jobin jogs daily and is an alpine skier. He, his wife, and his children live in Cap-Rouge, Québec.

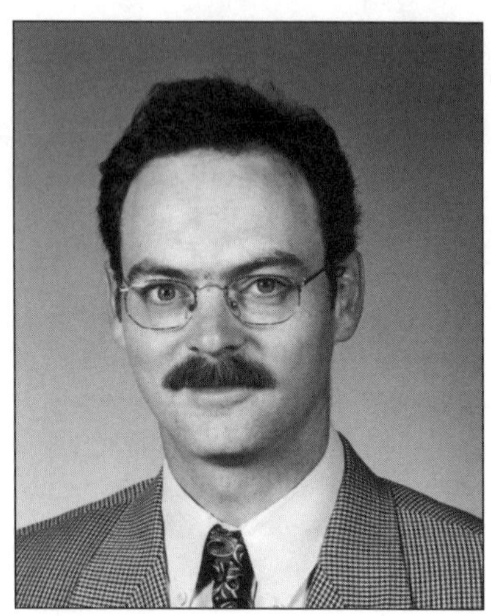

François Maltais

François Maltais, MD, is a respirologist at the Pneumology Center at Laval Hospital in Québec. He is adjunct professor of medicine at Laval University and director of the Pulmonary Rehabilitation Program at Laval Hospital.

A member of the Québec, Canadian, and American Thoracic Societies, Dr. Maltais is certified in internal medicine and in pulmonary medicine. He has been awarded numerous research grants from private and public foundations including the Medical Research Council of Canada (MRC) to investigate such topics as peripheral muscle dysfunction, strength training, and exercise training in COPD among many others.

Dr. Maltais enjoys mountain biking and downhill skiing. He lives with his wife and children in L'Ancienne-Lorette, Québec.

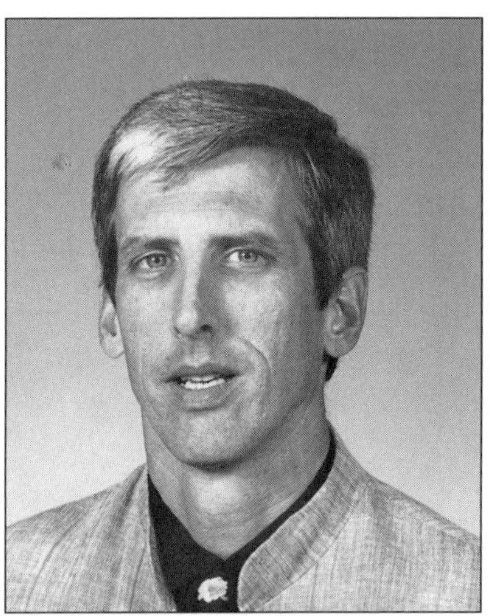

Pierre LeBlanc

Pierre LeBlanc, MD, is clinical professor in the department of medicine at Laval University, where he is in charge of teaching respiratory physiology. He is a member of the American Thoracic Society and the Canadian Thoracic Society. Dr. LeBlanc has published highly significant and often-quoted research concerning mechanisms of breathlessness during exercise in cardiorespiratory patients.

Dr. LeBlanc is an avid cyclist and enjoys cross-country skiing. From 1975 to 1976, he was a member of the Canadian track and field team. He, his wife, and his children live in Cap-Rouge, Québec.

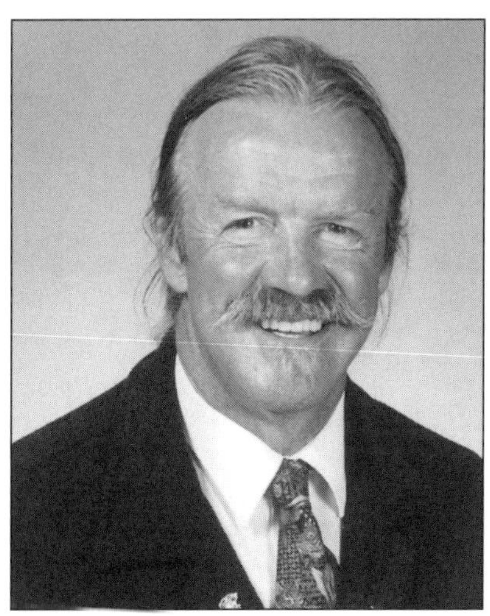

Clermont Simard

Clermont Simard, PhD, is professor of Physical Education and Special Populations at Laval University. He founded the International Federation for Adapted Physical Activity in 1976, for which he was specially honored by Spain's University of Lleida in 1999.

Dr. Simard is a fellow of the ACSM and was president of the First Québec International Symposium on Cardiopulmonary Rehabilitation in May 1999. His many years of research have focused on adapting physical activity to populations with special needs, the impact of disuse on muscular metabolism and function, the aging process and physical activity as they affect quality of life, and on means of helping older adults live more autonomous lives.

Dr. Simard and his wife make their home in St.-Nicolas, Québec.